Fundamentals of Radiology

Fundamentals of Radiology

FOURTH EDITION

Lucy Frank Squire, M.D.

Professor of Radiology, and Director of Undergraduate
Radiology Education, State University of New York
Health Science Center at Brooklyn

Consultant in Radiology, Massachusetts General Hospital
Boston, Massachusetts

Robert A. Novelline, M.D.

Associate Professor of Radiology, Harvard Medical School

Director, Emergency Radiology, and Director, Undergraduate
Radiology Education, Massachusetts General Hospital
Boston, Massachusetts

With drawings and diagrams by
Francis Cunningham and Shelley Eshleman

Harvard University Press

Cambridge, Massachusetts, and London, England

First edition entitled *Fundamentals of Roentgenology*.
Copyright © 1964 by the Commonwealth Fund
Second, third, and fourth editions entitled *Fundamentals of Radiology*.
Copyright © 1975, 1982, 1988 by the President and Fellows of Harvard College
Printed in the United States of America
10   9   8   7   6   5   4   3

This book is printed on acid-free paper, and its binding materials
have been chosen for strength and durability.

Library of Congress Cataloging-in-Publication Data

Squire, Lucy Frank, 1915–
   Fundamentals of radiology / Lucy Frank Squire and Robert A.
Novelline : with drawings and diagrams by Francis Cunningham and
Shelley Eshleman. — 4th ed.
   p. cm.
Includes index.
ISBN 0-674-32926-0 (alk. paper)
   1. Diagnosis, Radioscopic.   2. Diagnostic imaging.   I. Novelline,
Robert A.   II. Title.
   [DNLM: 1. Radiography.   WN 100 S774f]
RC78.S69 1988
616.07′572—dc19
DNLM/DLC
for Library of Congress   87-33875
                CIP

To Dr. Richard Schatzki,
with grateful appreciation
for his inspiration
and example

Preface

In undertaking the preparation of this textbook, we have been concerned with providing an instruction manual that will help medical students learn how to look at x-ray films and other diagnostic images, and relate abnormal radiologic findings to pathophysiology with logic and confidence. We have *not* wanted to provide a compendious reference work in which one might hope to be able to look up the "radiologic signs by which diseases are diagnosed"; for that is not the way in which radiology is practiced today, since few single "signs" are pathognomonic for a particular disease. With the many imaging modalities presently available, plain films, conventional tomography, computed tomography, ultrasonography, magnetic resonance and special procedures, for example, are all used in various combinations as complementary aids to diagnosis—in tandem, always, with the clinical picture.

This kind of algorithmic approach, selecting certain of the imaging modes and deciding that others are inappropriate, must be learned gradually against a basic understanding of medicine. During the preclinical years in school, familiarity with radiology can be an excellent aid in learning other disciplines such as anatomy, physiology, and pathology. Later the young clinician will be helped in solving virtually every diagnostic problem if he understands enough about radiology to want to discuss and rediscuss the details of his patients' imaging studies with the consulting radiologists who have performed and interpreted those studies.

This fourth edition of *Fundamentals of Radiology* has, again, eliminated a good many obsolete illustrations or replaced them with better ones. Many new examples of useful computed tomography studies have been added throughout the book, as well as new sonograms and magnetic-resonance images. The uses of nuclear medicine have been more thoroughly addressed. After a basic introduction to film viewing in the first twelve chapters, gastrointestinal radiology, and the imaging of the abdominal organs in all its current complexity in most of the common disease conditions, are explained for the more advanced student in Chapters 13 and 14, followed by two final chapters on bone radiology and neuroradiology. Unknowns to test the student's advancing knowledge are included in the basic chapters, with the answers provided at the back of the book. Specific credit references appear with our grateful thanks, and both illustrations and text have been indexed to facilitate finding items for review. It is best to read the book first from cover to cover, since concepts and methods are cumulatively treated.

As with previous editions, we provide our addresses below in the hope that readers will take the time to communicate their critical response to this book and let us know how we and other writers can better serve their needs.

Lucy Frank Squire, M.D.
1 West 72nd Street
New York, NY 10023

Robert A. Novelline, M.D.
Department of Radiology
Massachusetts General Hospital
Boston, MA 02114

Acknowledgments

Our gratitude goes first to all the students who have helped us in a multitude of ways in the preparation of this fourth edition. Their enthusiasm, imagination, critical good judgment, and hard work have certainly made possible a volume much better suited to their needs.

We are extremely grateful as well to all our friends, colleagues, and associates at the two medical schools and throughout the world who have so generously contributed illustrative material during the past three decades. Their contributions are noted individually in the credits section at the back of the book.

The Eastman Kodak Company and the editors of *Medical Radiography and Photography* made available extensive files of published and unpublished materials and supplied us with prints of top quality, without which the character of the illustrations would not have been possible; we are deeply appreciative of this help.

We are indebted to our department chairmen, Dr. Joshua A. Becker at the State University of New York Health Science Center at Brooklyn and Dr. Juan M. Taveras at Massachusetts General Hospital, for their constant support.

Naomi Gershon and Donna Markham have given us invaluable assistance in patiently committing the manuscript to word processors during the two years we have worked on the fourth edition. Gordon Squire has helped continuously in a variety of ways, including many hours of proofreading and photocopying.

Although the authors must shoulder the responsibility for collating, organizing, and revising any teaching and learning manual such as this one, we have been continuously aware of our good fortune in having so many helpers and contributors. We thank each and every one and send them our warm regards.

L.F.S.
R.A.N.

Contents

Fundamentals of Radiology

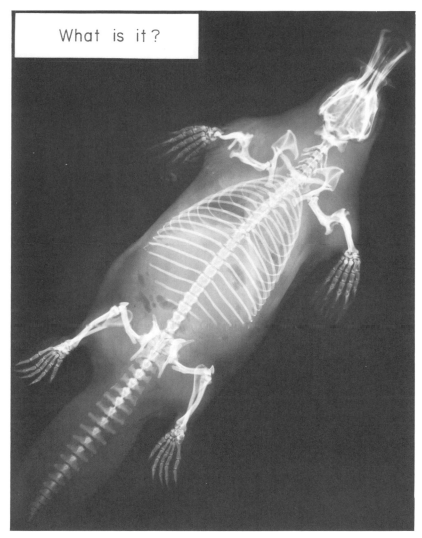

Figure 1-1. Its name is *Ornithorhynchus anatinus,* and you have never seen an x-ray portrait of it before. Nevertheless, there is one creature and one only in the animal kingdom which could give this x-ray appearance, and you can reason out its identity.

CHAPTER 1 Introduction and Basic Concepts

As you probably already know, x-rays are produced by bombarding a tungsten target with an electron beam. They are a form of radiant energy similar in several respects to visible light. For example, they radiate from the source in all directions unless stopped by an absorber. Like light rays, a very small part of the beam of x-rays will be absorbed by air, whereas all of the beam will be absorbed by a sheet of thick metal. The fundamental difference between x-rays and light rays is in their range of wavelengths, the wavelength of all x-rays being shorter than that of ultraviolet light. The useful science of radiology is based on this difference, since many substances which are opaque to light are penetrated by x-rays. It was this attractive property which caught the attention of Professor Roentgen of the University of Würzburg on a cold November night in 1895, when he first observed certain physical phenomena he could not explain.

Roentgen had been experimenting with an apparatus which, unknown to him, caused the emission of x-rays as a by-product. Accustomed to the darkened laboratory, he observed that whenever the apparatus was working, a chemical-coated piece of cardboard lying on the table glowed with a pale green light. We know now that fluorescence, or the emission of visible light, can be produced in a variety of ways by complex nuclear energy exchanges. But in 1895 Roentgen recognized at first only the fact that he had unintentionally produced *a hitherto unknown form of radiant energy which was invisible, could cause fluorescence, and passed through objects opaque to light*. When he placed his hand between the

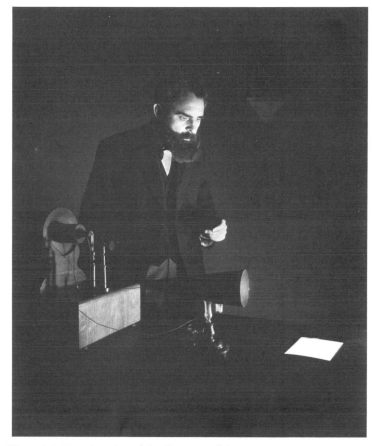

Figure 1-2. Staged version of the discovery of the roentgen ray.

source of the beam and the lighted cardboard, he could see the bones inside his fingers within the shadow of his hand. He found that the new rays, which he named x-rays, penetrated wood. Using photographic paper instead of a fluorescing material, he made an "x-ray picture" of a hand through the door of his laboratory.

1

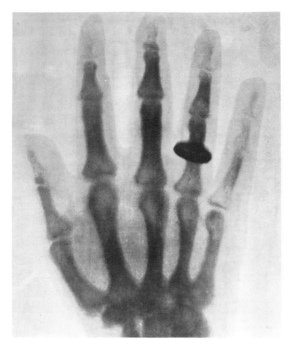

Figure 1-3. What Roentgen saw when he placed his hand between the tube and the fluorescing cardboard on the laboratory table. Areas not in the shadow of his hand fluoresced vigorously. Fewer x-rays reached the areas under the bones, so they were not so luminous.

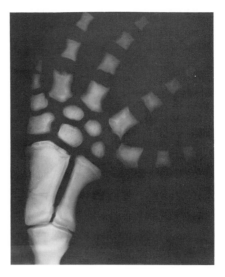

Figure 1-4. Radiograph of a hand . . . well, actually not a hand. Guess what it might be. (Note: Throughout this book you will find rhetorical questions and unanswered propositions. Sometimes they will be found answered in the text immediately following; sometimes, if you read straight along, you will find the answer several pages later buried in the text or incorporated into the legend of a related illustration. It is our intention to help you learn by reasoning.)

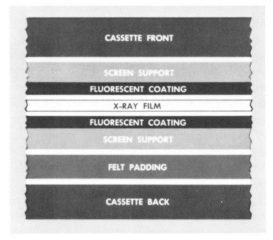

Figure 1-5. Cross section of a cassette, or modern film holder. The x-ray film in use today consists of an acetate sheet coated on both sides with photographic emulsion, and the cassette is constructed so that plastic fluorescent screens are applied in contact with each side of the film. In this way light rays reinforce the photochemical effect on the film of the x-rays themselves. This effectively speeds up the exposure, shortening the time, and reduces the blurring effect of the patient's motion.

Six years later the first Nobel Prize in physics was awarded to Roentgen for his discovery, and by then this remarkably systematic investigator had explored most of the basic physical and medical applications of the new ray.

The idea of being able to see through opaque objects caught the public fancy all over the world, and a great deal of nonsense was written on the subject in many languages within the first decade after its discovery. There is a fascinating file of cartoons and articles in the Library of Congress documenting this fever. It was even predicted that the mind would be explored by the radiologist, but in time others seem to have preempted that field.

Are you quite sure you can imagine exactly what Roentgen saw when he first observed that he could "see through his hand" with the help of the new ray? In order to grasp this clearly, you must first understand the important difference between what one sees fluoroscopically (Figure 1-3) and what you see today in an x-ray film of the hand, such as the one in Figure 1-4. You should call this a *radiograph,* not an x-ray.

When light hits photographic film, a mysterious photochemical process takes place in which metallic silver is precipitated in fine particles within the gelatin emulsion, rendering the film

2

black when it is developed chemically. Places on the film that are not exposed to light remain clear. When a "positive" paper print is made of this "negative" film, the values are reversed: the black, silver-bearing areas prevent light from reaching the photosensitive paper, while clear areas in the film permit the paper to be blackened.

The x-ray film you will see in medical school is equivalent to the negative film you may have worked with in your own photographic darkroom. X-rays, like light rays, precipitate silver in a photographic film, but they do so much less rapidly than light. A patient cannot be expected to hold still long enough for films to be made using x-rays alone, and too much exposure to radiation is both dangerous and technically undesirable. Therefore, an ingenious reinforcing technique has been worked out using a special film container, or *cassette*.

The cassette contains a fluorescent screen, which is activated by the x-rays and in turn emits light rays that reinforce the photochemical effects of the x-rays themselves on the film. In this way the silver-precipitating effect of the x-rays combined with that of the light rays they generate work together to blacken the film. When an object interposed between the x-ray beam source and the cassette has absorbed the rays, no light activation of the fluorescent screen will take place; neither x-rays nor light rays will reach the film, and no silver will be precipitated.

In Figure 1-6 a woman's left hand has been placed over the cassette and exposed to a beam of x-rays. Notice that the film not covered by any part of the hand has been intensely blackened because very little of the beam was absorbed by the *air*, which was the only absorber interposed there between x-ray tube and film. The fleshy parts of the hand (or *soft tissues*, as they are called by the radiologist) absorbed a good deal of the beam, so that the film appears gray. Very few x-rays reached that part of the film directly under the *bones*, because bones contain large amounts of calcium. All *metals* absorb x-rays to an extent depending on atomic number and thickness. No x-rays at all were able to pass through the gold ring, and the film underneath it was not altered photographically.

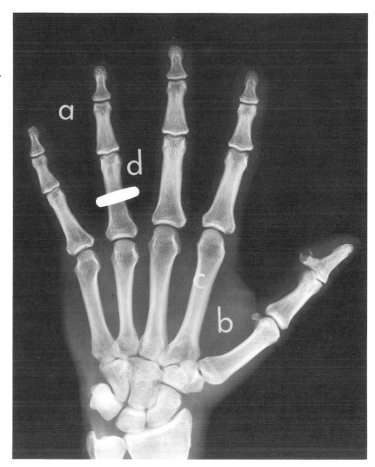

Figure 1-6. Modern radiograph of a hand. *a*, Blackened area where only air is interposed between beam and film. *b*, Soft tissues absorb part of the beam before it reaches the film. *c*, Calcium salts in bone absorb even more x-rays, leaving film only lightly exposed and relatively little silver precipitated in the emulsion. *d*, Dense metal of ring absorbs all rays; no silver is precipitated. (Note: This, like all x-ray illustrations in textbooks and periodicals published in this country, is a doubly reversed print, so that what you see here is what you will see whenever you hold a film of the hand against the light.)

What Roentgen saw, on the contrary, was the reverse of all the light-dark values you have been looking at in the film of the hand. X-rays reached the coated cardboard in abundance all around his hand so that the *background* fluoresced vigorously, while the shadow of his hand emitted less light and appeared gray-green. The cardboard underneath the bones of his fingers appeared darkest of all, since it received almost no activating rays. (Compare Figure 1-3.)

Figure 1-4 is not a human hand but a whale's flipper reduced photographically.

3

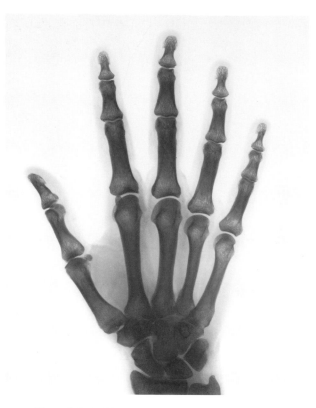

Figure 1-7. Positive print of a radiograph of the hand, made by singly reversing the values. This is also approximately as the hand would look on the fluoroscopic screen.

Fluoroscopic light is very faint unless it is amplified electronically. Today all fluoroscopic rooms are equipped with such "image intensification" machines, functioning in a lighted room. You may not see much fluoroscopy in your lifetime, but you will see many thousands of x-ray films. For this reason we suggest that you make a practice of thinking in terms of the white and black values that relate to the usual x-ray film as you saw them in the hand in Figure 1-6. Think of dense objects as white and of those more easily penetrated as gray or black. All the illustrations in this book are printed like Figure 1-6, and you will find that American journals and books print x-ray illustrations in this way.

While it is essential to understand which are the more dense (or *radiopaque*) substances and which the more transparent (or *radiolucent*) ones, your concern, even as you first begin looking at radiographs, should not be only with density. One often makes quite reasonable and useful deductions from the *form and shape* of radiographic shadows. If you figured out that Figure 1-1 was, and could only be, a radiograph of a duck-billed platypus, you have experienced the sort of educated guessing one uses all the time in radiology. One guesses imaginatively and then subjects one's own guess to a rigorous logical analysis based on radiologic and medical data. Putting together expected density and expected form, you will soon find that you can predict the appearance of the radiograph of an object or structure.

Begin, then, by applying imagination and judgment to a variety of nonmedical objects. Try to predict the type of shadow that would appear on the film if you x-rayed an egg.

Figure 1-8 is a radiograph of a woman's purse. Although the cloth from which the purse was made offered almost no obstruction to the x-rays, anything made of metal inside it, including the frame of the purse, absorbed the rays and left a white profile on the film. You will be able to identify from their outlines alone a paper clip, a bobby pin, a safety pin, a pair of rimless spectacles, coins, a lipstick case, two locker keys (overlapped), a nail file, and a metal pencil. You can almost construe the girl: a poverty-stricken, myopic individual who is taking two lab courses but wears makeup. One might, of course, be mistaken about the state of her finances: folding money, even in pounds sterling, would be quite radiolucent.

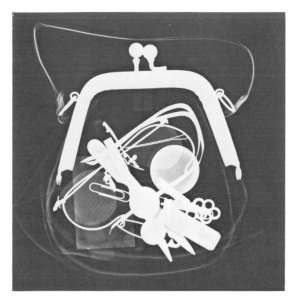

Figure 1-8

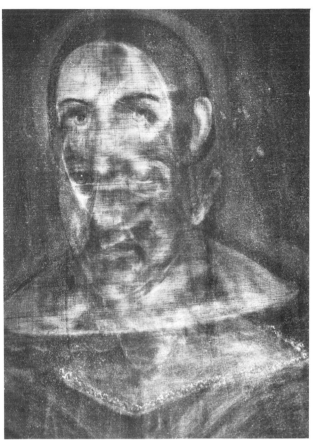

Figure 1-9. Radiograph of a portrait in oils painted over an earlier portrait. Only the woman with the pale eyes was visible on viewing the painting.

Pure metals are relatively radiopaque and so are their salts. Consequently, so also are the mixtures of oil and brilliantly colored metallic salts responsible for the whole field of oil painting. The radiography of paintings and other works of art is a fascinating and technically useful branch of the science. Frauds, inept reconstructions, masterpieces painted over by amateurs, may sometimes be detected by x-ray studies.

In Figure 1-9 two painters have used the same canvas—or, dissatisfied with his portrait of the man whose eyes appear as the lower pair, the same painter may have done the portrait of the woman with the light eyes and severely dressed hair, covering over the earlier portrait. Only the lady was visible as one looked at the painting.

Variations in the precise metallic composition of artists' colors used at different times in history may help in the identification and dating of such works of art. The pigments in use since about 1800 have been made of the salts of metals with much lower atomic numbers than the older pigments and for that reason will x-ray quite differently.

Thus a modern forgery of an old master, no matter how adroit a copy, will have an entirely different radiograph from the original. On the other hand, a copy made by a pupil of the master or another artist of the same school, painting at about the same time in history with the same hand-ground, earth-mineral colors, could be expected to x-ray in about the same way.

The characteristic use of brushstrokes, which, even better than his signature, often stamps the work of a great artist, may also help to identify a concealed painting covered over by a lesser artist. You would be able to imagine the radiograph of a contemporary canvas with the vigorous, heavy brushstrokes of Van Gogh showing through, for example.

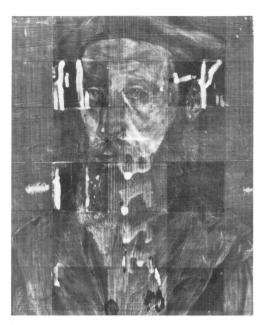

Figure 1-10

Remember too that any radiograph of a painting represents the summation of not only the various paint densities but the x-ray shadows of the canvas itself and the supporting structures. The wooden frame on which the canvas is stretched will cast some shadow, and if there are any nails in the wood they will appear in the radiograph also. Figure 1-10 shows a radiograph of a painting supported on wooden strips. The curious white areas are wormholes that have been filled with white lead. The x-rays have been completely absorbed, you notice, by the white-lead *casts* of the wormholes, and under them no x-rays have reached the film to blacken it. The white areas on the film are actually, therefore, *shadow-profiles* of these white-lead casts. Remember this! It has an important parallel in barium work in medical x-ray studies of the gastrointestinal tract.

The industrial uses of x-rays are many and important. Flaws, cracks, and fissures in heavy steel can be shown by x-raying big equipment or building materials. Especially powerful machines are needed for this sort of work, ones which will produce a more penetrating beam of x-rays of very short wavelength, often called hard x-rays. X-rays of long wavelength, or soft x-rays, are used to study thin or delicate objects. Very soft x-rays are used to study tissue sections of bone 1 or 2 microns in thickness (microradiography), while very hard x-rays are used to penetrate deep into the body and destroy malignant tumor cells (radiation therapy). Between these two extremes fall the wavelengths that are used in medical x-ray diagnosis.

The *electromagnetic spectrum* is a scaled arrangement of all types of radiant energy according to wavelength. Within the range used in diagnostic radiology, the x-ray technician is trained to select and use the particular wavelength suited to the density and thickness of the part he is filming. He does this by varying the kilovoltage of his machine: the higher the kilovoltage, the harder or more penetrating the beam of rays produced. He can also vary the amount of radiation in the beam by altering the milliamperage used, and, finally, he can control the time of exposure. Thus, for instance, for a thin object like the hand he uses a soft beam for a short time, and for a dense object like the head, a hard beam and a long exposure.

6

Radiodensity as a Function of Thickness

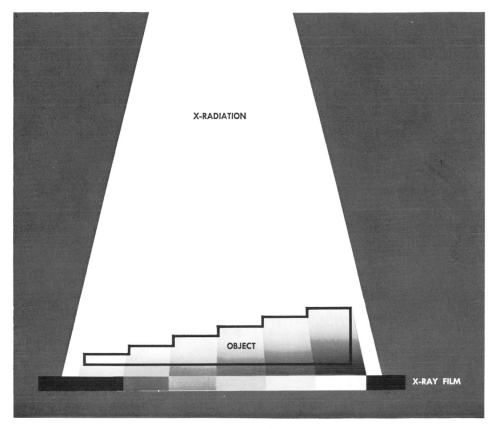

Figure 1-11. Radiodensity as a function of thickness of the object. Here the object to be filmed is of homogeneous composition and has a stepwise range of thickness. Gray shading indicates degree of absorption of the x-rays.

Thickness Kept Constant While Composition Varies

Having reasoned through all this, you must consider in greater detail the *relative radiodensities* of various substances and tissues. In order to do this most easily, let us eliminate thickness completely for the moment. Consider an imaginary row of 1-centimeter cubes of lead, air, butter, bone, liver, blood, muscle, subcutaneous fat, and barium sulfate. Can you arrange them in order of their radiodensity, decreasing from left to right?

If they were all pure elemental chemicals, you certainly could arrange them in order by looking up their atomic numbers. Only one of them is quite as simple as that, and a judicious guess will surely place first to your left as most dense the cube of lead, with an atomic number of 82. Are you hesitating between bone and barium sulfate? Barium has an atomic number of 56, and calcium in the bone cube has an atomic number of 20. Bone, however, is not even pure calcium salt. It has a functioning physiologic structure with holes and spaces to accommodate body fluids and marrow. It is composed of an organic matrix into which the complex bone mineral is precipitated. All such organic substances will reduce the radiodensity of the cube of bone, and it would consequently have even less radiodensity than a similar cube of packed bone dust. The cube of barium sulfate must be placed next to the lead cube, therefore, and after it, the cube of bone.

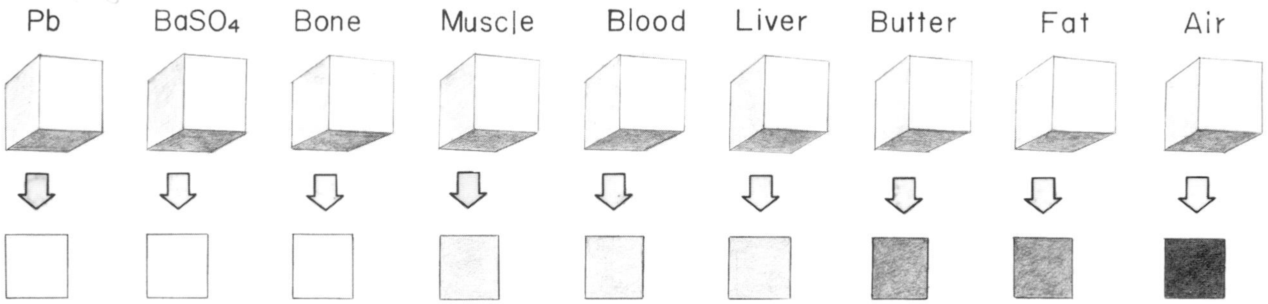

Pb	BaSO₄	Bone	Muscle	Blood	Liver	Butter	Fat	Air

Figure 1-12. Thickness kept constant while composition varies.

As to the most radiolucent of all, you can have no trouble with that: surely you will have put the cube of air far to the right, at the opposite end of the scale from the lead. The film under the air cube will be black, since the sparse scattering of air molecules offers almost no obstacle to the rays. The square of film under the lead, unaltered because no rays penetrated the cube to reach it, will be clear white, whereas that under the bone will show a tinge of gray.

Butter and subcutaneous fat have very similar x-ray densities. They are extremely radiolucent and must be placed next to air in the scale we are considering. Neither butter nor fatty tissue is homogeneous, since one is never quite free of water and the other contains both circulating fluids and a supporting network of fibrous connective tissue. Their squares on the radiograph would be almost the same very dark gray.

Between the three very dense cubes and the three very lucent ones there remain to be arranged the three cubes of blood, muscle, and liver. These will all x-ray an almost identical medium gray, and you can remember that all moist solid or fluid-filled organs and tissue masses will have about the same radiodensity, greater than fat or air but considerably less than bone or metal. Thus the muscular heart with its blood-filled chambers could be expected to x-ray as you see it on the chest film, a homogeneous mass much denser than the air-containing lung on both sides of it, but showing no differentiation between muscular ventricle wall and blood within the ventricle.

Remember that in the above discussion of relative radiodensities, we have kept thickness and form constant, as well as such technical factors as kilovoltage and time of exposure. We have planned this deliberately so that you might more easily build a working concept of the relative densities of different tissues. In practice, the radiologist adjusts the technical factors to accentuate these differences. Upon this useful spectrum of differing radiodensities of human tissues is based the whole field of medical radiography.

Once these considerations are learned, radiology becomes an exercise in logical deduction and an absorbing habit of mind. More important for you, it is also a delightful extra dimension in learning, a sort of custom-tailored illustrative tool related to nearly everything you will study in medical school. If you wish, you can use it to help you learn from the first day you begin to study anatomy, through your courses in physical diagnosis, pathology, medicine, and surgery, as a means of comprehending and remembering medical facts.

8

How Roentgen Shadows Instruct You about Form

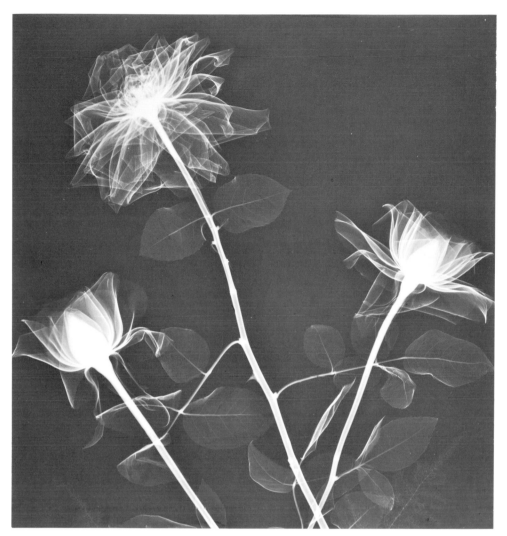

Figure 1-13

Consider now the contribution of *form*. Figure 1-13 is a radiograph of three roses, which we can use as an example of the basic logic of the roentgen shadows of complex objects. Flowers require only a very soft beam, of course, because they are both thin and delicate. A glance will tell you that one rose is full-blown and the other two more recently opened. You can deduce a great deal of information from the form, outline, shape, and structure of roentgen shadows. This is so true that in time you will learn to recognize with confidence the *identity* of certain shadows in medical radiographs because of their shape or form.

Now study the density of various parts of a single petal and compare the radiodensity, or whiteness, of the petals with that of the leaves. The leaves look less dense than the flowers and stems. Notice too that the veins within each leaf are denser than the rest of it. Veins of leaves have, of course, a structure independent of the cells composing the flatter part of the leaf. Stems are thicker and they also convey fluid. In both medical and nonmedical radiographs you can anticipate added density, in general, wherever there is fluid.

9

Radiographs Are Summation Shadowgrams

Another reason for the denser appearance of the petals compared with the leaves in Figure 1-13 is that they do not lie flat against the film but are curved and folded and overlap one another. This gives you a clue to a very important facet of radiologic interpretation. A sheet of any uniform composition, if it lies flat and parallel to the film, will have a uniform x-ray density and cast a homogeneous shadow. If it is curved, however, those parts which lie perpendicular to the plane of the film will radiograph as though they were much more dense.

This is perfectly simple. X-rays pass through a complex object and render upon the film not a picture at all but a "composite shadowgram," representing the sum of the densities interposed between beam source and film. Thus a sheet of rose petal which lies perpendicular to the film, or in the plane of the ray, is equivalent to many thicknesses of petal laid one upon another and, quite logically, is much more dense than a single sheet lying flat. Find the leaf which is turned on edge.

Curved sheets, considered geometrically, arrange themselves into groups of planes, if you will, and should be so considered in imagination when you are interpreting an x-ray film. Of course, in nature, and consequently in medicine, the curved plane is common and the symmetrical plane rare. In the radiograph of any curved-plane structure, therefore, learn to think in terms of those parts of it which are *relatively parallel to the film* and those which are *roughly perpendicular to it*.

Observe, finally, that the shadow of the stem of the rose in Figure 1-13 has a form you will find characteristic of any *tubular structure* of uniform composition. The margins are relatively dense because they represent long, curved planes radiographed tangentially, and the center area between them appears as a darker, more radiolucent streak. Rose stems are not truly hollow as one looks at them with the naked eye, but the central core, like that of tubular bones, is filled with a structure having less radiodensity. Hence that stem looks hollow and tubular on the film, just as a hollow tube containing air would look.

By this time you have several important principles clearly in mind, although you have learned them largely from examples. *First,* you know that x-rays are radiant energy of very short wavelength, beyond light in the electromagnetic spectrum, and that they penetrate, differently according to their wavelengths, substances opaque to light.

Second, you know that a beam of x-rays penetrates a complex object like the hand in accordance with the relative radiodensities of the materials which compose the object. You know that it produces on the film a composite shadowgram representing the sum of those radiodensities, layer for layer and part for part. You know that radiodensity is a function of atomic number and of thickness.

Third, you have realized that the parts of an object may become recognizable as to form, and their structure deduced, according to whether they are constructed most like solid or hollow spheres, cubes, or cylinders, or like plane sheets lying flat or curved upward away from the film.

Because we believe that the working of problems and puzzles will greatly increase your enjoyment of this book, we have included some in virtually every chapter. They are geared to the chapter in question both in subject matter and in difficulty. In general, they are presented with a few details about the patient, and you should imagine yourself the intern or practicing physician in charge of that patient. Often, especially in the early chapters, you are asked not for a diagnosis but rather for an impression of variation from the normal of a particular structure. You will see that this will help you to gauge as you go along just how roentgen shadows can be reasoned out and used as a mnemonic device in learning medicine. We think it will also persuade you that you know more and can reason better than you had realized (a comforting thought). The answers are provided at the back of the book, and the unknowns are numbered 1-1, 1-2, 1-3, etc., 2-1, 2-2, 2-3, etc., according to the chapter in which they appear.

10

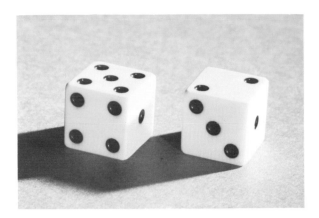

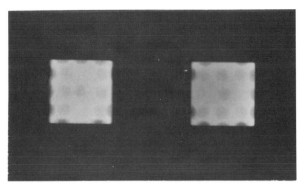

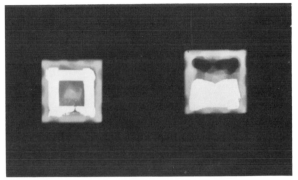

Figure 1-14 (*Unknown 1-1*). Sometimes the radiologist figures in criminology as an adjunctive source of information. The lucky throw you see in the innocent-looking pair of dice in the photograph was actually not luck at all but planned economy. Below are two radiographs, one of a pair of loaded dice and one of a pair of unloaded dice for which they could be switched. It is simple enough to decide which are the loaded dice, but can you figure out precisely what has been done to them?

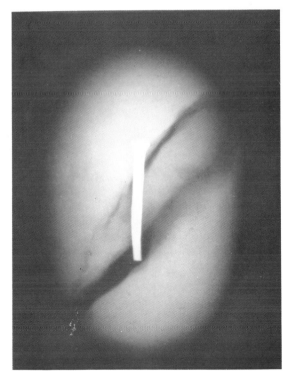

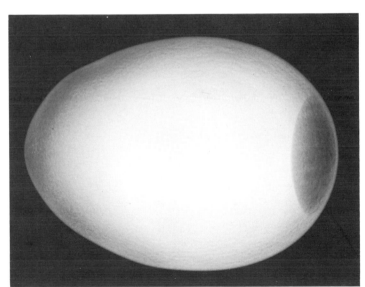

Figure 1-16. Not an unknown. This is a radiograph of the egg referred to earlier. You no doubt anticipated its shape, but did you predict the air pocket at the blunted end? Note how the density of the shell increases peripherally, as with any hollow sphere.

Figure 1-15 (*Unknown 1-2*). This is not a familiar object, and though you can figure out what its structure is from this, its radiograph, you will be very gifted indeed if you can say where it was when found.

CHAPTER **2** **An Invitation to Think Three-Dimensionally**

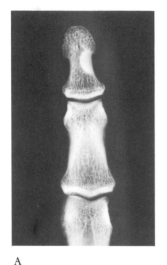 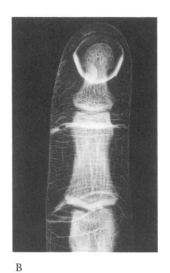 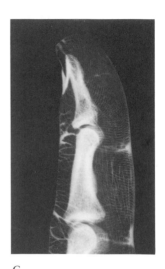

A   B   C

Figure 2-1

Changes in Roentgen Shadows When You Change Your Point of View or the Technique Used

These three radiographs of a finger illustrate at once how important it is for you to learn to think in three dimensions about x-ray shadows, reconstructing form from two views at right angles. Note that the soft tissues in A are seen as a faint uniform gray outline encompassing the bones. In B and C, however, the skin with its wrinkles and folds as well as the crevice between the cuticle and nail all seem to become visible. This is because they have been coated with a creamy substance containing a metallic salt.

Actually, the skin itself is no more visible than it was before, but the radiopaque cream collecting on its patterned, irregular surface forms a visible coating which marks the position of the skin. A and B were made in the *frontal projection;* C is made from the side and is called a *lateral view.*

Although A probably looks very flat to you and B and C give an illusion of depth, you will have realized that you can look at a medical x-ray film and *think about it three-dimensionally* even though you do not see it that way. The radiograph is a composite shadowgram and represents the added densities of many layers of tissue. One must think in layers when looking at any radiograph.

The most striking contrasts in radiodensity exist in the region of the chest, where air-filled lungs (radiolucent) on both sides of the muscular fluid-filled heart (relatively opaque) occupy the inside of a bony cage (a fretwork of crossed radiopaque strips). It is practical to discuss the chest first in this book and to outline for you a system by which you can study chest radiographs.

12

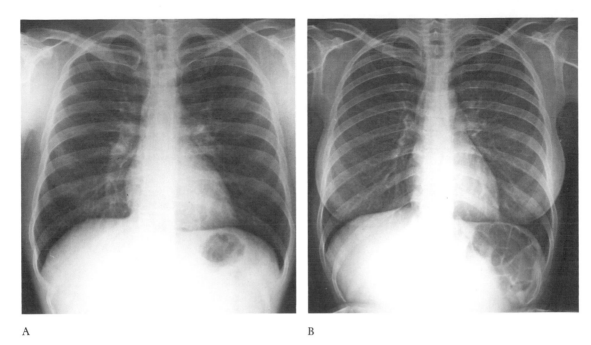

A   B

Figure 2-2

The Routine Posteroanterior (PA) Film

In Figure 2-2A imagine the structures through which the x-ray beam has passed from back to front: skin of the back; subcutaneous fat; lots of muscle encasing the flat blades of the scapulae, vertebral column, and posterior shell of the rib cage; then the lungs with the heart and other mediastinal structures between them; the sternum and anterior shell of the ribs; pectoral muscles and subcutaneous fat; breast tissue and, finally, skin.

Note the crescents of density that are added in Figure 2-2B, where the x-rays have had to traverse the female breast in addition to all the other tissue layers. Below the shadow of the breast and above that of the diaphragm the film is blacker where more rays have reached it.

One of the problems that will worry you as you begin looking at chest films will be how to put them up on the light boxes against which they are viewed: since they are transparent, you can look through them from either side. *Always place them so that you seem to be facing the patient.* Naturally this is only possible with PA and AP (anteroposterior) views.

X-ray films are usually marked by the technician to indicate which was the patient's right side—or, in the case of films of the extremities, whether it was his right or left leg, for example. In chest films one can usually be somewhat independent of the marker because the left ventricle and the arch of the aorta cast more prominent shadows on the left side of the patient's spine. Always view a chest film, then, so that the patient is facing you with his left on your right, and remember that when one says "left" in speaking of a finding on the film, one invariably means the *patient's* left. When you read "the right breast is missing" you are going to check, automatically, the breast shadow to your left.

Most of the chest films you see will have been made with the beam passing in a sagittal direction "posteroanteriorly," the x-ray tube behind and the film in front of the patient. This is the standard PA chest film, and films of all kinds are called PA views *if the beam passes through the patient from back to front.* It has become customary to make a PA chest film of any patient who is able to stand and be positioned.

13

PA and AP Chest Films Compared

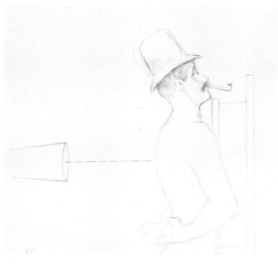

A

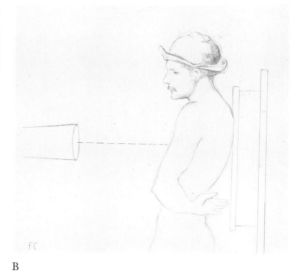

B

Figure 2-3. A (*above left*): Posteroanterior beam produces a PA chest film, the conventional view you see most often. B (*above right*): Anteroposterior beam produces an AP film. Note that the film is named for the direction the beam takes through the patient. (Drawings after Cezanne.)

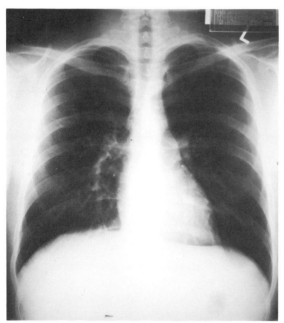

Figure 2-4A. PA chest film.

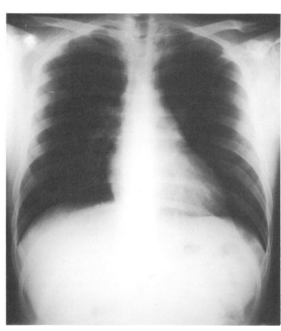

Figure 2-4B. AP chest film (same patient).

Less satisfactory but often valuable AP films of the chest are made with a portable x-ray machine when the patient is too sick to leave his bed. The patient is propped up against his pillows and the film is placed behind him, the exposure being made with the x-ray tube over the bed. Thus the ray passes through the patient "anteroposteriorly." You will be seeing such portable AP films of your very sick patients, and although they do not compare in quality with the PA films made with better technical facilities in the x-ray department, they do offer important information about the progress of the patient's disease. Sometimes a patient who cannot stand is not too sick to be taken in his bed to the x-ray department and filmed AP with the equipment available there, a better film being obtained in this way than is possible with the portable unit.

An AP film is not precisely comparable with the standards for normal which your eye will have set up for you based on the larger number of PA films you see. This is because the divergence of the rays enlarges the shadow of the heart, which is far anterior in the chest, and the position of the patient leaning back makes the posterior ribs look more horizontal. This is all particularly true at the shorter tube-film distances used in portable radiography at the bedside. Remember that, in addition, the diaphragm will be higher and the lung volumes less than in a standing patient.

The Lateral Chest Film

After the standard PA film, the next most common view of the chest is the "lateral." It is marked with an R or an L *according to whether the right or the left side of the patient was against the film.* Most often a *left* lateral is made, because the heart is closer to the film and less magnified. Note how the ribs all seem roughly parallel, some pairs superimposed by the beam, forming a single denser white shadow. Mark how far the vertebral column projects into the chest. Large segments of lung extending farther back on either side of the spine are superimposed on it in the lateral view. You may not be able to tell whether you have a right or left lateral in your hand if the technician has forgotten the marker.

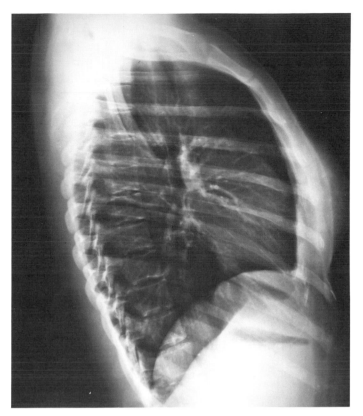

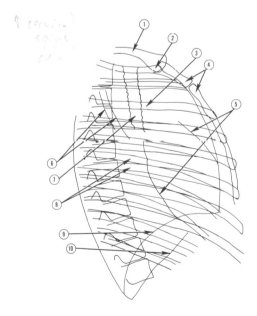

Figure 2-5 (*above*). Right lateral chest film.

Figure 2-6 (*below*). Labeled drawing of Figure 2-5: *1*, clavicle; *2*, medial end of the first rib; *3*, pair of third ribs superimposed; *4*, manubriosternal junction; *5*, anterior and posterior surfaces of the heart; *6*, scapulae; *7*, air in the trachea; *8*, pair of sixth ribs not superimposed; *9* and *10*, right and left hemidiaphragms.

15

The Lordotic View

Here is a patient who was admitted to the hospital with a persistent cough, one episode of blood-streaked sputum, weight loss, and a daily fever. The routine PA chest film in Figure 2-7 is not strikingly abnormal at first glance, but there was a strong clinical suspicion of pulmonary tuberculosis, so a special projection called a *lordotic view* was made. Because the patient stands leaning backward in exaggerated lordosis, the horizontal beam of AP x-rays foreshortens the chest by penetrating it at such an oblique angle that the anterior and posterior segments of the same ribs are superimposed. The result of this maneuver is, of course, to project the clavicles upward so that by looking between the ribs one can much more effectively visualize the lung tissue of the apex. Note that this case is a good exercise in the use of *bilateral symmetry* in examining films made with a sagittal beam. Now one is able to see that there *is* a fluffy white shadow in the upper part of the left lung, best seen in the second interspace. Note that there is nothing like it in the same interspace on the other side. Analysis of the patient's sputum confirmed the diagnosis of tuberculosis.

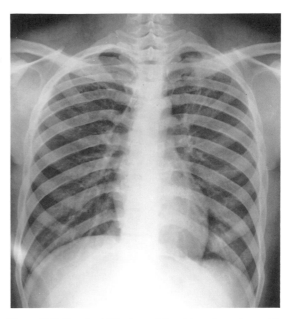

Figure 2-7. Standard PA view of the chest of a patient with cough, fever, weight loss, and hemoptysis.

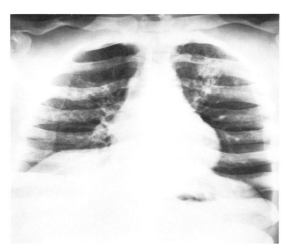

Figure 2-8. Special lordotic view of the chest of the same patient.

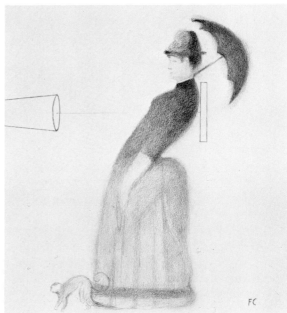

Figure 2-9. Position in which Figure 2-8 was made. (After Seurat.)

16

The chest film in Figure 2-10 offers you an opportunity to test your progress in three-dimensional thinking. There is an obvious metallic radiodensity. The shape of the metal object suggests it might be a bullet. This, in fact, is a film made on a soldier wounded in the Sicilian campaign during World War II. He was invalided out to a hospital, where the surgeons observed what you observe. They requested, as you are about to do, a lateral view to determine the location of the bullet. It might, of course, be in any of the structures whose roentgen shadows superimpose in this view on the origin of the fifth rib.

The importance of localizing a bullet is illustrated by the cross-section drawing. If the bullet is lodged in the spinal cord or the trachea, or in one of the major vascular structures at this level, there may be less hope of saving the patient. In point of fact, the bullet was located harmlessly in the anterior mediastinum, had not injured any vital structure, and was removed without incident. (For the lateral view see Figure 2-12, next page.)

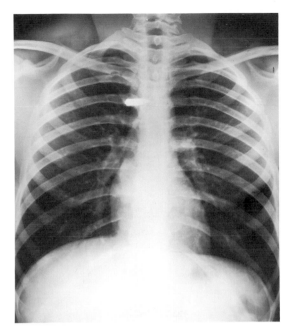

Figure 2-10

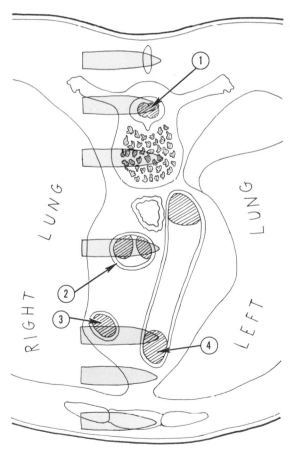

Figure 2-11
(1) Spinal cord
(2) Trachea at bifurcation
(3) Superior vena cava
(4) Ascending aorta

17

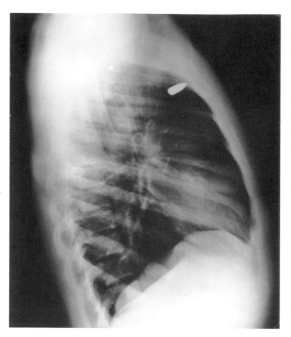

Figure 2-12

You can never know precisely where a foreign body is located from a single radiograph. A film made at right angles to the first is essential, and minute metallic foreign bodies in the soft tissues of the extremities are localized very accurately by a refinement of this procedure. Fractured bones can appear to be in good position, end to end, in one film, although a second film made at right angles shows that the fragments are separated and do not align. Often the making of such supplementary lateral films is a routine matter. At other times you will have to ask that they be made on your patients. Always ask for a right lateral chest film if you think the lesion is on the right, so that the structure to be studied is as close as possible to the film. In most clinics in this country a chest series includes a PA chest film and a *left* lateral. Can you decide why?

At about this point you will begin to say to yourself, "How am I going to know which views are important for me to understand and learn to use?" If, in the course of your training in medicine, you can familiarize yourself with the chest structures and their shadows *as seen in the standard PA and lateral views,* you will have built yourself a very useful and satisfying tool, and you should have no trouble in doing so. Do not feel confused or defeated if occasionally you see chest films which look like nothing you have ever seen before. Some of these will in fact be films of grossly abnormal chests. Others, however, will turn out to be films made by special or rarely used x-ray projections and procedures with which you are not yet familiar. You should rely comfortably on your acquaintance with the standard views, but not be incurious or resistant to the possibilities of other modes of examination.

There are all sorts of ingenious obliquities of projection and many fascinating special procedures in the armamentarium of the radiologist that you will want to know about. Two of them, the posteroanterior obliques of the chest, are sometimes used in studying the heart or hila of the lung. Detailed study of the ribs is obtained by obliques made anteroposteriorly. Others, designed for visualizing a particular structure in a particular way, also offer anatomic information not otherwise available. Sometimes these views or procedures are carried out at the discretion of the radiologist and on his initiation. At other times you will ask for them specifically or, better yet, discuss with a radiologist the advantages of their being used in the study of your patient's particular problem.

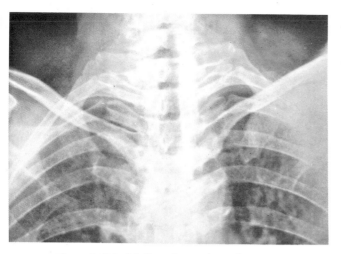

Figure 2-13A. PA film of upper bony thorax.

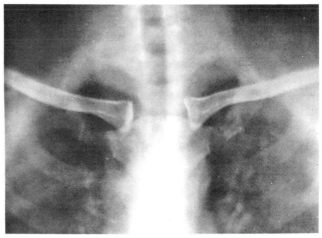

Figure 2-13B. Coronal tomogram of anterior part of bony thorax.

Tomography

The two films in Figure 2-13 were made of the same patient. A, on the left, is an ordinary PA radiograph; B is a special-procedure film called a tomogram. This type of study is going to be very useful to you throughout this book and will help you to visualize better the shadows which must be added together to make up the usual x-ray film. It is important, therefore, to understand how such radiographs are made.

Imagine that a frozen cadaver is sawed into *coronal* slices about 1 inch thick and that you then make a radiograph of each slice. Each film will have on it only the shadows cast by the densities of the structures in that slice. There will be no confusing superimposition of the shadows of structures from other slices to trouble you. How much simpler it would be, for example, to be able to study the manubrium and medial halves of the clavicles if they were not superimposed upon the shadow of the thoracic spine as they are in the standard PA chest film. On the next few pages you will find some radiographed slices of such a cadaver to study. They are arranged in order from front to back, the very first slice having been omitted. (It included the anterior chest wall, rib cartilages, and sternum.) You will find it helpful to refer back to these slices as you learn the x-ray appearance of various organs and structures. Now notice how well you can see in Figure 2-13B the shadows cast by the clavicles where they join the manubrium.

Tomographic studies (like those in Figure 2-13B above) effectively slice the living patient so that you can study the shadows cast by certain structures free of superimposed shadows. The term "tomogram" is a general one and there are different types of sectioning studies, the techniques of which depend upon the result desired, that is, the shadows intended for study and those one wishes to distort. On first acquaintance to mograms will look blurred and confusing to you, but in this book you will be shown many paired studies so that you have the usual x-ray film in the same projection for comparison. Whenever you are puzzled by one of them, try coming back to the cadaver slices on the next two pages to get your bearings, remembering that *only the structures in one plane will be in focus in the tomogram*. Remember too that the thickness of these particular cadaver slices may not match perfectly the chosen plane of the study you happen to be looking at, since the pivot point determining the plane of a tomographic study is calculated arbitrarily for a certain distance in centimeters from the surface of the body.

Coronal Slices of a Frozen Cadaver Radiographed

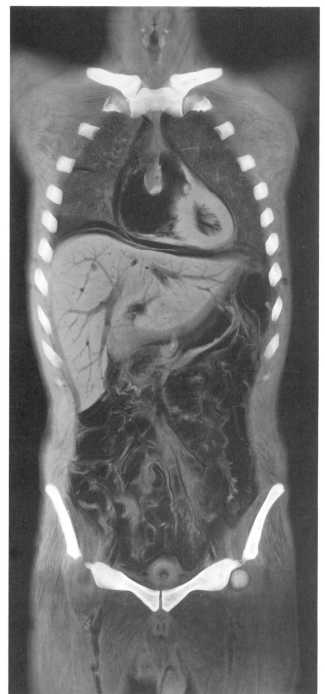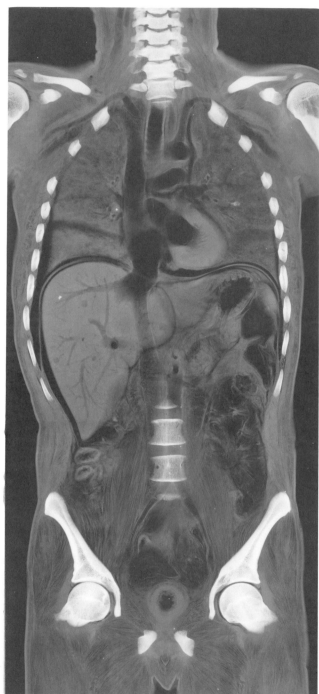

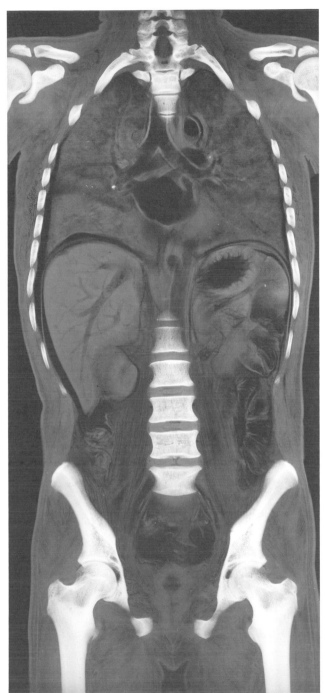

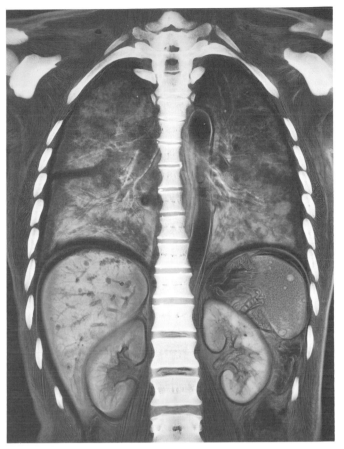

Figures 2-14 to 2-17. Radiographs of a series of coronal slices of cadaver, arranged from front to back. Identify the following:

Junction of manubrium and clavicles
Superior vena cava (empty and filled with air)
Fundus of stomach
   (Each locates the level of the slice just as a body-section tomographic study would identify the level of the slice by including certain structures and excluding others)
Symphysis pubis
Empty cavity of left ventricle
Trachea, carina, and major bronchi with air-filled left atrium immediately below

Note the change in shape of the liver from section to section. Note too that these are *unlike* tomograms because there are no blurred images of structures in other slices.

21

Problems

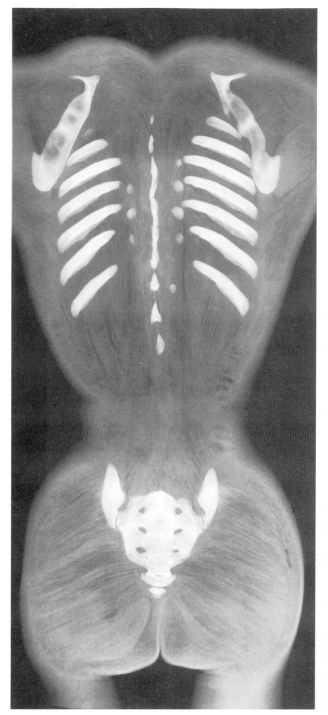

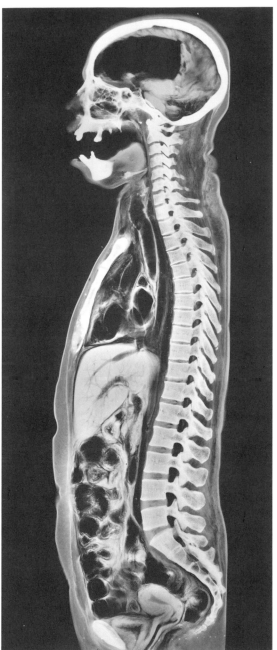

Figures 2-18 (*left*) and 2-19 (*right*). Figure out precisely what has been radiographed. (Answer: *upside down at bottom of page.*)

Answer: Neither is a tomogram. You know this because the images are sharp and clear, unlike the superimposed blurry images one sees as part of any plain tomographic study. (Compare Figure 2-13B.) These are both radiographs of cadaver slices. Figure 2-18 is a far-posterior coronal slice of the cadaver you have seen. This slice contains only the sacrum, posterior parts of the scapulae and ribs, the tips of the spinous processes of the vertebrae, and the muscles about

them. Figure 2-19 is a radiograph of a midline sagittal slice of another cadaver—a female, as you can see from the pelvic structures (uterus lying posterior to the urinary bladder and anterior to the rectum). The section was 1 inch thick, to include the bodies of the vertebrae and their spinous processes but none of their lateral structures. Note the two chambers of the heart that are sectioned (right ventricle and left atrium).

Conventional Tomograms Give You Radiographs of Slices of the Living Patient (here in the coronal plane)

Technically this is done by *moving both the x-ray tube and the film around the patient during the exposure*. They are moved about a pivot point calculated to fall in the plane of the object to be studied. In this way the shadows of all the structures *not* in the plane selected for study are *intentionally blurred* because they move relative to the film. Thus, in the diagram (Figure 2-20) the object to be studied, *b*, will be "in focus" in the film, while the shadow of an object at *a* will be magnified, blurred, and distorted to lie between *a′* and *a″* on the film. Only the structures in the plane of the pivot point will be recognizable (as in Figure 2-21C); the shadows representing organs in front of or behind it are distorted in such a way that shape and form are no longer recognizable and the blurred images are easy for your eye to ignore. Tomography is used as an adjunctive study whenever detail is needed of a structure superimposed on and obscured by other structures in the line of the x-ray beam.

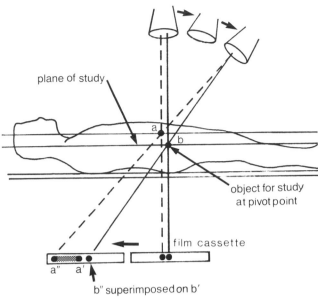

Figure 2-20. Tomogram for a coronal slice.

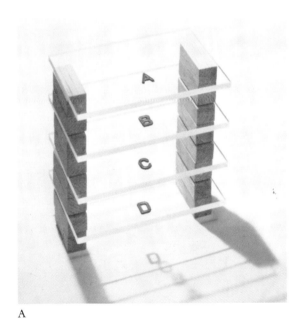

A

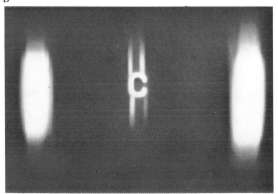

B

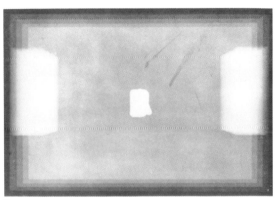

C

Figure 2-21. Demonstration of the effect obtained with tomography. A: Series of plastic shelves each holding a lead letter superimposed vertically. B: Conventional radiograph superimposes the shadows of the letters. C: Conventional tomogram at the level of C shows that letter clearly but distorts and blurs the others.

Computed Tomography

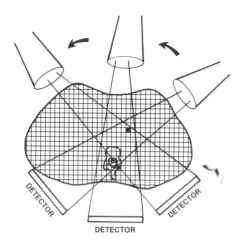

Figure 2-22. Simplified diagram of the principle of computed tomography.

Whereas x-rays were certainly a discovery, computed tomography can be said to be an invention, for it was developed in response to a need for better visualization of the brain than had been possible with ordinary x-rays. Computed tomography (CT) adds an important dimension for you in that it provides the equivalent of cross-sectional slice radiographs of the living body. These are the CAT (computerized axial tomography) scans known to the lay public and have become a vital source of additional radiologic information in medicine in the past two decades. You would not be able to function today as a physician without a sound understanding of radiology and the way in which it has been embellished by computed tomography.

You can begin by understanding the difference between plain radiographs, plain (or conventional) tomography, and CT. Remember that ordinary plain x-ray films are superimposition shadowgrams: the images of all superimposed structures appear on the film. *Conventional* tomography gives you sharply focused radiographic information about one plane of the patient upon which are superimposed (unfortunately) the *blurred* images of structures in slices on both sides of the plane chosen for study.

A CT scan, on the other hand, gives you focused radiographic information about one cross-sectional slice of the patient only, without any confusing superimposed images. Thus a CT scan gives you a schema of density values for a particular chosen slice of the patient, which should be studied with regional cross-sectional anatomy in mind. You will be able to learn the relationships between structures in the body much more accurately with the help of the added dimension CT provides.

An awareness of the relative x-ray densities of different tissues and organs and their interfaces with fat planes in the body helps you as you look at CT scans. In computed tomography a pencil-thin collimated beam of x-rays passes through the body plane chosen for study as the x-ray tube moves in a continuous arc around the patient. Carefully aligned and directly opposite the x-ray tube are placed special electronic detectors, a hundred times more sensitive than ordinary x-ray film. These detectors convert the exiting beam on the other edge of the body slice into amplified electrical pulses, the intensity of which depends upon the amount of the remaining beam of x-rays that has not been absorbed by the intervening tissues. Thus if the beam has passed mainly through dense areas of the body (such as bone), fewer x-rays will emerge than when the beam traverses mainly low-density tissue (such as lung).

If you conceive of a body slice as a flat mosaic of unit volumes, or voxels (see Figure 2-22), forming a geometric grid, you can see that a single denser unit volume (perhaps calcium containing, like the small black square in Figure 2-22) will absorb more of the beam than other less dense neighboring voxels.

As fast as it is received by the detectors, this information is conveyed to a computer, which then calculates the x-ray absorption for each voxel in the mosaic. The pictorial arrangement of absorption values makes up the final CT image. The absorption value is expressed in Hounsfield units (after one of the inventors of CT). Water was arbitrarily assigned the value of zero, while denser values range upward to bone (which can be +500 or more). Less dense structures range downward through fat to air (which can be −500).

24

The attenuation number so obtained for each voxel in the mosaic matrix slice is converted into a dot on a television monitor screen, the brightness of which depends on the density of that unit volume and so reflects its anatomic structure. The "picture" so produced is equivalent to a radiograph of that cross-sectional slice of the living patient.

It is conventional to view the CT scan so produced as though one were looking up at it from the patient's feet (Figures 2-23, 2-24, and 2-25), and it is important to remember that therefore the structures seen on your right are those on the left side of the patient's body, just as they are when you view an ordinary chest film. Permanent images are produced by photographing the TV screen. The CT scans in your patient's film envelope are documented on 14 × 17 inch x-ray film, each such film having a number of scan slices in sequence, so that you can look from one slice to the next above or below for additional information about a structure or an organ (as in the scans in Figure 2-23 just above the aortic arch and Figure 2-24 through the arch).

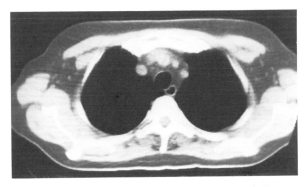

Figure 2-23. A CT scan made just above the aortic arch. You can identify the great vessels from the patient's right to left: right brachiocephalic vein being joined by the left brachiocephalic vein crossing just behind the sternum. The large brachiocephalic artery lies between it and the black (air-filled) trachea. Then, in the order in which they come off the aorta, come the left common carotid and left subclavian arteries.

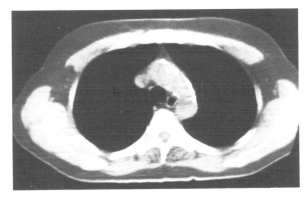

Figure 2-24. A CT scan made 2 centimeters lower through the arch of the aorta. You can identify the superior vena cava and partially calcified aortic arch, as well as the air-filled trachea and esophagus. (Remember, you are looking up from the patient's feet.)

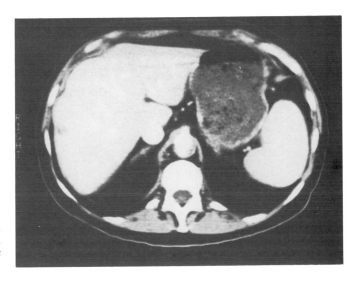

Figure 2-25. A CT scan made through the upper abdomen. Identify the liver, spleen, stomach containing fluid and food. You know the patient is supine (lying on his back) because the air-fluid level you see in the stomach must be horizontal.

The usual CT series of scans consists of contiguous 10-millimeter-thick slices through the region requested, but slices as thin as 1.5 millimeters can be obtained when finer detail is needed for diagnosis. The x-ray dose per slice varies from 1 to 4 rads (but only to the slice being imaged) and is comparable to the exposure for conventional x-ray studies of the area.

High-density materials such as barium or metal (a hip prosthesis or metal surgical clips) may produce artifacts like bright stars with sharply geometric radiating white lines that degrade the image obtained and interfere with the information available from it. Motion too degrades the image. The movement of abdominal organs during respiration is 1 or 2 centimeters, enough to distort the images of smaller structures.

CT scanners require only 1 to 10 seconds to complete a slice, and a patient who cannot hold his breath may have motion artifacts on his scan. Most patients can hold their breath for 5 seconds repeatedly, but of course unconscious, very ill, or dyspneic patients and small children requiring CT studies may produce motion degradation of the image. Mild sedation and reassurance by you as well as by the radiologist may help, but the *gantry*, or housing for the equipment, is huge and may be frightening. It behooves you to inspect the CT room in your x-ray department so that you can explain to your patient beforehand that the procedure is as painless as having his photograph taken, in spite of the look of the machine.

Body CT scans can be produced with the patient supine or prone or lying on his side. Other planes of imaging, especially of the head and extremities, are possible, but you will need to learn to think of most CT body scans as transaxial and supine, since the patient is most comfortable and relaxed lying on his back.

It is important for you to realize that CT should be considered most of the time as a sophisticated study for special problems, usually arranged following consultation with the radiologist. Other less expensive procedures like plain films and ultrasound are used when the information obtained is comparable.

The important exceptions to this principle are in traumatized patients and central nervous system emergencies. In head trauma the superior capacity of CT to recognize intracranial hemorrhage often makes ordinary skull films a dangerous waste of time. Patients with abdominal trauma too are taken straight to the CT suite for serial scans from the diaphragm through the pelvis, supplying a rich gain of emergency information about hemorrhage and organ rupture that can save lives. CT much more efficiently informs managing clinicians about the order in which treatment procedures should be undertaken.

Depending on the clinical condition under investigation, contrast media may be used during CT scanning to enhance the difference in density of various structures. The GI tract can be illuminated by giving the patient dilute oral contrast material, which will help to distinguish stomach and bowel from other soft-tissue structures and masses. Intravenous administration of water-soluble contrast material will produce a temporary increase in the density of vascular structures and highly vascularized organs. This is referred to as enhancement and is extremely useful. For example, a great vessel and the tumor mass encasing and constricting it will appear as one homogeneously dense mass unless the vessel is enhanced with contrast material, when its narrowing will be apparent.

Other Important Imaging Modalities

The application of CT and other important imaging procedures will be addressed as we go along, but you need a brief mention here of several other imaging modalities that are used to reveal the three-dimensional form and composition of anatomic structures.

Ultrasonography also gives you an image of a slice of the body by directing a narrow beam of high-energy sound waves into the body and recording the manner in which sound is reflected from organs and structures. Ultrasound does not produce an image that is as sharp and clear as CT, but it has four singular advantages: it does not employ ionizing radiation and produces no biological injury; it can be employed in the transaxial plane or sagittally or at any chosen obliquity as required by the anatomic region being investigated; it is far less expensive than either CT or magnetic resonance; it can even be performed portably at the bedside of very sick patients. As it is employed most widely in studying the abdomen, a more detailed discussion will be deferred until the chapters on the abdomen.

Like ultrasound, *magnetic resonance* (MR) does not use ionizing radiation as ordinary x-rays and CT do. The rapid development of magnetic-resonance imaging makes it essential for

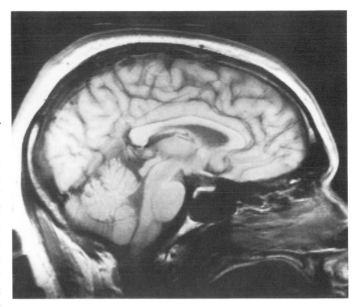

Figure 2-27. Magnetic-resonance image made midsagittally through the brain.

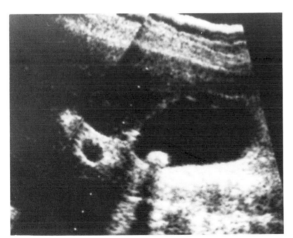

Figure 2-26. Longitudinal (parasagittal) sonogram showing a solitary gallstone sitting on the posterior wall of the gallbladder. The patient has been studied lying on his back. At the top of the cut you see the anterior abdominal wall and layers of muscle. No reflected sound waves are returned to the scanner by the fluid filling the gallbladder or from the shadowed area behind the gallstone.

you to have some idea of its uses in clinical medicine as well as the exquisite visualization it renders possible for anatomic structures in the living patient. This technique for imaging places the patient within the bore of a powerful magnet and passes radio waves through his body in a particular sequence of very short pulses. Each pulse causes a responding pulse of radio waves to be emitted from the patient's tissues. The location from which the signals have originated is recorded by a computer, which then produces a two-dimensional picture representing a predetermined section or slice of the patient.

The thickness of the section can be chosen as well as its orientation. In addition to the transverse sections of the body which you are now accustomed to expect from CT, magnetic-resonance imaging can be carried out in the sagittal and coronal planes as well as in various desirable degrees of obliquity.

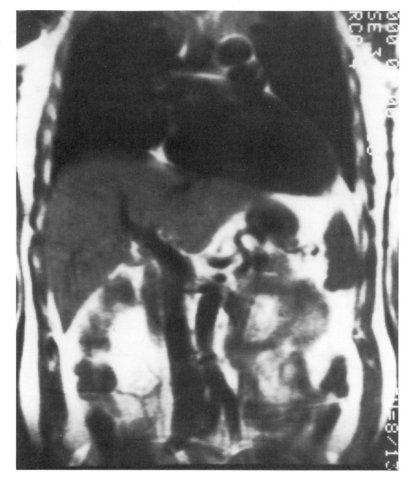

Figure 2-28. Magnetic-resonance image made coronally through the body. You will be able to identify the liver, portal vein, vena cava, aorta, fundus of stomach, and spleen.

Different body tissues emit characteristic MR signals, which determine whether they will appear white, gray, or black on the final scans. Tissues which emit strong MR signals appear white in MR scans, whereas those emitting little or no signal appear black. The operator can vary the technique used by changing the sequence of pulses so that particular tissues can be seen better. This may vary the appearance of the scan, but in general *air and cortical bone as well as rapidly moving fluid (blood) will appear black, whereas fat will appear white.* Slowly moving blood, however, may produce a detectable signal by MR. Consequently some venous structures and arteries imaged during diastole may return signals and appear in various shades of gray, as you will see in the chapter on the heart.

28

Finally, *nuclear imaging,* another branch of radiology, offers physiologic information of importance in modern medicine which you must be aware of and to some extent familiar with. This branch of radiology is based on the visualization of particular living organs and tissues because an injected radioactive isotope takes up residence there briefly. It does so because the selected chemical substance to which the isotope has been attached is normally involved in the physiologic metabolism of that organ or will remain there long enough to be imaged. An image is obtained because the radioactive isotope emits gamma rays for a brief period of time. The emitted rays are recorded by a *gamma camera* during the period of gamma emission. A few hours or days later, the isotope will stop emitting detectable rays as it returns to a stable state. Its return to stability is measured in terms of its *half-life,* that is, the period until it is seen to be emitting half as much radiation as it did initially. Isotopes chosen for tagging are those which will remain in the organ to be studied long enough to produce a usable image but with relatively short half-lives so as to minimize radiation to the patient's tissues.

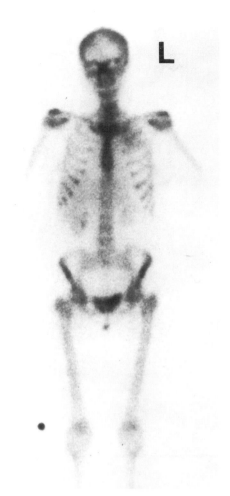

Figure 2-29. Normal technetium bone scan. Compare with Figure 2-30.

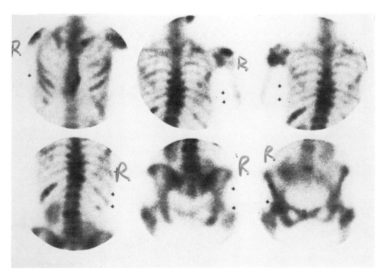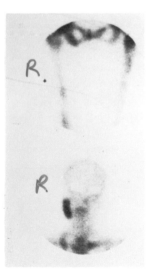

Figure 2-30. Series of technetium bone scans in a patient with breast carcinoma. Note uptake of the isotope as dark patches, and asymmetry of distribution of the metastases. Some of these scans are made with the gamma camera positioned anteriorly and in others posteriorly, in order to place various bony parts nearer the scanner.

Technetium has proved to be the most useful radioactive tracer and is linked to various physiological substances that will seek different organs. One of these, deposited temporarily in bone, is called a bone seeker. The image obtained shows areas of more or less intensity of radiation related to portions of the bone having increased turnover. Thus "hot spots" showing markedly increased activity of bone will be seen as dense black areas on a gamma camera or rectilinear scan of the whole skeleton (see bone scan, Figure 2-29). Unfortunately, these are very nonspecific and do not tell us the cause of the increased bone turnover. If they are located in symmetrical joint areas, for example, they may be being caused by acute arthritis, and if they are located eccentrically like those in Figure 2-30, they may be assumed to indicate the location of bone metastases from the patient's known or suspected cancer.

Technetium may also be linked to a sulfur colloid that is normally picked up by the liver and will remain there long enough to be imaged as a densely homogeneous, liver-shaped area of activity on the isotope scan of the abdomen. With any such radiopharmaceutical used, there may be areas on the scan where "cold spots" indicate decreased physiological uptake. These also are nonspecific in that they indicate only an area of less metabolic turnover. Thus a large solitary cold spot in the otherwise homogeneously imaged liver might indicate the location of a large tumor metastasis or of a benign cyst.

The man whose liver you see imaged in Figure 2-31 was known to have had a normally homogeneous scan two years ago, when his carcinoma of the colon was resected surgically. Now he has multiple cold spots and must be presumed to have metastases to the liver, a very common location for tumor spread. An ordinary x-ray film of the patient's abdomen might show his liver to be enlarged, but would not differentiate the tumor-invaded areas from normal metabolically active liver tissue around them. Isotope scans, like all other radiologic images, must always be interpreted in tandem with clinical information about the patient.

As we proceed through this book, other important procedures using radioactive isotopes will be described. Remember for now that nuclear medicine gives you less precise anatomic information but much more important physiological information, which will help you to understand and remember metabolic processes, both normal and abnormal.

Realize that in the usual isotope scan, the image obtained is produced by gamma radiation from the *entire thickness* of the organ, not from a single slice of it as in CT, MR, and sonography. Realize also that just as *fluoroscopy* in plain radiography consists of continuous or intermittent observation of tissues penetrated by x-rays and produces *dynamic* radiographic information, so too any of the other imaging modalities we have been discussing can be used dynamically. The motion of the fetal heart is routinely monitored by "real-time" sonography as evidence that a quiet fetus is, in fact, alive. Dynamic studies using rapidly sequenced CT scans during the intravenous injection of contrast material produce time-lapse information about the vascularity of a liver mass. Similarly, sequential isotope scans are in use to document flow patterns such as blood flow through the heart chambers in a patient suspected of having a congenital heart anomaly.

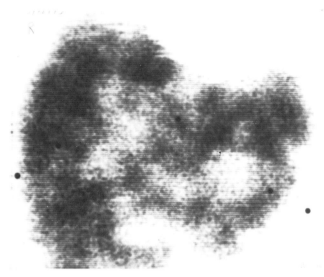

Figure 2-31. Liver isotope scan shows many areas of no uptake, metastases from carcinoma of the colon.

As a student, you certainly can learn to recognize some of the basic pathophysiological changes imaged on plain films of the chest, abdomen, and bones. You cannot expect to learn to recognize all of the innumerable more subtle plain radiographic changes the radiologist identifies. Neither will you be able to "interpret" the findings the radiologist recognizes in the many supplementary modalities such as CT and ultrasound. A four-year residency in radiology is scarcely enough time in which to learn to do that.

It is important, though, for you to learn while you are in medical school how to use the help the radiologist can give you in planning which procedures ought to be included in your diagnostic workup plan, and the order in which they should be undertaken.

Now we are ready for the time being to return to plain radiographic studies in common use, and we will begin with the chest film.

CHAPTER 3 How to Study a Chest Film: The Bony Thorax and Soft Tissues

Hardly anyone ever reads the preface to a book, but if you read ours, you know that the goal of this book is threefold: to help medical students understand x-ray shadows as an aid to learning in the other disciplines, to equip them with a basic knowledge of the reasons for the roentgen appearance of some of the common disease conditions they will meet as physicians, and to help them learn how to use the radiologist as a valued consultant early in the patient's workup. It is our hope that those who study this book will develop a habit of mind in which every shadow on the radiograph arouses the responsive question, "*Why* does it look like that?"

One glance at a chest film often is enough to "see" a very striking abnormality. Having seen it, the observer must reason out its structural identity, seldom quite so obvious, and attempt to deduce its nature in accordance with a knowledge of the patient's illness. While the single-glance approach has its value, it is full of danger to the patient, because the presence of a very obvious abnormality tends to suppress psychologically your search for more subtle changes. And the subtler changes are quite often more important to the patient than the obvious ones.

Let us say that you correctly interpret the shadow of a large mass in the lung on Mr. B's chest film (Figure 3-2A) as being consistent with the cancer you thought he might have when you questioned and examined him. You will have failed him if you neglect a deliberate quest for any possible secondary involvement of his bones, since quite a different program of treatment may then become appropriate. Figure 3-2B illustrates the point by showing in more detail, with a more penetrating x-ray beam, the extent of his bone destruction.

The system generally employed by the radiologist is to *look at* various structures in a deliberate order, concentrating on the anatomy of each while excluding the superimposed shadows of other structures. Even as an exercise in intellectual discipline, this is not as difficult as it sounds.

Prove it to your own satisfaction by trying to *look at* one clavicle or one rib on any of the chest films in this chapter, thinking of its normal anatomic proportions and excluding other shadows overlying it which you know are not part of the bone you are studying.

The best way to be systematic about studying any film is to adopt a definite order in which you look at the structures whose shadows appear there. For a chest film you will *look at* the bony framework and then, just as deliberately, *look through it* at lung tissue and the heart.

Begin with the scapulae. Then look at the portions of humerus and shoulder joint often visible on the chest film. Inspect the clavicles, and then finally study the ribs, quickly but in pairs from top to bottom. When you can, always compare the two sides for symmetry. The spine and sternum are, of course, superimposed upon each other and upon the dense shadows of the mediastinal structures in the PA view so that, at the kilovoltages used for lung study, little of the beam penetrates and the film remains less well exposed down the midline.

Remember that the technique used for chest films has been designed for study of the lung; what you see of the bones is incidental. Ideal techniques for studying these same bones will be quite different. In a PA chest film, for example, the scapulae and posterior ribs are as far as possible from the film. Therefore they are enlarged and distorted to some extent. In addition, on the chest film the scapulae have been intentionally rotated to the sides as much as they can be by placing the hands on the hips, palms out, with the elbows forward. Try it. In the PA view of the chest this maneuver prevents the superimposition of the scapular shadows upon the upper lung fields, and only the medial margin of the scapula will be seen overlapping the axillary portions of the upper ribs. Decide whether the scapulae were properly rotated in Figure 3-1.

32

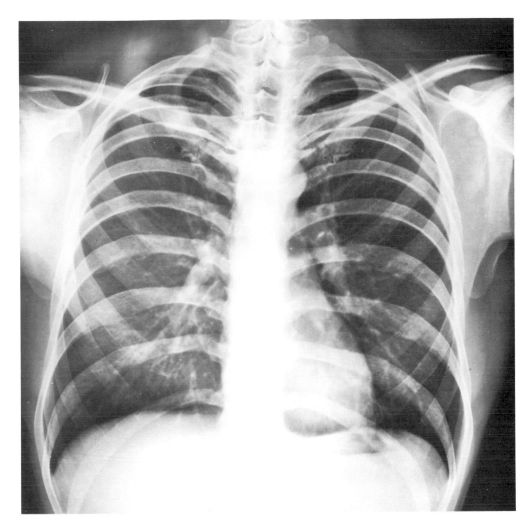

Figure 3-1. Normal PA chest film.

Figure 3-2. A (*left*): PA chest film of Mr. B, admitted with cough, chest pain, hoarseness, and a fist-sized mass in the left supraclavicular region. B (*below*): Detail study of the thoracic inlet made AP with a more penetrating beam. Left posterior first rib and parts of the first two thoracic vertebrae have been destroyed by tumor.

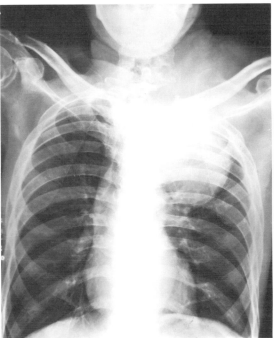

A

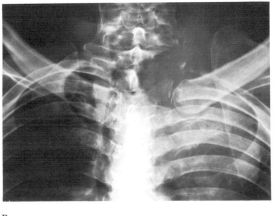

B

33

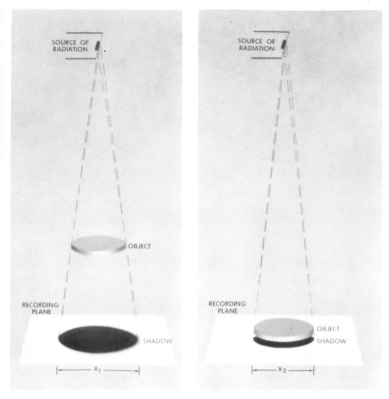

Figure 3-3. Effect of projection in enlarging the roentgen shadows of objects far away from the film.

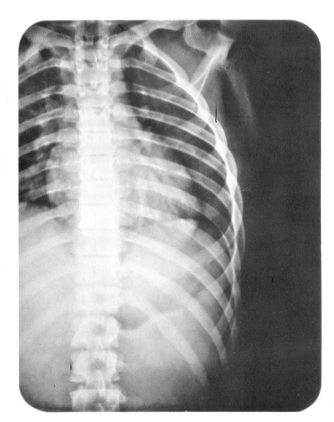

Projection

Do not discount the factor of *projection* in altering the appearance of structures far away from the film. You need not be confused by such changes, however, once you are familiar with them. In Figure 3-3 you have a diagram illustrating the effect of projection, in which you can equate the "object" with the scapula in any AP and PA chest film. You can equate it also with the anteriorly placed heart in the AP film, Figure 3-4. Note that the heart in this film appears to be larger, with less sharp margins, than the hearts in the PA chest films you have seen up to now. Note also the slight difference in the width and shape of the posterior rib interspaces compared with those on the usual PA film.

The routine chest film measures 14 × 17 inches, and its cassette film holder is placed with the long dimension vertical. In broad-chested persons little of the *shoulder girdle* and *humerus* will be seen, but in slender, smaller individuals you may actually have all of the shoulder and most of the upper arm to study. Figure 3-5 is a radiograph of the shoulder made AP. Figure 3-6, next to it so that you can look back and forth, is a photograph of the bones of the shoulder. Notice how you seem to see the coracoid *through* the spine of the scapula because they superimpose, just as you see the head of the humerus and the acromion additively.

The man in Figure 3-7 had fallen from a horse and had his arm immobilized in plaster (*a,a*), which you see more densely wherever the ray came through it tangentially. Since there are several fractures and several fragments, this is what is called a *comminuted* fracture. Note the folds and wrinkles in the plaster and the point in the axilla where the cast ends (*b*).

The woman in Figure 3-8 could not comb her hair or tie her apron strings without intense pain in her shoulder. She had tenderness over the insertion of the supraspinatus tendon and, as you see, she has *calcification* in that area and around the shoulder joint—dense white shadows not present on any of the x-rays of normal shoulders you have seen so far. These findings (*b*) are typical of "bursitis" or calcific peritendinitis of the shoulder.

Figure 3-4. AP view of the chest made with the posterior ribs close to the film. The heart, far from the film, is projected and looks larger than normal. Compare also with Figures 2-4A and 2-4B.

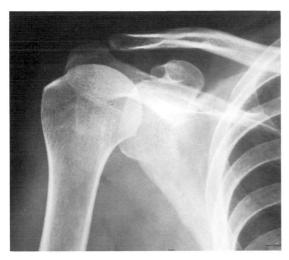

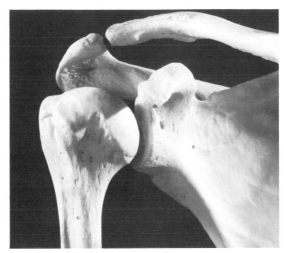

Figure 3-5. Identify the clavicle, acromioclavicular joint, head and greater tuberosity of humerus, glenoid, acromion, and coracoid process.

Figure 3-6. Photograph of the bones of the shoulder.

Note the dense white triangular shadow medial to the midhumerus (*a*) in Figure 3-8. It is common in radiology and is called an *overlap shadow*. In this instance it is created by the added densities of heavy breast and soft tissues of the upper arm. The confusion arising from the unexpected density of the shadow at *a* will be easy for you to resolve if you remember that *thickness* as well as *composition* determines radiodensity. Although fat, skin, and muscle ought to be less radiodense than bone, the shadow cast by a thick mass of these tissues will approach that of bone, as you see in this figure. Note, on the other hand, that a small amount of air imprisoned in the axilla is black on the film, probably because it was a long pocket of air x-rayed end-on.

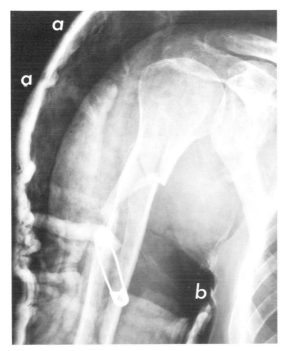

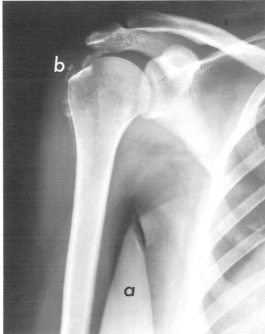

Figures 3-7 (*left*) and 3-8 (*right*). Two patients with shoulder pain.

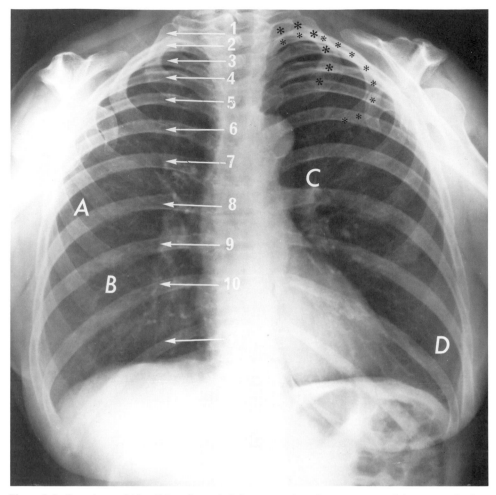

Figure 3-9. Counting and identifying ribs and rib interspaces is an important part of the systematic chest film survey. (See text for instructions.) Note, incidentally, that the breast shadows in this patient come well below the level of the diaphragm and do not obscure the lower lung field; in many female patients they do.

Systematic Study of the Rib Cage

Using the bilateral symmetry of each pair of ribs in Figure 3-9, and beginning at the origin of the first rib at its junction with the first thoracic vertebra, trace each rib as far as you can anteriorly to the beginning of the radiolucent (and hence invisible) costal cartilage. The ribs are useful to the radiologist because he locates an abnormal shadow by its proximity to a particular rib or interspace on a film he is describing. Anyone reading his written report can identify in this way the precise shadow he is discussing. Thus *A* in Figure 3-9 could be described as lying in the seventh interspace on the right, close to the axilla (that is, the outer third of the space between the posterior halves of the right seventh and eighth ribs). If you do not locate it there, count again;

you are probably getting lost in the overlap tangle of ribs 1, 2, and 3. To avoid this, identify the first rib carefully by finding its anterior junction with the manubrium and following this rib *backward* to the spine. Then count down the posterior ribs. *B* would be said to be located in the ninth interspace on the right. Note that the word "interspace" always implies the space between *posterior* segments of adjoining ribs, unless the anterior is specified. Try your hand at designating the location of *C* and *D*, covering the left half of this figure and the spine with all its numbers. (Have you noticed anything peculiar about this film? Is there anything missing? Compare it with Figure 3-1.)

36

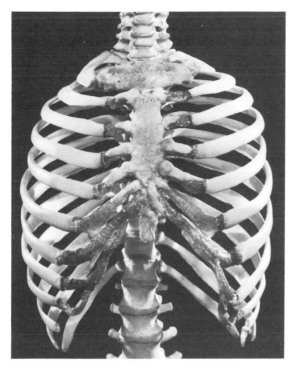

A: Anterior and posterior ribs.

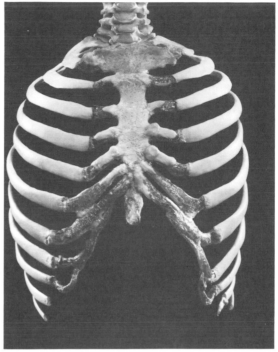

B: Anterior ribs only.

Figure 3-10. The bony thorax photographed in such a way as to help you visualize chest films three-dimensionally. Imagine the location of the diaphragm in each figure. B and C were photographed with the thoracic cage stuffed with black velvet.

The *ribs* confuse everyone beginning to look at chest films. The miracle is that one can discern anything useful about the heart and lungs through such a crosshatched pattern of shadows. Three-dimensional thinking will be easier if you try to concentrate first on the posterior halves of the ribs and then on the anterior. In Figure 3-10B and C the same thorax was photographed from the front and from the back after the cavity had been stuffed with black velvet to give you the illusion you seek in trying to study the posterior ribs while excluding from your mind the anterior ones.

Warning! Remember to think in terms of *coronal* slices and the summation shadows they produce, as in the cadaver in Chapter 2. The transaxial shadows used in CT are useful too in three-dimensional thinking, and we will return to them presently.

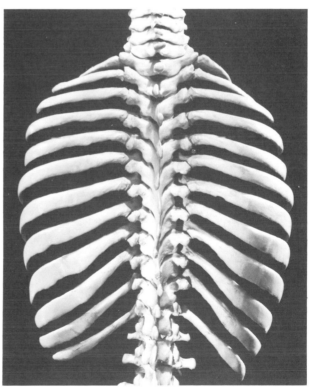

C: Posterior ribs only.

Rotation Produces Confusing Shadows

Because of their curiously curved shape, the shadows of the two *clavicles* will appear symmetrical on the chest film only if there is no rotation of the chest. In a perfectly true PA film the beam passes straight through the midsagittal plane. The arms and shoulders of the patient are arranged symmetrically, either hands on hips or arms overhead, and the technician checks for rotation and corrects it before making the exposure. Turned even a few degrees, the clavicles will exhibit a remarkable degree of asymmetry. This fact will prove very useful to you, because a glance at the clavicles will tell you whether or not the beam has passed through the sagittal plane and whether you are therefore looking at a true PA or AP film without rotation.

Even slight rotation is undesirable in a chest film, because the heart and mediastinum are then radiographed obliquely and their shadows appear enlarged and distorted. If you think of the mediastinum as a disc of denser structures flat-tened between the two inflated lungs and normally x-rayed end-on in a PA chest film, it is easy to see how rotation of this disc will produce a wider shadow. If it were a valid finding, enlargement of the heart or widening of the mediastinal shadow would be an important piece of roentgen evidence for disease. One has to be able to disregard apparent enlargement due to rotation, therefore, and the best clue to rotation is asymmetry of the shadows of the two clavicles. Learn to watch them, mentally noting their symmetry or lack of it, in your systematic survey of the chest film.

Now look back at Figure 3-9. Did you notice that there were no clavicles? The patient was born without them and is an ideal subject on whom to learn to count ribs. Compare this with any normal chest film and observe that you can mentally subtract the shadow of the clavicle when you want to in order to study or count the first three ribs.

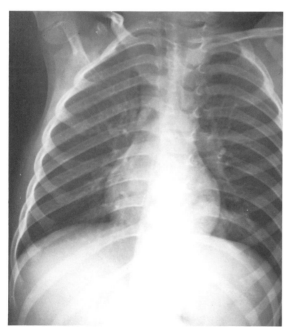

Figure 3-11. Chest film made when the patient was accidentally somewhat rotated. Note the marked asymmetry of the clavicles.

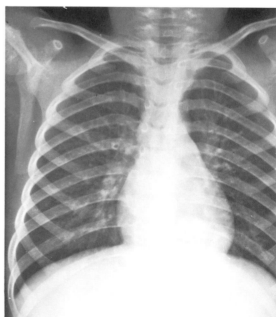

Figure 3-12. Same patient refilmed precisely PA.

38

Problems in Studying Ribs and Clavicles

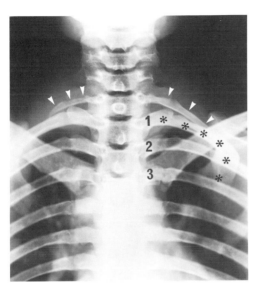

Figure 3-13 (*Unknown 3-1*). If you think the ribs are correctly labeled here, how do you account for the structures indicated by the white arrows?

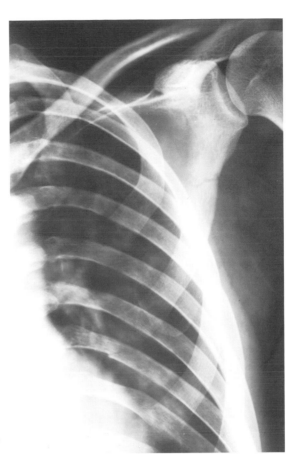

Figure 3-14 (*Unknown 3-2*). This patient has been filmed after an automobile accident. Which rib is fractured?

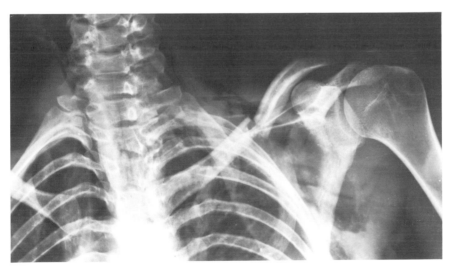

Figure 3-15 (*Unknown 3-3*). The figure is obviously not a true PA film, for the very good reason that the patient was in a great deal of pain. Study the bones using any normal shoulder girdle for comparison. Then study the soft tissues outside the chest cage around the shoulder girdle. How can you account for the dark streaks?

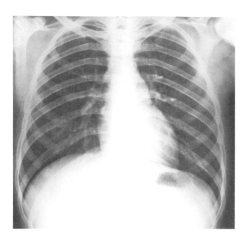

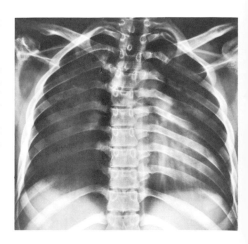

Figure 3-16 (*left*). Regular chest film made PA at 6 feet with the patient standing.

Figure 3-17 (*right*). AP film of the chest exposed for study of the spine. Patient lying down; Bucky diaphragm used. Ideal exposure for a chest film today is somewhere between these two and allows faint visualization of the intervertebral spaces through the heart.

Importance of Exposure

The thoracic spine is not well seen in the chest films you have been looking at because its density added to those of the mediastinal structures and sternum together absorb almost all the rays and few reach the film to blacken it. This is true of the techniques commonly used for studying the lung. Seeing detail through very dense parts of the body requires a different technique. More penetration can be achieved in several ways. One is by increasing the exposure factors (kilovoltage, milliamperage, and time) to produce a beam of x-rays of shorter wavelength, so-called harder rays. A film made in this way is often called an overexposed film, intentionally overexposed in order to increase the penetration of dense structures.

Unfortunately, when x-rays impinge on matter of any kind, secondary x-rays are generated which radiate in all directions as from many point sources of light. This is called scattered radiation and is, of course, added photographically to the primary beam, additionally blackening the film. Since there are thus multiple sources of radiation, a blurred and distorted image is produced. Moreover, increasing the exposure factors to produce a harder and more penetrating beam also increases the amount of scattered radiation. Thus, a simple overexposed film will usually be lacking in contrast and sharpness.

Scattered radiation can be eliminated by an ingenious device called a *Bucky diaphragm*. Interposed between the patient and the film, it is a flat grid composed of alternate very thin strips of radiolucent and radiopaque material (wood and lead, for example). Only the most perpendicular rays pass through the lucent wood strips. The oblique rays, representing most of the scattered radiation, strike the sides of the lead strips and are absorbed.

If the interposed grid is motionless, of course, the lead strips will appear on the film as fine white lines. To prevent this, it is only necessary to move the grid across the film throughout the exposure; no lines will appear.

You will find that in an obese patient, or in any patient whose spine, mediastinum, skull, or heavy long bones must be studied by x-ray, Bucky-technique films will have been made automatically by the technician. Every film you see of the abdomen will have been made in this way also.

The PA chest film in Figure 3-16 was made expressly for the purpose of studying the lung. Figure 3-17 was made AP (so that the spine toward which the study was directed would be close to the film), and a Bucky diaphragm and the appropriate exposure technique were used to produce it. Notice how well you can see the structure of the vertebrae with their interposed

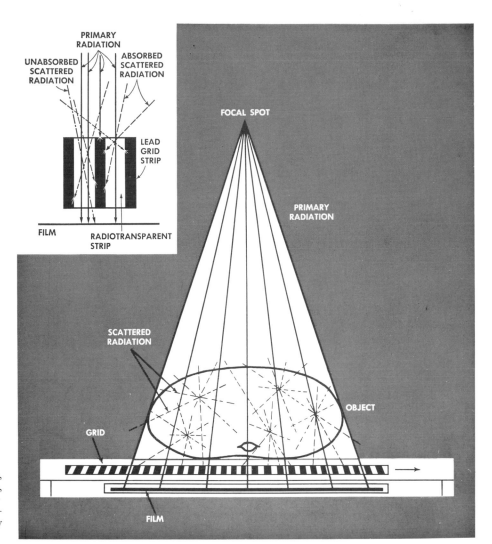

Figure 3-18. The Bucky diaphragm, plus increased kilovoltage and time, give the desired increased penetration and clearer detail to radiographs of thick parts of the body (see text).

cartilaginous discs, which should be just visible in a routine chest film. Note also that here you can see the ribs below the diaphragm, scarcely visible in most regular chest films. This film would be useless for studying the lung, all the delicate detail being lost.

Therefore, as you look at any chest film you should try to estimate whether it is exposed correctly or overexposed or underexposed. Correct PA exposure for routine chest films allows you to see the more radiolucent intervertebral spaces but not the detailed anatomy of the vertebrae. This is important for the following reasons: if a film is underexposed you will be tempted to overinterpret vascular shadows in the lungs, whereas in an overexposed film minute densities of importance may be missed because they are "burned out."

Soft Tissues

Mammography

Just as the lung detail is burned out with these techniques, so also are the soft tissues of the chest lying outside the thoracic cage. Having completed your survey of the bones, you should now *look at* these soft tissues, studying breast tissues, supraclavicular areas, axillae, and the subcutaneous tissue and muscles along the sides of the chest where it is seen in tangent. You will be able to study the soft tissues in any film exposed for study of the lungs, and they often give you vital information about the patient. Are the soft tissues scanty, indicating perhaps that the patient has lost weight? Are the normally symmetrical triangles of dark fat in the supraclavicular region disturbed in any way? Look back at Figure 3-2A and at Unknown 3-3. Always be sure to check whether there are two breasts: a chest film showing one missing breast often means that the patient is being studied for recurrence of cancer, and attention should be directed toward bones and lung field for evidence of metastases. The lung field under a missing breast appears a little darker than the other lung field because of the missing tissue of the breast and sometimes pectoral muscles removed at the time of the mastectomy. Look forward a few pages, identifying the female patients, and see if you can find one with a breast missing on the left.

The breast itself may be studied radiographically with a special technique called *mammography,* in which the breast is the only part placed between the beam source and the film. This technique is widely used for early detection of breast cancer. Cancer of the breast would not be recognized on a regular chest film. Your radiologist will help you to determine when mammography is indicated for your patient. As a general rule, women younger than 35 are not now routinely studied by mammography if they are asymptomatic with no reason to suspect a malignant mass, because of the radiation exposure involved. If a mass is palpated or questioned on physical examination, or if the patient's breasts are difficult to examine, most physicians would want mammography done. Older women often have routine screening mammograms. In them the relatively larger amount of fat in the breast makes the recognition of malignant nodules much easier even when none can be palpated.

So much, then, for the first step in studying a chest film: a systematic survey of the bones and soft tissues. You are ready now to look past the bones at the shadow of the lung itself.

Unknowns

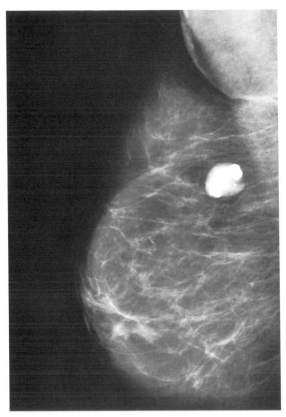

A

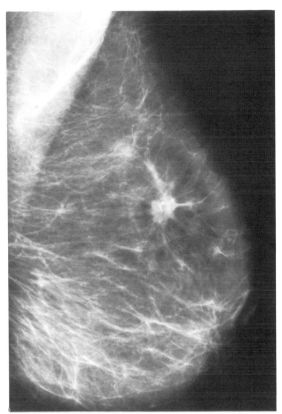

B

Figure 3-19 (*Unknown 3-4*). Mammograms of the two breasts of a woman who had discovered a mass in her right breast (on your left above). Her physician confirmed the mass and considered it suspicious for carcinoma (the left breast was normal on physical examination). Find the mass and describe it on the telephone to your chief. (See Answers to Unknowns for resolution of case.)

Figure 3-20 (*Unknown 3-5*). The patient was asymptomatic. Is this a normal film?

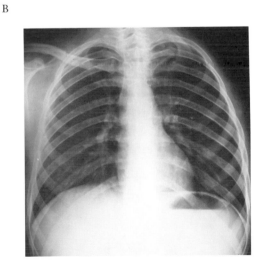

CHAPTER 4   The Lung Itself

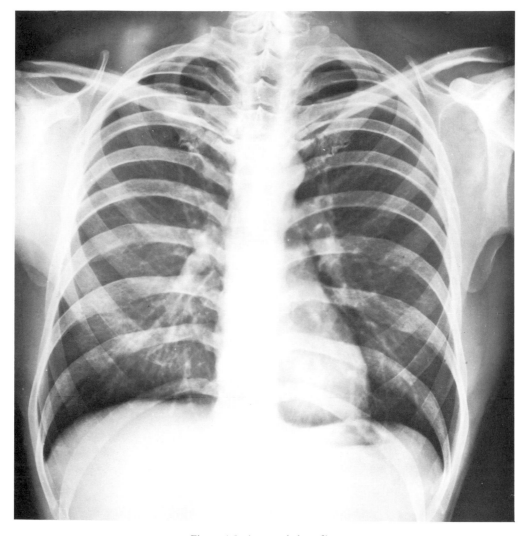

Figure 4-1. A normal chest film.

The Normal Lung

Look now past all those distracting shadows of the ribs and soft tissues at the roentgen images which belong to the lung itself. Because of its contained air the normally expanded lung is largely radiolucent, as we have said, but nevertheless you do see in Figure 4-1 traceries of branching gray linear shadows. What precisely are they? You can reason it out.

Reflect first that logically any structure of greater radiodensity suspended in the middle of a radiolucent structure like the lung will absorb some of the x-rays and cast a gray shadow on the film, a patch of film where less silver has been precipitated.

If this structure is spherical and of uniform composition, it will cast a round shadow. If the surface of the mass is knobby and irregular, knobs will be present in the outline, as in Figure 4-2. If the suspended dense structure is cylindrical, like a blood-filled vessel traversing lung substance, a tapering linear gray shadow results; and if the vessel branches, the shadow will be seen to branch.

When a vessel passes through the lung in a direction roughly parallel to the film (and perpendicular to the ray), its tapering and its branching will be accurately rendered on the PA film. But if it passes through the lung in a more nearly sagittal direction, it will then line up with the beam, absorbing more x-rays so that its shadow will appear as a dense round spot. The situation is analogous to the rose leaf on edge in the first chapter. You can find such end-on vessels in Figure 4-1, or in any chest film.

That the normal "lung markings," as the radiologist calls these linear shadows, are indeed vessels and not bronchi and bronchioles is also quite logical. The bronchial tree, being air filled and thin walled, casts little or no shadow when it is normal. It is practical, therefore, to think of the normal lung markings as wholly vascular.

The tracheobronchial tree may be *rendered visible,* of course, with relatively harmless radiopaque fluids instilled via a tracheal catheter into the lung of a living patient, who later coughs up or absorbs and excretes the opaque substance. This procedure, called *bronchography,* is carried out under local anesthesia to depress the cough reflex. It is rarely used clinically today except for staging bronchiectasis.

Figure 4-2. The mass suspended in this air-filled lung casts a shadow recording its knobby outline.

Figure 4-3A. The tracheobronchial tree coated with opaque material, a bronchogram. Vessels filled with blood are only faintly seen.

Figure 4-3B. A regular chest film. Note that the air column is seen in the trachea, but the rest of the tracheobronchial tree is not visible at all. Note the faint vascular shadows.

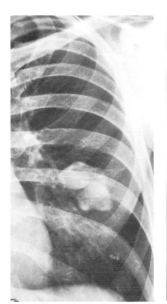

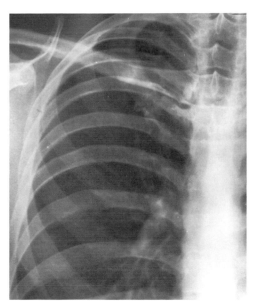

Figure 4-2 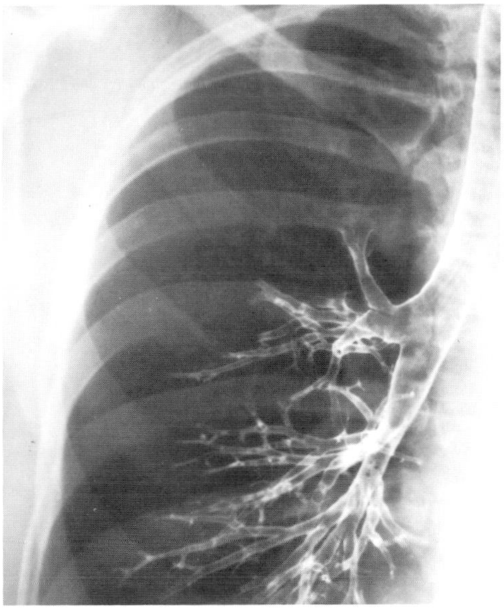   Figure 4-3A   Figure 4-3B

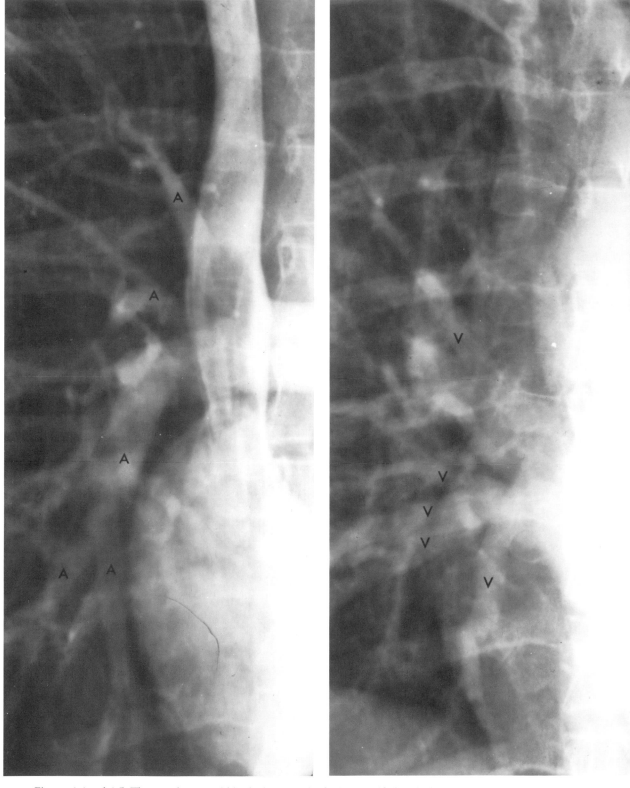

Figures 4-4 and 4-5. The vascular tree within the lung may be further opacified in the living patient, so that the vessels are more clearly seen than they are on the plain chest film. Radiopaque fluid miscible with blood may be injected quickly into an antecubital vein or through a filament catheter, so that a particular volume of blood passing through the right heart to the lungs is "seen" as a series of dense white "casts" of the cardiac chambers and the pulmonary vessels in sequence. Multiple rapid-filming devices or x-ray movies have been used to record the passage of the visible bolus of blood from the heart to the lungs, back to the heart, and out to the body tissues. Figure 4-4 shows an opaque-filled bolus of blood coming into the right heart from the superior vena cava and out into the lung via the pulmonary arteries. Figure 4-5, a film made a second or two later, shows the veins returning that bolus of opacified blood to the left atrium.

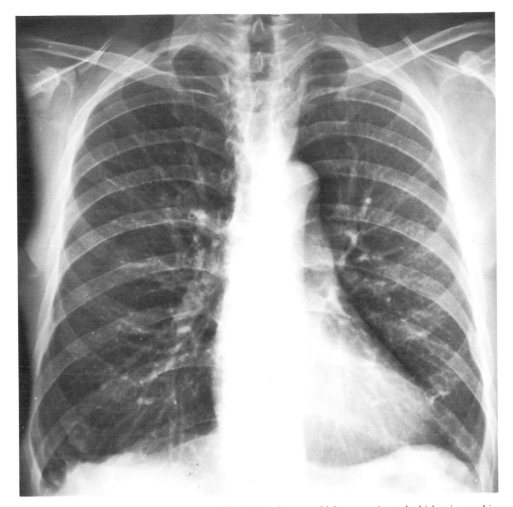

Figure 4-6. A normal chest film. Note how difficult it is to be sure which are arteries and which veins on this "plain film" without added contrast material.

Much less dramatic but nonetheless important information is available from any simple PA chest film as you study the vascular shadows in the lung, marked only by the blood they contain. Notice first that the largest vessels at the hilum of the lung cast the heaviest and widest shadows, just as you would expect. This Medusa-like tangle of arteries and veins on either side of the heart shadow is referred to by the radiologist in his reports as the "hilum" or "lung root." The right hilar vessels seem to extend out farther than those on the left, but this is only because a part of the left hilum is obscured by the shadow of the more prominent left side of the heart. Measured from the center of the vertebral column, the vessels will be found to be symmetrical except for the slightly higher takeoff of the left pulmonary artery, which hooks up over the left main bronchus rather abruptly (Figure 4-7). For this reason the left hilum on any normal chest film is a little higher than the right.

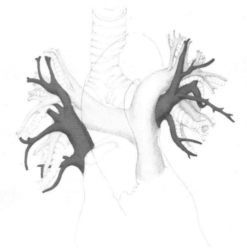

Figure 4-7. The anatomical composition of the hilum. The aorta has been rendered as though transparent. The tracheobronchial tree is indicated with cartilage rings; arteries are light and veins dark.

47

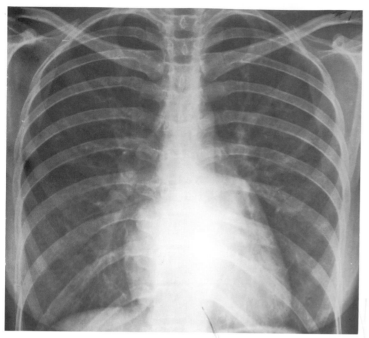

Figure 4-8. Engorged hilar root shadows in mitral stenosis. Note upper lobe vessels, which are enlarged in mitral disease. Compare with Figure 4-1.

Variations in Pulmonary Vascularity

Compare the normal hila in Figure 4-1 with a few abnormal hilar shadows. The lung root may be enlarged because of engorgement of its *veins,* for example, in any condition in which there is obstruction to the return of oxygenated blood from the lung to the left side of the heart. Such a condition exists in acute left heart failure after a myocardial infarction. More chronically, the same condition exists in rheumatic heart disease with mitral stenosis, where the gradual narrowing of the mitral valve results in back pressure in the pulmonary veins. Figure 4-8 shows the appearance of the hilum in moderately advanced mitral stenosis. Note the enlargement of the lung root and its obviously fat and tortuous branches, compared with the slim, straight vessels in Figure 4-1.

Dilatation of the *arteries* in the hilum will also become familiar to you in types of congenital heart disease in which an abnormal opening in the septum reroutes blood from the left chambers back into the right chambers and to the

lesser circulation, thus overloading the right heart and pulmonary arteries. A patent ductus arteriosus with a shunt of blood from the aorta to the pulmonary artery, and septal defects between the atria, commonly give this picture. Figure 4-9 shows an example of the marked hilar arterial engorgement seen in congenital heart disease of this type.

There is often actually some enlargement of both veins and arteries, and it is not usually possible for you to say from the plain radiograph which vessels predominate. In judging the appearance of the hilum in the patient whose film you see for the first time, you will decide simply that you are looking at vascular trunks of normal caliber or that they are enlarged.

The vascular trunks of the hilum normally branch and taper out into the lung field in all directions. They are so fine in the far peripheral lung close to the chest wall that you can sometimes no longer see them depending on the technique used. If you mask off between two pieces of paper first the hilum and medial half of the lung and then the lateral half, you will be struck by the decreased number of trunks laterally. But this will not surprise you when you

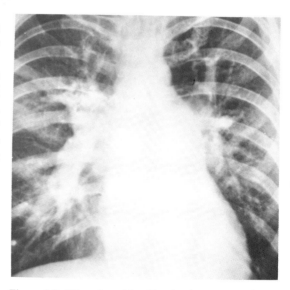

Figure 4-9. Hila enlarged by dilated pulmonary arteries in a patient with interatrial septal defect. The normal quantity of blood returning to the right atrium from the vena cava is augmented by blood shunted through the defect from the left atrium. This results in recirculation of blood through the lungs, overload of the pulmonary circulation, and dilated arteries.

recall that the lung is much thicker medially where it bounds the mediastinum than at its lateral extremity, and that there are many more vessels superimposed on each other in the medial half of the lung field on the radiograph. If you similarly divide the lung field on the x-ray film into upper and lower halves, you can see at once that there are many more branching vascular trunks in the lower half of the lung than there are in the upper half. This too is a function of thickness, and to think three-dimensionally about the vascular tree within the lung at this point is to recall the pyramidal shape of the lung with its broad base against the diaphragm and its apex coming to a point under the arch of the first rib.

You will be disturbed from time to time by the juxtacardiac portion of the lower right lung (the right cardiophrenic angle). Many vascular trunks overlap there in the PA view, because those for the anteriorly placed middle lobe are superimposed on those for the posteriorly placed lower lobe. One is easily misled into supposing that there is some increased density in this area, when in fact none exists. You can prove this to your own satisfaction by reviewing in films on this page and preceding ones the appearance of the portion of the right lung lying just above the diaphragm and to the right of the heart. Observe that even in normal films (see Figure 4-1) the area looks more heavily traversed by vessel trunks than you expect it to be. Part of the difficulty is the visual trick your eye plays; you are probably comparing the lung on the two sides of the heart, but because of the shape of the heart, the lung tissue just beyond the left border of the heart is not actually comparable to the problem area on the right, which we have been discussing. The point is easily proved by measuring from the midline: the truly comparable part of the left lung field lies closer to the midline, obscured by the shadow of the heart itself. In Figures 4-10 and 4-11 you have abnormal and normal cardiophrenic angles to compare.

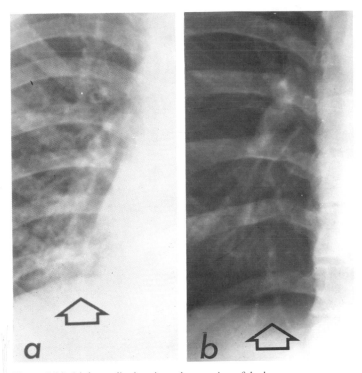

Figure 4-10. Right cardiophrenic angle, a section of the lung field often difficult to assay because of the large numbers of vessels superimposed. In *a* a fluffy density is filling in the area which is seen to be clear in the normal, *b*. The man in *a* had pneumonia.

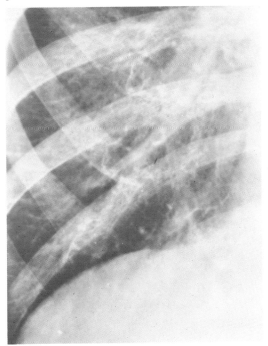

Figure 4-11. Cardiophrenic angle and lower right lung field in mild cardiac failure. The shadows of the engorged veins in the hilum superimposed on those of the arteries give a matted, thickened look to the hilum and lung field. Note Kerley's B-lines—horizontal, laterally placed linear or beaded densities which represent engorged lymphatics or the thickened interlobular septa in which those lymphatics lie.

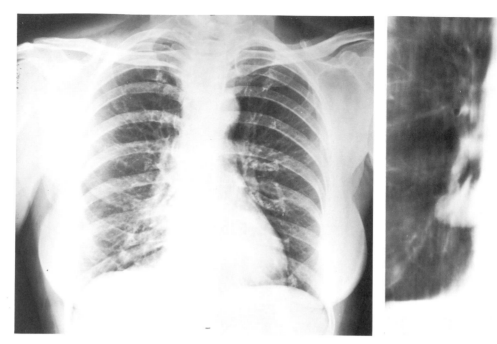

Figure 4-12. Ill-defined thickness in the lower part of the right hilum in a patient with cough and bloody sputum proved on tomography, Figure 4-13 (*right*), to be a smooth round mass below a clearly normal right pulmonary artery. Finding at surgery: benign tumor.

Often enlargement of the hilum is not vascular in nature. There are many *lymph nodes* in the hilum and mediastinum, lost among the heavier shadows of vessels and normally too small to be seen. They may enlarge, however, and become visible, either singly or in groups (when they respond to an inflammatory process in the lung, for example, or are secondarily invaded by tumor). They may be seen as overlapping round shadows or, when they are matted together, they may cast a confluent shadow.

Primary tumor masses occurring near the hilum are common. If you are thinking three-dimensionally about the lung root on the radiograph, you will also realize that tumor masses in the peripheral lung tissue in front of or behind the hilum may cast shadows which superimpose on that of the hilum in the PA chest film. Figures 4-12 and 4-14 are examples of this sort of problem. In Figure 4-12 the mass is just below the right hilum, and in Figure 4-14 it is either behind or in front but superimposed on a true left hilar mass of tumor-invaded nodes. A variety of special procedures can help to distinguish the nature of such masses. Tomograms were immensely useful in the past, and you should think of those in the illustrations used here as radiographs of a slice of the patient made through the level of the hilum in the coronal plane. Computed tomography is the preferred method of evaluating the hilar structures today. CT, offering you a cross-sectional slice, will show you whether such a mass lies anterior to or posterior to the hilum.

Hilar enlargements due to tumor tend to be rounder and smoother in outline and are more frequently unilateral. Masses which prove to be clusters of enlarged nodes, you will find, look like a radiographed bunch of grapes, with many overlapping round shadows. Vascular hilar enlargements, on the other hand, taper into the lung field and are almost invariably bilateral. You are going to see exceptions, of course, but these very rough generalizations will provide you with a temporary working rule. With contrast CT hilar enlargement due to tumors or nodes can be routinely distinguished from vascular hilar enlargement. Remember too that you must expect to see hilar enlargements that are *combinations* of tumor and nodes (as in Figure 4-14) or vessels and nodes.

50

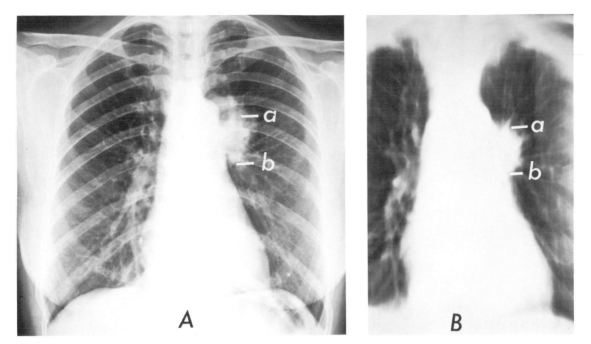

Figure 4-14. Left hilar mass, normal right hilum. Note that the tomogram, B, was made through the hilum. It shows a cluster of enlarged nodes in the hilum (*a-b*), but it excludes the upper part of the original shadow in A, overlapped on that of the nodes and representing the primary tumor behind or in front of the hilum. Thus the abnormal shadow on the plain film is actually two densities overlapping. Computed tomography would show at what level the primary mass lies, precisely how large it is, and what structures it involves.

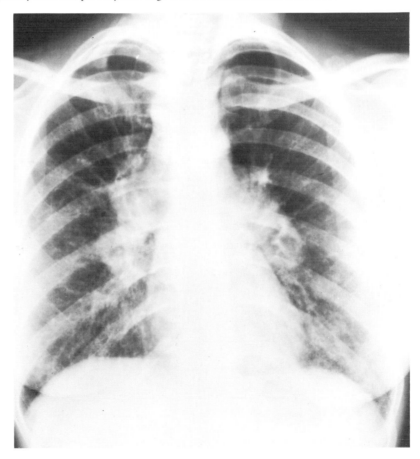

Figure 4-15. Bilateral hilar adenopathy in a patient with sarcoidosis.

Limitations and Fallibility

Finally, remember that sometimes a very innocent-looking hilum is not actually normal and may conceal among its vascular shadows tumor-involved nodes not yet large enough to be seen on the films. Retrospective studies of chest films in large groups of patients who were found to have tumor-involved hilar nodes at CT have shown a number of perfectly normal-appearing hilar shadows. The radiologist can do nothing about this except to report that your patient *seems* to have normal hilar shadows on the chest film, and both you and he have to consider that the presence of normal-sized but tumor-involved nodes would make a difference in the treatment of the patient.

You learn the limitations of other modes of inquiry constantly in medical school, and you must be aware that despite its great usefulness the radiographic inquiry also has some limitations, even in the hands of the most expert interpreter. When he can help you solve a specific problem, the radiologist will do so. When he knows he cannot help you, *or that a simple negative report is likely to be misinterpreted as a clean bill of health for the structure in question,* it is his obligation to warn you of that fact and to suggest other studies when they may produce additional information. Today, for example, he will suggest CT for the patient with lung cancer to determine whether there are enlarged mediastinal nodes present. It is this type of problem which, more than anything else, makes it imperative that you not rely entirely on the written report but supplement it with a personal conference with the radiologist while viewing the films yourself. Without sufficient clinical information the radiologist cannot truly serve the best interests of the patient, cannot offer you a report framed around the difficulties of a particular human being with a particular set of symptoms.

A Look at the Pulmonary Microcirculation

In Figures 4-4 and 4-5 you have seen the entire pulmonary arterial and venous systems visualized at arteriography. By advancing the arterial catheter farther toward the lung periphery, we can visualize the microcirculation. The study display on the next page shows normal circulation with injected contrast material, as well as three abnormal arterial patterns. The abnormal patterns show dramatic changes in the terminal arterial branches. In Figure 4-17 you see pulmonary arterial hypertension with occlusion of multiple small terminal arterial branches, producing a "pruned tree" appearance. By contrast, in Figure 4-18 you see hypervascularity in a patient with a left-to-right cardiac shunt and marked enlargement of all the terminal branches as compared with the normal. This is a result of the increased volume of blood passing through the lung. You could have predicted these changes from your knowledge of pathology and physiology, just as you can predict that the chest film of the patient in Figure 4-17 would show fewer vascular lung markings than normal, and that of the patient in Figure 4-18 an engorged pulmonary bed with many more lung markings (vessels). Figure 4-19 shows multiple small pulmonary emboli blocking the terminal arteries.

Variations in the Pulmonary Microcirculation

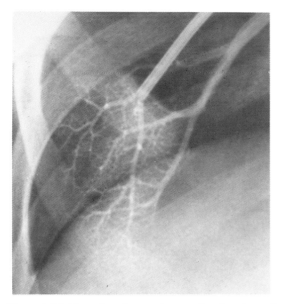

Figure 4-16. Normal wedge arteriogram showing the capillary bed in the lung.

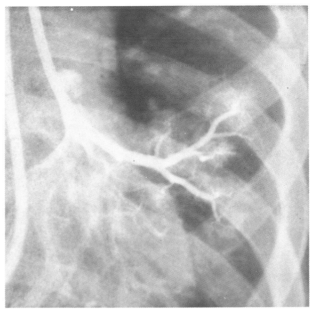

Figure 4-17. Patient with pulmonary arterial hypertension. From the narrowing of small end-arteries and sparse branching this has been called the "pruned-tree" arteriogram. Pulmonary flow is reduced 50 percent.

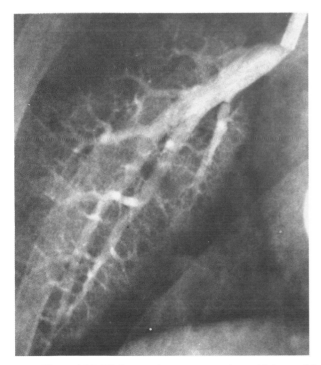

Figure 4-18. Wedge arteriogram on a patient with interatrial septal defect and a left-to-right shunt so extensive that the pulmonary flow was increased to 470 percent of the systemic flow.

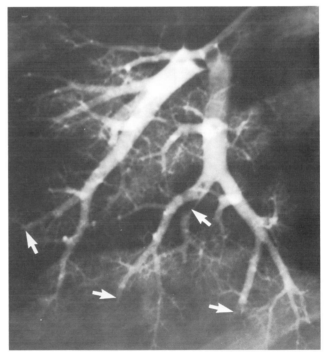

Figure 4-19. Balloon occlusion pulmonary arteriogram (BOPA) at the base shows multiple small emboli as intraluminal filling defects or sharp cutoffs (*arrows*).

53

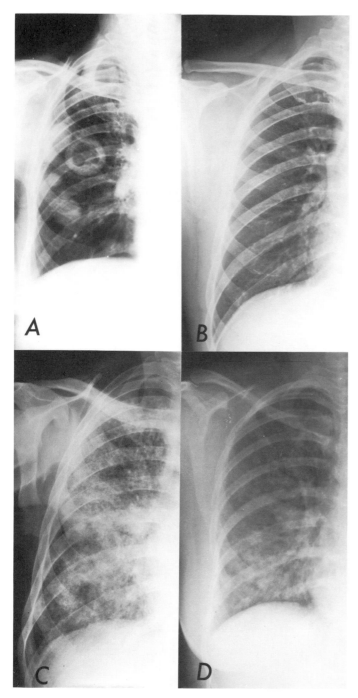

Figure 4-20. (See text.)

Solitary and Disseminated Lesions in the Lung

Imagine now the *alveolar portion of the lung* folded like a conical cuff around three sides of the hilum. You have looked at the peripheral lung when it was normal and seemed completely radiolucent in the lateral third of the PA film, where it is not superimposed on hilar trunks. What shadows will be added, then, if the vascular tree is normal but the alveolar lung is sprinkled with minute tumor nodules, patches of pneumonia, or small areas of collapse, or where it is threaded and reefed in by scar tissue from old infections, or flooded with interstitial fluid?

Look briefly over the eight lung fields on these two pages and then come back to the text. Are there any normals? Which ones seem to have changes in the lung so widespread that you think at once of some generalized process involving *all* lung tissue? Which show fewer than six isolated areas of abnormality?

Now consider them one by one. In A, several round shadows hang in an otherwise normal lung, their margins smooth and sharp, since they are surrounded by well-aerated lung tissue on all sides. One of them appears circular with a darker central area because it has a hollow, air-filled cavity inside it. (More x-rays pass through this part than through the shell tangentially.) The radiologist may not be able to tell you whether these are tumor nodules growing in the lung or multiple abscesses with breakdown. He *can* help you to assess the probabilities for one or the other diagnosis on the basis of their appearance, their growth rate from film to film over a period of time, and the clinical story.

B, the right lung of the patient seen in E, is normal and can be used as a norm for studying the others.

Both C and D show innumerable patches of increased density which, on the original film, involved both lungs. (G is the left half of D.) Unfortunately, many different conditions produce a picture similar to these two films. Some are common, others rare. From the film alone, without any knowledge of the acuteness of the patient's illness or of his occupational background, or even of the tentative clinical diagnosis, one cannot guess at the most probable diagnosis. One can describe the abnormal shadows—no more.

When you know, however, that the man in C had inhaled beryllium salts in a fluorescent-lamp factory over a period of time, you *can* say that his chest film shows shadows just like those seen in autopsy-proven cases of berylliosis where myriad small granulomas and a lacework of scar tissue produce such roentgen shadows in the lung. On the other hand, if you know that the woman in D and G was pulled out of the water several hours ago, half drowned, her film becomes intelligible because this is a picture often seen after such mishaps. Many small areas of collapse from inhaled water and bronchial secretions produce this sort of patchy density. In addition, from the violent struggle in the water there is usually some pulmonary edema with extra fluid in the interstitium of the lung about the vessels, and extensive hemorrhage.

Any chest film is only a point on a curve in the course of the patient's disease. *Change* from film to film in a day or a week or a year often alters the whole spectrum of diagnostic possibilities considered on viewing the original film. You may still not be able to be sure what the patient has, but you can then be sure of a good many things that he has not. To know that the man in C had shown the changes you see there for several months before this film was made, and that his lung picture did not change appreciably before he died, would strongly affirm your conviction that he had a chronic lung injury, probably related to his known industrial exposure. The half-drowned woman got well in a few days, and you could predict she would. In fact, H shows her left lung two days after G. Slightly enlarged vessel shadows seem the only remaining abnormality.

In case you have not been able to find anything wrong with E, look again at the ninth interspace. This solitary nodule had not changed since a chest film one year before, and at surgery it proved to be a benign tumor. In F the entire lung is sprinkled with minute areas of a density rightly suggesting calcium and representing the healed scars of an old infection, unchanged for many years. It has been estimated that such lesions must be at least 2 millimeters in size to be visible by x-ray.

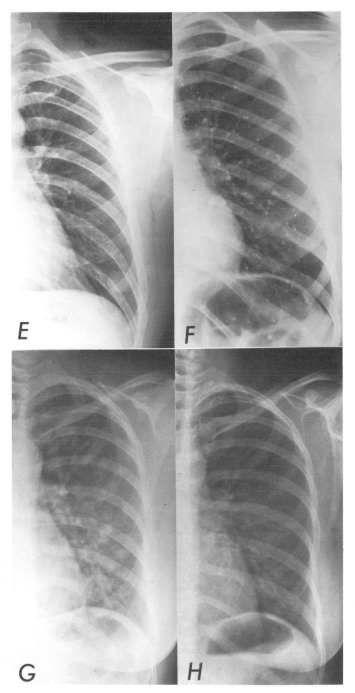

Figure 4-21. (See text.)

55

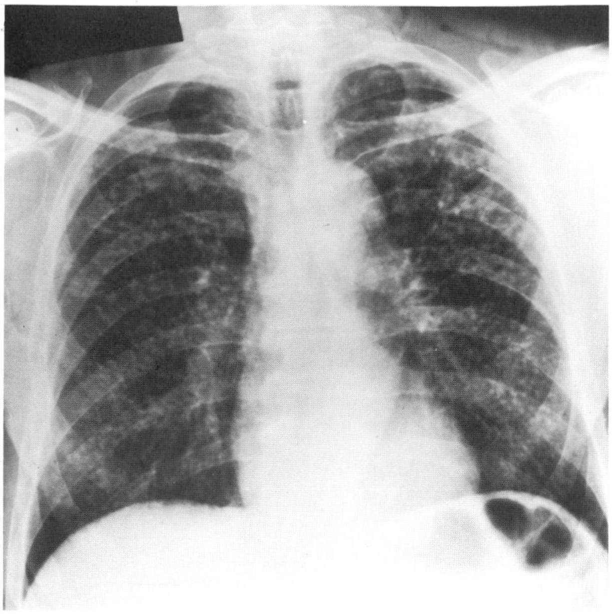

Air-Space and Interstitial Disease

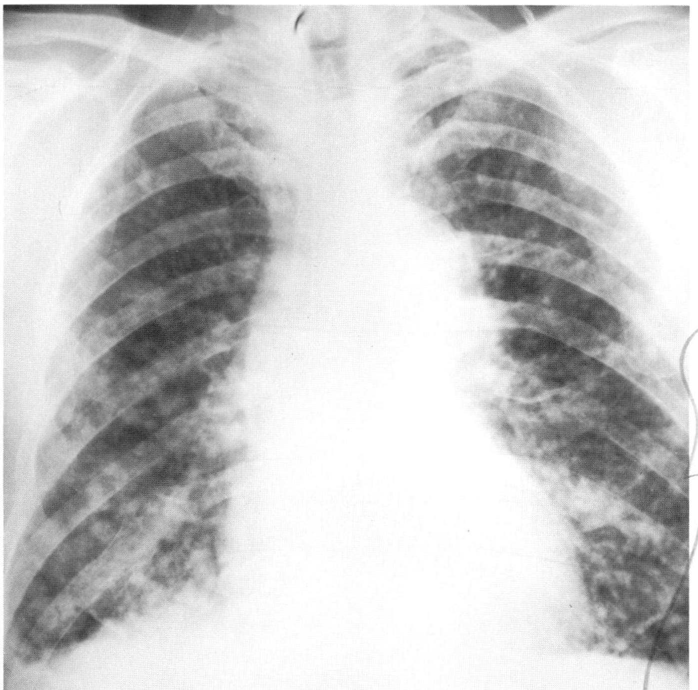

Two basic patterns of disease in the lung do differ significantly in their roentgen appearance. *Air-space disease* involves the alveoli, which fill with fluid or exudate that displaces the air in them. These areas of alveolar filling (whether large and single, multiple or coalescing as the disease progresses) appear dense, white, and radiopaque on the chest film. Various kinds of pneumonia do show air-space disease, but it is by no means pathognomonic as a picture of pneumonia, and many other disease processes can produce this picture.

Interstitial disease is distributed through lung tissue that is otherwise well aerated. Any interstitial process will ultimately produce either linear strands of density or spherical densities, small or large, seen to be superimposed upon the normal radiating pattern of vessel trunks. You have already seen some examples of interstitial disease (Figures 4-20 and 4-21) in this chapter, and in the next chapter you will be studying air-space disease as an illustration of lung anatomy.

Unfortunately, neither process can be interpreted as a pathognomonic finding independent of clinical information about the patient, and positive diagnosis usually depends on other modes of investigation. Taken together with the patient's history, physical findings, and laboratory data, a presumptive or working diagnosis is made with the help of the confirmatory radiologic findings.

Beware of leaning too heavily on your decision that the chest film shows either air-space or interstitial roentgen findings, because in a number of pathologic states they may coexist. For example, in cardiac failure with or without pulmonary edema, the abnormal densities on the chest film are initially produced by the presence of interstitial fluid surrounding the vascular trunks and advancing along interstitial planes into the lung. In time this fluid spills over into alveoli and produces clusters of densities that gradually coalesce. Thus in cardiac failure interstitial and air-space disease are often seen together.

Figure 4-22

Figure 4-23

56

Remember that *bilateral disseminated interstitial disease* is a very nonspecific pattern on the chest film. In fact, there are over one hundred disease conditions which may produce it. Often the picture taken together with the clinical data add up to a high probability that one specific disease process is involved. The radiologist needs as much relevant clinical information as you can provide on the requisition for a chest film.

Now try to decide on a most probable diagnosis for the figures on this page spread *before you go on to the next page spread.*

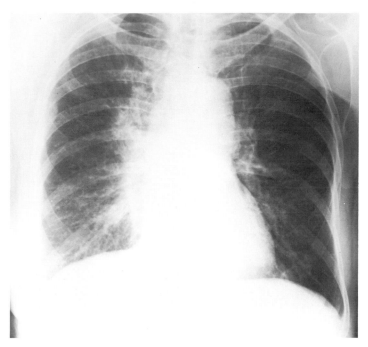

Figure 4-24

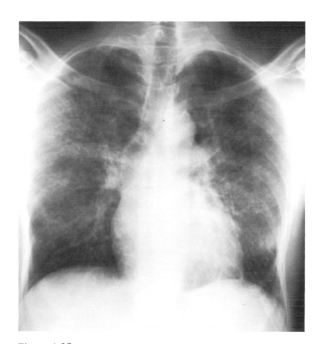

Figure 4-25

Answers

The clinical story in patients with *bilateral disseminated interstitial disease* helps to narrow the differential diagnosis to one or two most probable entities. All four of the patients on the preceding page spread have bilateral disseminated interstitial disease in their lungs. While they do show differences, none has a pathognomonic pattern. Figures 4-22 and 4-25 show similar streaky linear lesions; 4-24 also has linear infiltration mainly extending outward from the hilum, and 4-23 shows more nodular interstitial lesions. None of this helps you much toward a diagnosis, and the radiologist interpreting the films can only describe the findings.

When you inform him, however, that the man in Figure 4-22 had worked in a silicon-laden atmosphere without respiratory protection for years, silicosis becomes by far the most likely explanation.

You ought to have informed the radiologist on your requisition for the patient in Figure 4-23 that he has been treated for several years for carcinoma of the prostate. When you know that (and that earlier chest films were normal), metastases to the lung become the almost certain explanation.

There *is* a clue on the film of the patient in Figure 4-24: she has only one breast. This radiating perihilar pattern is sometimes seen in lymphangitic spread of breast cancer from the mediastinum outward into the lung, choking the lymphatics with tumor. It is *not* a pathognomonic pattern, since carcinoma of either stomach or pancreas can produce the same findings by extension to the mediastinum first and then outward along the lymphatics into the lung. These patients often present with sudden extreme dyspnea. This was the presenting complaint of the patient in Figure 4-24, and although she had her mastectomy five years ago, she has no symptoms suggesting either stomach or pancreatic cancer, so that lymphangitic spread from breast cancer becomes the most probable diagnosis.

Finally, the young man in Figure 4-25 also has bilateral disseminated interstitial disease. He has no industrial history of importance, as he is a clerk in a brokerage office. He has no peripheral nodes to suggest sarcoidosis nor any symptoms to prompt us to think of scleroderma, although both can give such findings in the lung. When we learn, however, that he is in a high-risk group for exposure to HIV virus, the diagnosis of pneumocystis carinii pneumonia due to acquired immune deficiency syndrome (AIDS) then becomes very probable. That diagnosis was made presumptively and confirmed bacteriologically and at autopsy.

Remember to give the radiologist *all* the clinical information you have when you write out the requisition, so that he can best advise you.

Review Problems

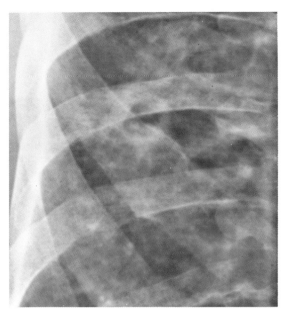

Figure 4-26 (*Unknown 4-2*)

Unknown 4-1 (no figure)

It is eleven o'clock at night. You receive a telephone report that an admission PA chest film on a patient you have just examined shows the shadow of a straight pin overlying the dark shadow of an air-filled trachea. The patient, a woman in for elective foot surgery tomorrow, talked comfortably when you were with her. What should you do?

Unknown 4-2 (Figure 4-26)

A 23-year-old medical student gives you a two-week history of cough, fever, weight loss, and bloody sputum, but he was able to go to classes today. Figure 4-26 shows a detail of his right midlung field. He tells you that an insurance chest film was entirely negative three months ago. Compare what you see here with the eight lung fields you have just studied. What sorts and shapes of abnormal shadows do you see? How would you be inclined to interpret them in terms of pathological changes that might cast such shadows? Weighing all factors (history, possible pathological condition, and roentgen appearance), which of the following very general categories of lung disease do you think most probable in this patient:
(1) Acute inflammation one day old
(2) No disease
(3) Subacute inflammation one month old
(4) Chronic lung insult related to employment
(5) Metastatic tumor spread in the lung (is this interstitial or air-space disease or both?)

Unknown 4-3 (Figure 4-27)

A young man known to be an intravenous drug abuser (heroin) is admitted with high fever, sweats, and coughing. Is this interstitial or air-space disease or both?

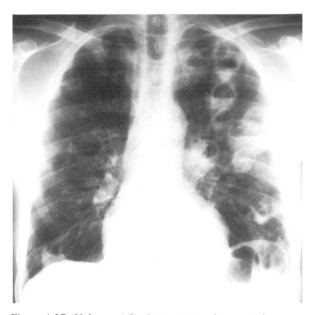

Figure 4-27 (*Unknown 4-3*). A young man known to be a drug abuser (heroin).

59

CHAPTER 5   The Roentgen Signs of Lung Consolidation; Air-Space Disease; Interstitial Disease; The Solitary Pulmonary Nodule

Consolidation of a Whole Lung

By massive lung consolidation we mean, for practical purposes, that a whole lung, a whole lobe, or at least one entire bronchopulmonary segment is solid in that it is almost entirely airless. The solid part will cast a uniform shadow of approximately the same density as the heart shadow, and its projection shadow will relate to the shape of the part involved. Although this sounds as though a theoretical situation were being proposed, the fact is that in everyday radiologic practice shadows of this kind are common. Hardly a day passes in a big general hospital without there turning up, for example, a radiograph in which by a logical analysis of the abnormal shadows on the chest film one can recognize a consolidated lobe in a patient with clinical lobar pneumonia. Likewise a shadow which can only represent a solid right upper lobe may be recognized in a patient already suspected of having lung cancer. To understand first the roentgen appearance of whole-lung consolidation and then that of consolidation of only one lobe is the orientation of this chapter.

In Figure 5-1 we have diagrammed for you the roentgen findings you must anticipate when one or the other *whole lung* becomes solid but does not change in size or shape. Begin by noticing that in A the normal heart shadow (white) is thrown into relief by the normally aerated lung (black) on either side of it. So also the two domed diaphragmatic shadows covering the liver and spleen are seen in relief because there is air in the lung above them. The stomach bubble under the medial half of the left hemidiaphragm may be seen in the upright patient as the shadow of radiolucent air imprisoned in the fundus of the stomach above a horizontal fluid level.

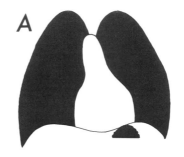

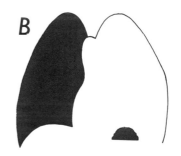

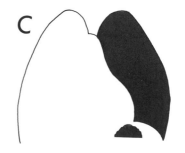

Figure 5-1

60

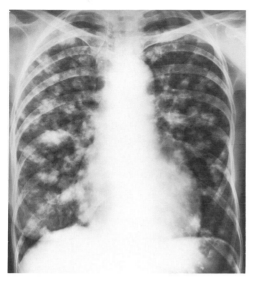

Figure 5-2

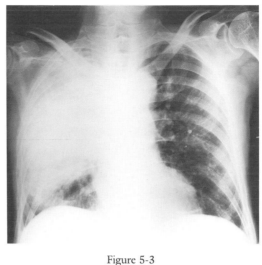

Figure 5-3

Now suppose that the entire left lung becomes consolidated, as in B. The heart, mediastinal structures, and dense lung are all of the same density (white) and their shadows merge into one, so that the left side of the heart profile disappears. They also merge with the shadows of the spleen and left lobe of the liver, and the outline of the left diaphragm is therefore lost, its location indicated only by the rays which reach the film through the air in the stomach. Look back at the cadaver sections in Chapter 2 to check these relations of stomach, spleen, and diaphragm.

If the left lung remains normal and the right solidifies, the chest film will look like C. The liver, right lung, and heart being nearly identical in density, their shadows now merge.

Disappearance of profiles or interfaces normally seen, then, on a chest film of this sort implies solid change in the lung next to them because the usual air-solid roentgen interface no longer exists. It is interesting to realize that even a lung that is riddled with small disseminated nodules of tumor will still contain enough air to behave like a well-aerated lung with respect to profiles. The patient in Figure 5-2 proved at autopsy to have both lungs generously sprinkled with metastatic interstitial tumor nodules; yet you do see

the heart shadow and both diaphragms because of the air in alveoli around the disseminated lesions.

Contrast with it Figure 5-3, in which pneumonia consolidating the entire upper part of the right lung results in loss of the upper part of the mediastinal and heart shadows, but preserves the shadow of the right diaphragm and of the lower right heart.

Any consolidation against the mediastinum will result in loss of a part of the mediastinal border, therefore, and any consolidation of the base of the lung will erase the shadow of the diaphragm or a segment of it. Because the heart is in the anterior half of the chest, consolidation which erases the border of the heart must, of course, be located in the anterior part of the lung. Thus you will not be surprised the first time you observe for yourself that although the diaphragmatic shadow on one side is absent and the lower part of the lung on that side appears dense, the border of the heart is seen clearly through it, thrown into relief by juxtaposed air-filled *anterior* lung. When you see this you will reason accurately that the *lower* lobe, in contact with the diaphragm, is solid, whereas the rest of the lung is normal.

Consolidation of One Lobe

Right Lung

In the drawings of seemingly transparent lung on this page you can see exactly why a solid lower lobe erases the shadow of the diaphragm and how the upper lobes, which do not touch the diaphragm, apply themselves, full of air, against the heart in the anterior part of the chest and preserve its profile on the PA film. You can also see at once how, with consolidation of the upper and middle lobes on the right, the right heart border would disappear but the profile of the diaphragm would be preserved by the well-aerated lower lobe.

The oblique planes of the two major fissures are important to remember, for their location will often be visible to you in the lateral view and bear a significant relationship to an area of abnormality. The fissures normally contain two layers of visceral pleura in contact and are seen in the normal chest film only when the pleura, x-rayed tangentially, appears as a thin line of density outlined on both sides by lung. The *minor fissure* on the right should be thought of as roughly horizontal, extending forward and laterally from the middle of the major fissure to form the floor of the right upper lobe and the roof of the right middle lobe. On the PA view it is frequently seen as a thin line extending straight laterally from the hilum.

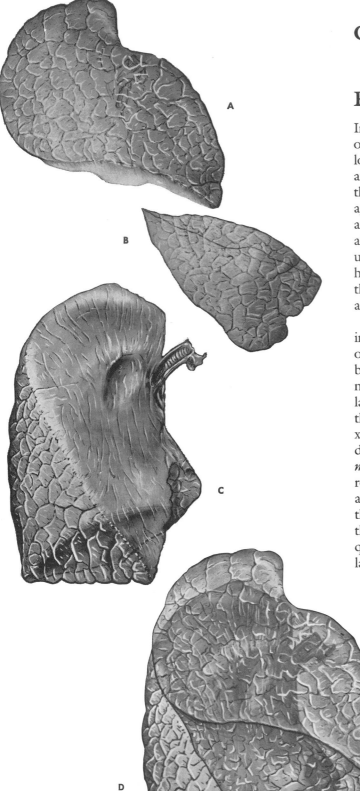

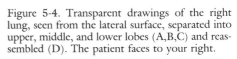

Figure 5-4. Transparent drawings of the right lung, seen from the lateral surface, separated into upper, middle, and lower lobes (A,B,C) and reassembled (D). The patient faces to your right.

E: see facing page.

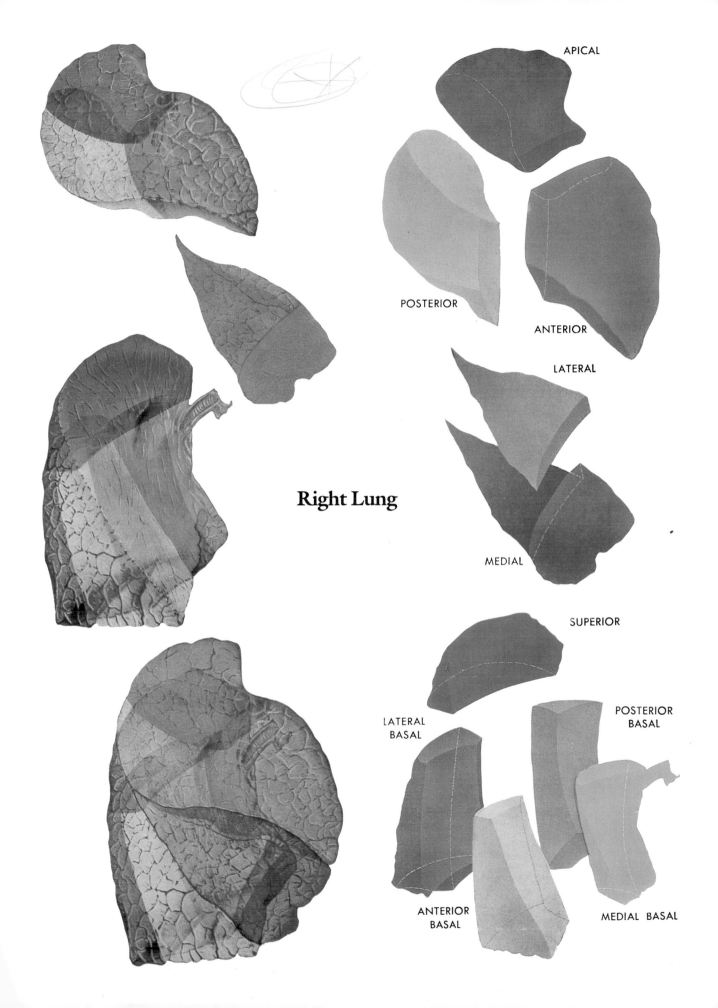

APICAL

POSTERIOR

ANTERIOR

LATERAL

MEDIAL

Right Lung

SUPERIOR

LATERAL
BASAL

POSTERIOR
BASAL

ANTERIOR
BASAL

MEDIAL BASAL

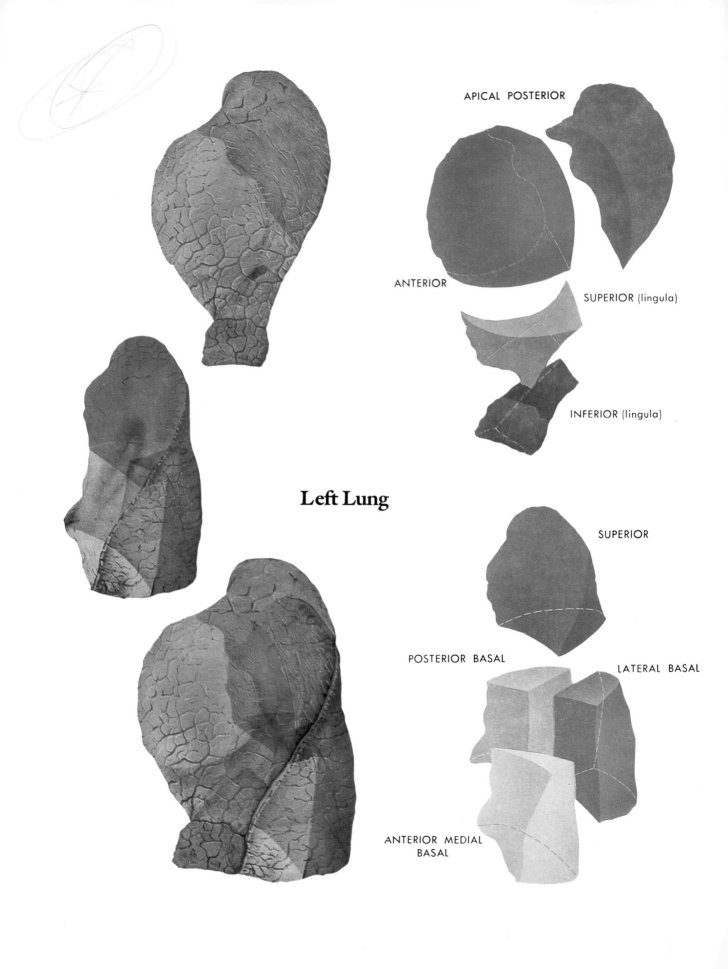

APICAL POSTERIOR

ANTERIOR

SUPERIOR (lingula)

INFERIOR (lingula)

Left Lung

SUPERIOR

POSTERIOR BASAL

LATERAL BASAL

ANTERIOR MEDIAL
BASAL

Exercise: Left Lung

Take pencil and paper and reproduce the outline of Figure 5-1A several times. Make diagrams predicting the block of density you would expect to see on the *PA* film if each lobe of the five became consolidated. Then try to predict the appearance of the block of density you would see on the *lateral view* to go with each PA. This will be easier if you begin with the right upper lobe, producing a density extending from the horizontal plane of the minor fissure upward to the apex. Work out for yourself these predictable shadow profiles, check them, and you will never forget them. As you reason each one, note which borders of the heart, diaphragm, and mediastinum can be expected to disappear with each block of density.

Remember that a dense sphere within the lung will project as a circular shadow on either PA or lateral view, but that *asymmetrical wedges* of different sorts will project quite differently according to the direction of the ray passing through them. The middle lobe best illustrates this point, since it is a long wedge x-rayed end-on in the PA view and appears as a much smaller shadow than when its full length is seen in the lateral view of the chest. The shadow profile in each instance is to be learned as an exercise in reasoning, independent of anatomic *surface* markings. Decide whether the consolidated middle lobe is going to be more dense-appearing on the PA or lateral chest film. Think sensibly in terms of summation shadowgrams and of the shape and location of the lobe.

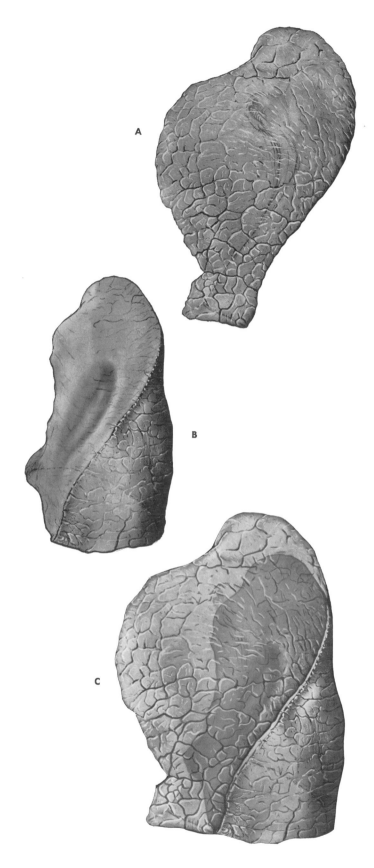

Figure 5-5. Transparent drawings of the left lung, seen from the lateral surface, separated into upper and lower lobes (A,B) and reassembled (C). The patient faces to your left. Note the similarities and differences between the middle lobe on the right and its analogue, the lingular segment of the upper lobe on the left. Density in either will obscure the lower part of the heart profile in the PA view.

D: see facing page.

The Diagrams You Should Have Drawn
for the Lobes of the Right Lung

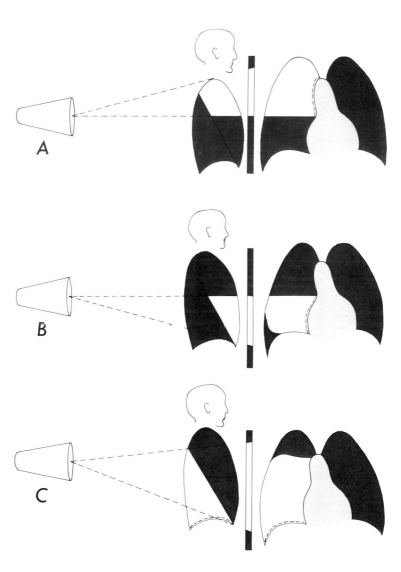

Figure 5-6. Projection shadows of each of the three lobes on the right. In A, the right upper lobe is consolidated, its inferior margin outlined by the air-filled middle lobe lying beneath the minor septum. In B, the middle lobe alone is dense; note that in the PA view it does not extend into the costophrenic sinus against the lateral insertion of the diaphragm. In C, on the contrary, the lung tissue filling the right costophrenic sinus is seen to be dense because the right lower lobe is dense. The heart shadow has been rendered in gray in these diagrams in order to clarify the shape of the lung mass shadows, but in an actual radiograph its density would merge with that of the middle lobe in B. Disappearing borders are outlined by dotted lines.

66

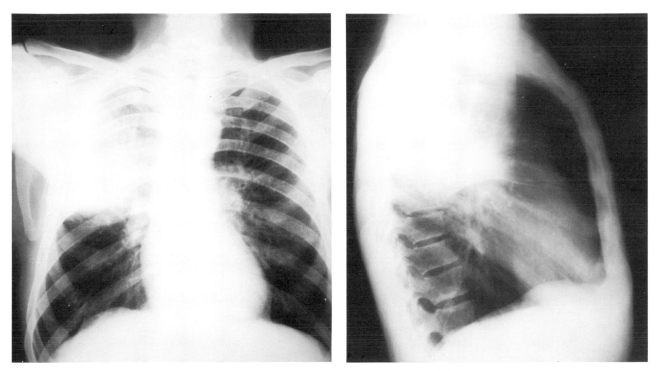

Figure 5-7. PA and right lateral view of a patient with right upper lobe pneumonia. The anterior segment is incompletely consolidated.

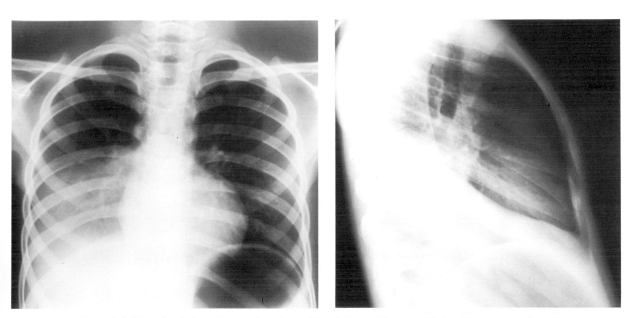

Figure 5-8. PA and right lateral view of a patient with right lower lobe consolidation. Note preservation of the heart profile in the PA and absence of the right diaphragmatic profile in the lateral. The wedge of density in the lateral view represents overlap of the consolidated lower lobe on the heart.

The Diagrams You Should Have Drawn
for the Lobes of the Left Lung

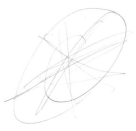

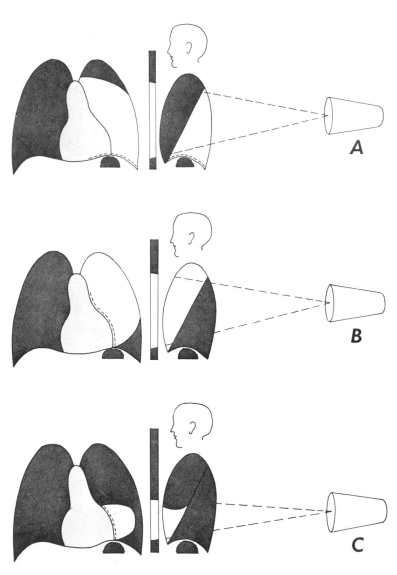

Figure 5-9. Projection shadows of the two lobes on the left. In A, the left lower lobe is consolidated; the diaphragmatic shadow disappears (*dotted lines*), since the roentgen shadows of the lower lobe and the spleen are merged; the approximate location of the left diaphragm may be indicated by the stomach bubble if one is present; the left heart border does not disappear but is seen through the dense lower lobe because air in the lingula of the left upper lobe anteriorly still throws it into relief. In B, the entire left upper lobe is consolidated and the left heart border is lost, but the diaphragm is seen because of lower lobe air above it. In C, only the lingular portion of the left upper lobe is solid, erasing the left heart border. Predict the radiographic appearance of the PA and lateral views in a patient with left upper lobe consolidation which spared the lingula.

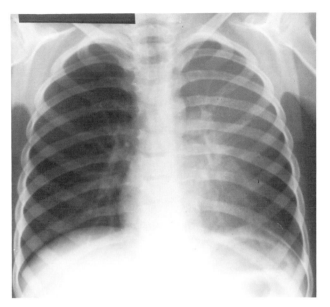

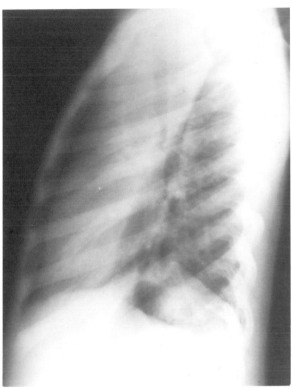

Figure 5-10. PA and lateral views of a patient with left upper lobe consolidation in pneumonia.

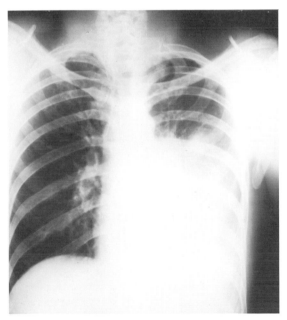

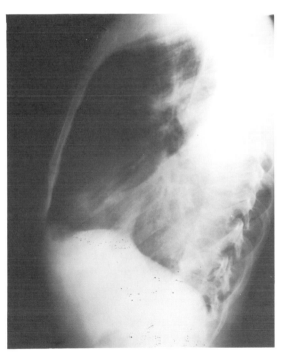

Figure 5-11. PA and left lateral views of a patient with left lower lobe consolidation (clinically pneumonia). Note absence of left diaphragm in the lateral view. On the original PA the left heart border could be faintly seen.

Consolidation of Only a Part of One Lobe

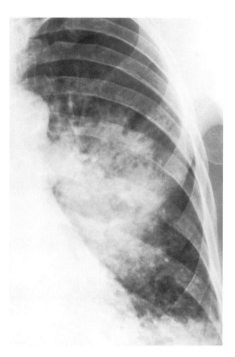

Figure 5-12. Here only a part of the left lower lobe is involved. It is a patch of pneumonia not in juxtaposition with the diaphragm, so the diaphragmatic profile is present. You know that this patch of consolidation is not anterior either because you see the heart profile so well.

When massive densities involve an entire lung or an entire lobe, you have certain clues which tell you how much of the lung is consolidated, and sometimes these same clues help you to determine the location of a patch of consolidation in the lung which does not occupy an entire lobe or bronchopulmonary segment, but only a part of one. Consolidation of all the lung tissue against the diaphragm will cause the outline of the diaphragm to disappear entirely, but a patch of dense lung against the lateral half of the diaphragm will cause the disappearance of only the lateral half of its outline, leaving the medial half visible.

Tomorrow you may see a chest film in which the lower left hemithorax appears dense, but if you can nevertheless see the entire diaphragmatic profile, you will know that there must be air filling the lower lobe. If on the other hand you cannot see any part of the diaphragm, but still see the left heart border through dense lung, you will know that there must be air in the upper lobe. You will not call either picture consolidation of the entire lung.

Neither will you be prompted to call a patch of partial consolidation like that in Figure 5-12 involvement of a whole lobe, but will think of it as involving most of a bronchopulmonary segment in the posterior part of the chest, since the heart border is so well preserved.

Now that you can recognize and locate anatomically areas of massive consolidation in the lung, as contrasted with the scattered small areas of density you saw in the last chapter, you are probably somewhat impatient to know how one labels them. As we have said, pneumonia and tumor can both produce solid areas in the lung giving the findings outlined above. It is current parlance to speak of "air-space disease" as opposed to "interstitial disease," and to attempt to differentiate them from each other on the PA chest film. It is true that the consolidation of lobar pneumonia *should* be thought of as pure air-space disease. It is also true that other abnormalities of lung in which the entire pathologic change is interstitial *do* produce linear strands of density on the radiograph. Yet the student who rigidly attempts to classify all disease as either air-space or interstitial from the roentgen appearance is in for a very disappointing and frustrating experience, because only some diseases pathologically show pure air-space or pure interstitial change. Other pulmonary processes (tuberculosis is one) may involve both interstitium and alveoli concurrently.

Lung that is airless because it has collapsed can produce much the same appearance as consolidation except that there will be evidence for change in size and shape of the lung part involved. Collections of fluid in the pleural space can also produce dense areas in the thoracic cavity, of course, obscuring the otherwise healthy lung it envelops and causing the disappearance of the diaphragmatic outline.

In both pneumonia and tumor, moreover, some atelectasis and pleural fluid are common in addition to the primary consolidation in the lung itself. One has to remember that these processes go together pathologically and, since they may cast very similar shadows, are often impossible to differentiate from each other from only the films on the initial study. In the next chapters you will learn how to determine the presence of pleural effusion and how to analyze the particular signals indicating that a lobe has collapsed. Then you will add them to the signs of consolidation we have covered above and interpret chest films systematically on each level.

In Chapter 3 you set up a system for beginning to study a chest film by surveying the bony structures and the soft tissues. In Chapter 4 you added the systematic survey of the hilum and its tapering vessels and the parenchyma of the lung itself. In Chapter 5 you have added a survey to make sure that no large patches of lung appear dense and that the heart borders and both diaphragmatic outlines are present, checking for *disappearance of profiles normally seen*. You are building gradually the sort of careful analysis of a chest film that will help you now in using roentgen data and serve you all your life in understanding the films on your own patients. Do not be impatient for diagnostic labels.

Unknowns: Air-Space Disease

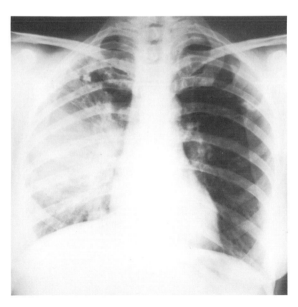
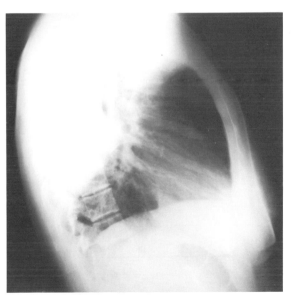

Figure 5-13 (*Unknown 5-1*). Clinically this young woman had pneumonia. Precisely what part of the right lung is consolidated? Is this air-space or interstitial disease?

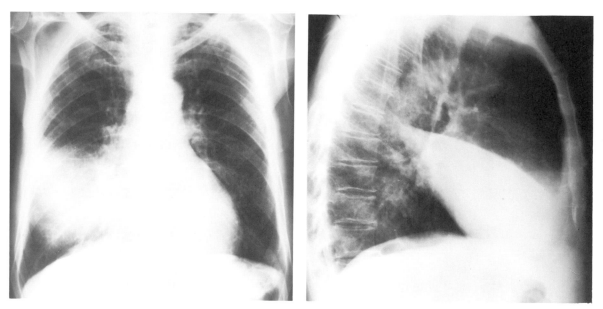

Figure 5-14 (*Unknown 5-2*). What part of the lung is consolidated here?

The Solitary Pulmonary Nodule

A special management problem arises with the small solitary mass density in the lung. You have seen one such mass in Figure 4-21E which, when resected, proved to be a benign tumor. Any such finding on a chest film must be subjected to serious consideration, for it may be either benign or malignant, a primary early carcinoma or a single metastatic focus from any of a number of distant primaries. One must be certain that it is indeed a single pulmonary mass, the presence of others having been excluded by CT or full chest conventional tomograms. Another step in the workup of the patient is to examine any earlier chest films that can be located. If the mass was not there in the previous films or has grown, it requires investigation. It may still be either inflammatory or neoplastic.

On the other hand, if the mass is unchanged or contains calcium which is central, densely particulate, or seen all around the periphery of the nodule, it is likely to be a benign granuloma and can be serially observed at intervals of three to six months. When calcification in such a mass is *eccentric,* however, it is more suspect and should be removed surgically. With CT important additional information can be obtained about solitary pulmonary nodules. Early metastases to the mediastinum can be demonstrated which are not seen on plain films (see Figure 5-16A and B). Enlarged nodes containing metastases render surgery for the mass in the lung futile, of course, and the patient has been saved an unnecessary thoracotomy. Radiation or chemotherapy then becomes the correct management, and many of these patients undergo a percutaneous needle biopsy of the nodule, performed under fluoroscopy, to provide tissue diagnosis.

72

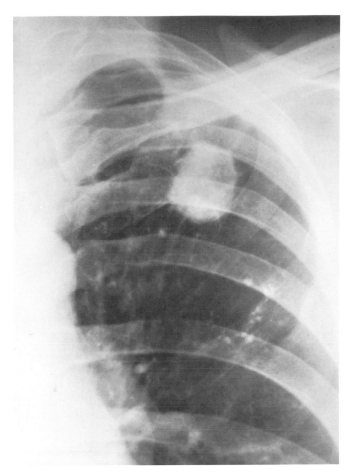

Figure 5-15 (*right*). A densely calcified solitary pulmonary nodule which is most probably a granuloma and might safely be watched. Contrast its density with that in the patient in Figure 5-16.

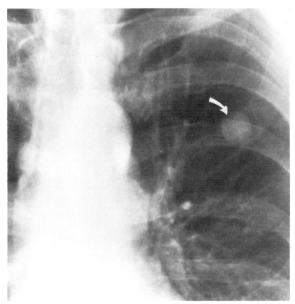

Figure 5-16A. Patient with a solitary pulmonary nodule discovered during an annual checkup. A film made one year before was normal. The nodule does not appear to be calcified.

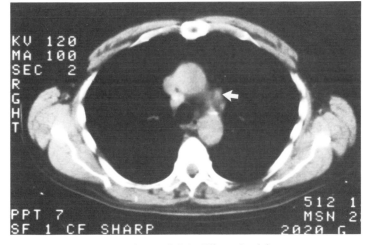

Figure 5-16B. CT scan made at a slightly different level does not show the pulmonary nodule but does show enlarged lymph nodes in the space between the ascending and descending aorta on the left, not present on normal CT scans at this level. This patient proved to have a lung cancer with mediastinal metastases.

CHAPTER 6   The Diaphragm and the Pleural Space; Pleural Effusion and Pneumothorax; Pulmonary Embolism

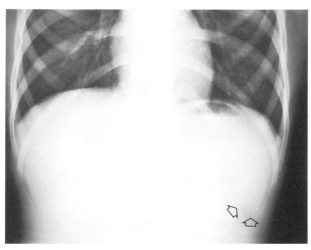

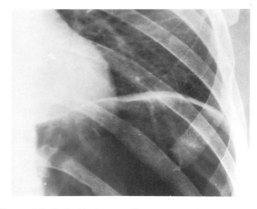

Figure 6-2. Left diaphragm filmed erect after an injury in which large amounts of air were admitted to the peritoneal space. The spleen and stomach are displaced downward. Note the vascular trunks in the lower lobe posteriorly extending well below the level of the crown of the diaphragm and superimposed on the subdiaphragmatic air. These lower lobe vessels are not seen in Figure 6-1 because they are behind the spleen.

Figure 6-1. Normal hemidiaphragms. Note stomach bubble with fluid level under left hemidiaphragm. Arrows mark the tip of the spleen. The spleen and fluid-filled stomach form a continuous shadow. Only the crown of the left hemidiaphragm, tangential to the x-ray beam, is seen. It has the wall of the stomach plastered against its inferior surface. The sloped curving anterior and posterior parts of the diaphragm are oblique to the beam and hence not seen at all. The right diaphragm is closely applied against the liver. Only the interface for its superior surface is seen.

The region of the diaphragm on the chest film affords some fine exercises in the logic of roentgen shadows. Just as you see the profile of the heart, dense between two lucent lungs, so you see the dome of the diaphragm because of a change in the sum of all superimposed densities. The sum of the shadows just below the *level* of the dome of the diaphragm on the radiograph includes a part of the lung posteriorly and the dense liver or spleen, solidly applied against its inferior concave surface. Above the level of the dome of the diaphragm the sum of all the densities is dominated by that of the lung, which offers little obstruction to the beam. Hence, on the chest film the diaphragm and its subtended organs are silhouetted, white against the lucency of the lung field above, *even though their shadows are added to that piece of lung which dips into the posterior sulcus.*

Anatomically composed of a thin sheet of muscle attached to xiphoid, lower six costal cartilages, ribs, and upper lumbar vertebrae, the diaphragm itself contributes little to the white shadow on the chest film which we mean when we refer to the "diaphragm." If free air in the peritoneal space interposes between spleen and diaphragm, as it did in the patient in Figure 6-2, the thin sheet of muscle alone is seen with air both above and below it. As usual when a curved, shell-like structure is x-rayed, what you see is that part of the diaphragm which is traversed in tangent by the beam. Although it appears to be linear, you will think in terms of roentgen densities and know it to be a domed shell dividing chest from abdomen. Under the fluoroscope it would be seen to contract downward and flatten with inspiration and to relax upward as the patient breathes out.

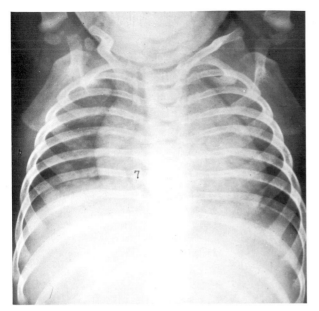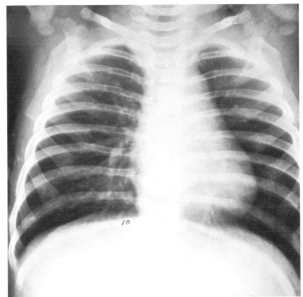

Figure 6-3 (*left*). The diaphragm at expiration. Figure 6-4 (*right*). Same patient at inspiration. Note absence of stomach bubble; the patient was lying down.

On most chest films made with the patient standing, the fundus of the stomach will be seen high against the diaphragm, usually containing swallowed air and fluid gastric juice (or lunch). A typical stomach bubble (Figure 6-1) shows a straight line marking the fluid level, above which air provides a radiolucent pocket through which more rays may pass. The same film made with the patient lying down and the beam still directed sagittally will show no level because the beam will strike the fluid level perpendicularly. Notice that in Figure 6 1 you seem to see the thickness of the diaphragm itself because there is air above and below it, but what you are actually looking at is the diaphragm plus the wall of the stomach.

A potentially hollow viscus that is completely filled with fluid and surrounded by dense viscera will not be distinguishable radiologically, but any hollow viscus that contains air will appear on the film as a dark shadow. While you are about it, take time to consider what you can do with air and a fluid level in radiography. Any hollow structure, normal or abnormal, which contains or can safely be made to contain both a gas and a fluid, will show a fluid level provided the beam crosses the plane of that level. Thus, by tilting the patient in several directions and always projecting the beam horizontally across the surface of the air-fluid interface, the entire inside

of a cavity can be visualized piece by piece. This can apply to the inside of the stomach, the inside of an abscess cavity, the inside of the ventricles of the brain or of the pleural space when it contains both fluid and air. Air thus becomes a useful *contrast substance*, forming a radiolucent cast of the hollow structure containing it, just as barium sulfate and other safely inert substances form radiopaque fluid casts of the hollow structures into which they are introduced.

Compare a chest film made at expiration (Figure 6 3) and one made when the same patient has taken a deep breath (Figure 6-4). Poorly aerated alveoli and crowded-together vessels naturally decrease the radiolucency of the lung to some extent. Note too that the flexible mediastinum and fluid-filled heart have been compressed upward by the high diaphragms in Figure 6-3, so that they cast an appreciably wider shadow and appear to be enlarged. This will be true of any film made at expiration and is an additional reason why it is important for you to determine the level of the diaphragm in the course of your survey of any chest film. The patient must be cajoled into taking a deep breath if he is at all capable of it, and before you attempt to draw any conclusions from his chest film, you must check the position of his diaphragm and decide whether he has done so.

75

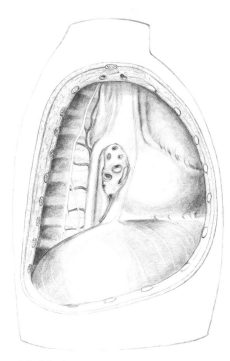

Figure 6-5. Diaphragm and costophrenic sinus with lateral chest wall cut away.

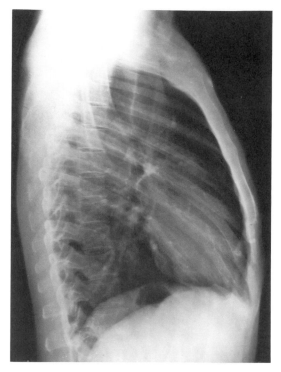

Figure 6-6. A normal right lateral chest film. Note the two diaphragmatic profile shadows curving down posteriorly. Which is the left diaphragm? Note vascular trunks curving down posteriorly below the level of the crown of the diaphragm. Here it is easy to say that the left is the higher diaphragm since the stomach bubble is close underneath it. You do not see its anterior segment: the heart, in contact with it, ablates its interface. What appears to be continuing left diaphragm is actually the anterior segment of the right diaphragm, always seen continuously from the posterior sulcus to the anterior chest wall.

Because the stomach bubble (present only if there is air in the stomach) normally lies close against the undersurface of the left diaphragm, it should be included in your systematic survey of a chest film. The interposition of anything between the diaphragm and the fundus of the stomach will displace the bubble downward. It may be deformed by the presence of tumor in the stomach. Both its appearance and its location are significant.

For example, when any massive density in the chest just above the left diaphragm causes the disappearance of the normal diaphragmatic outline, as you have seen in the last chapter, the location of the stomach bubble may tell you where the diaphragm is. In the lateral chest film the presence of the stomach bubble close under one diaphragmatic shadow determines which is the left diaphragm (Figure 6-6).

Although the anatomist thinks of and sees the diaphragm as a single sheet of muscle and tendon, dividing chest from abdomen, the radiologist sees it on the PA chest film and at fluoroscopy as two curved shadows on either side of the heart. He speaks of the "left and right hemidiaphragms," in spite of the fact that he knows that usage to be anatomically and semantically imprecise. It is convenient to refer to the two halves of the diaphragm in this way because they often respond independently to unilateral disease in the chest above or in the abdomen below.

The two hemidiaphragms, then, as seen on PA adult chest films, normally are smooth curves taking off *from the midline at the origin of the tenth or eleventh rib.* You should make a practice of counting down the posterior ribs close to the spine to determine the level of the diaphragm. Try it on a few of the chest films you have seen (being sure to identify the first rib by tracing it backward from the sternoclavicular junction). If you determine the level of the diaphragm on a few actual patients' films seen in the course of

76

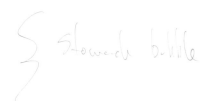

your clinical day, you will find that hospitalized patients tend to show considerable variation in that level. The well person who is merely having a checkup efficiently obeys the request of the technician to "take a deep breath"; but the anxious, tired, pain-beset hospitalized patient may fail to do so, even though he has a fractured ankle to be set and nothing at all wrong with his chest or abdomen. The result is of course that the lower part of his lung close to the diaphragm will be poorly inflated with air and consequently more dense on the chest film, giving an appearance of abnormality where, in fact, none exists.

The diaphragm may be elevated by large collections of fluid in the peritoneal space, as in the patient with heart failure or cirrhosis of the liver. With distension of many loops of large or small bowel in intestinal obstruction, the diaphragms are usually high and may also be limited in their downward motion, responding reflexly to abdominal pain. For the same reason they are normally high and "splinted" in their motion for a few days after abdominal surgery. You would expect them to be high in the third trimester of pregnancy and they are.

On the other hand, the diaphragm may be depressed and flattened in any condition that greatly increases the volume of the structures within the thoracic cage. Thus, in emphysema, with irreversible trapping of air in the lung and gradually increasing overexpansion, the diaphragms are low and flat. They may show serrated margins because then the insertions into the lower ribs become visible. Likewise, with the added volume of large collections of pleural fluid or of tumor masses in the lung, the diaphragm may be depressed.

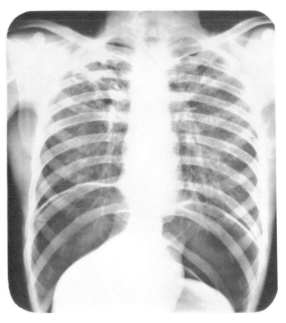

Figure 6-7 (*Unknown 6-1*). Determine the level of the diaphragms in this patient with bilateral upper lobe tuberculosis. Did the patient take a deep breath?

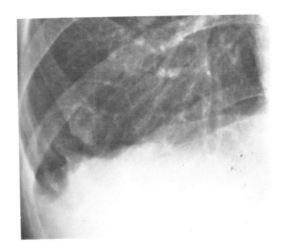

Figure 6-8. A low, flattened, serrated hemidiaphragm is often seen in older patients, most of whom have some degree of emphysema.

77

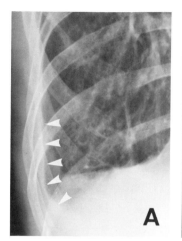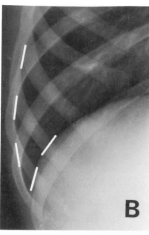

Figure 6-9. A: The old thickened pleura, caught tangentially by the beam of x-rays here, is actually a cuff of scarred tissue curving away from you and toward you over the surface of the lung, and represents parietal and visceral pleura densely adherent to each other. The pleural space in this area is obliterated, and with it the costophrenic sinus. This is not to be confused with a small pleural effusion. B is a normal costophrenic sinus, for comparison.

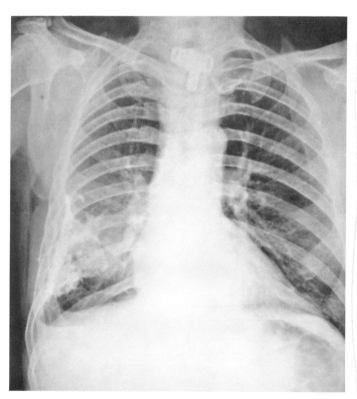

Figure 6-10. Calcification of an extensive plaque of thickened pleura. Note air in soft tissues in the lateral chest wall. This was a draining sinus in this patient with chronic inflammatory pleural disease, which explains the obliterated costophrenic sinus.

Pleural Effusion

The pleura is a closed empty envelope, one side of which invests the surface of the lung, dipping into its fissures. The other side is applied against the inner surface of the thoracic cage. Too delicate to be seen radiographically under normal circumstances, it may become visible when it has been thickened by inflammation and catches the beam of x-rays tangentially against the chest wall. The two thicknesses of pleura in the *minor fissure* may frequently be seen as a thin white line extending straight laterally from the right hilum, because the minor fissure is normally horizontal. Both the left and right *major fissures* and the minor fissure on the right may be seen on the lateral chest film whenever they happen to line up with the beam. The major fissures are too oblique to be seen on the PA chest film.

The pleural space, although normally empty and collapsed, *may come to contain either fluid or air or both,* any of which will alter the appearance of the chest film. A massive collection of fluid on one side can displace the mediastinum toward the opposite side, depress the diaphragm, partially collapse the lung, and render the entire hemithorax dense and white. Air in large or small amounts may gain access to the pleural space by rupture through the pleural surface of the lung, or after trauma when the lung is punctured by the ends of fractured ribs. Air may be introduced into the pleural space intentionally for diagnostic purposes following a pleural tap. If the amount of pleural air is large, the lung will be seen partially collapsed against the mediastinum. Any amount of air in the pleural space allows you to see some part of the surface of the lung that you do not see in the normal chest film because the lung lies closely in contact with the chest wall. Detection of a small pneumothorax depends on seeing the veil-like pleural margin of the lung, beyond which no lung markings extend.

Large amounts of pleural air or fluid are easy to visualize; small amounts are much more

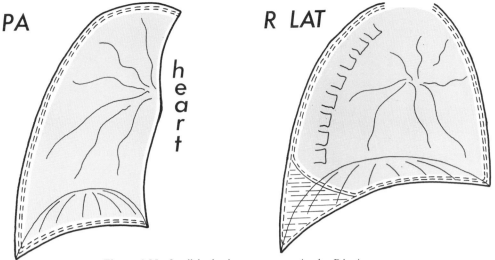

PA

R LAT

h
e
a
r
t

Figure 6-11. Small hydrothorax not seen in the PA view. *Broken lines* indicate layers of parietal and visceral pleura, between which the fluid lies.

difficult. If you look again at any normal diaphragm shadow in the PA projection, you will see that it dips laterally to form a sharp angle with the chest wall. The base of the lower lobe, cupped convexly over the diaphragm, dips into this recess at the sides and deep posteriorly. The *costophrenic sulcus* (or *sinus*), then, of which only the lateral part appears in the PA chest film, is a continuous ditch formed between the chest wall and the diaphragm. The lowest part of this ditch, when the patient sits or stands, is located far posteriorly on either side of the spine, as you have already appreciated from the lateral chest film. Into this ditch extends the base of each lower lobe against the posterior segment of the diaphragm, and pleural fluid gravitates into it. Thus the first hundred milliliters of pleural fluid which accumulate may not be visible in the lateral costophrenic sinus on the adult PA chest film, but *would* be seen in the lateral chest film obscuring the posterior portion of the diaphragm. Confirmation of a pleural effusion this small is usually made today with the help of ultrasound, which can also direct placement of the thoracentesis needle.

When enough fluid is present to fill the posterior sulcus, the lateral part of the sulcus begins to fill, and this will be noted on the PA chest film as a blunting or obliteration of the costophrenic sinus on that side.

Problem: What happens to the fluid in Figure 6-11 if, in preparing for a diagnostic tap posteriorly, the intern asks the patient to sit on a chair and lean forward? (Answer on next page spread.)

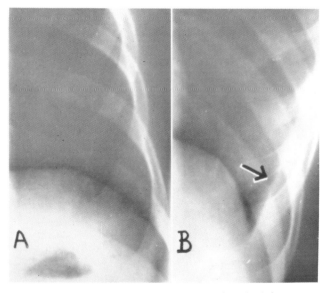

Figure 6-12. A: Patient erect. B: Patient tilted to the left. Fluid which is free in the pleural space can generally be dumped into the lateral costophrenic sinus, where it is easy to see.

79

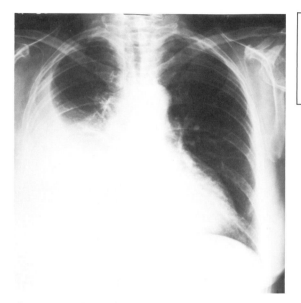

Figure 6-13. Pleural fluid engulfing the right diaphragm, surrounding the lung, and compressing the middle and lower lobes toward the hilum.

Answer to problem on preceding page: The fluid will flow forward into the lateral sulcus when the patient leans forward, something the intern must beware of in order to tap successfully.

As a greater amount of fluid collects, the density of it obscures the rounded shadow of the diaphragm entirely and it will be seen as an upward-curving shadow against the chest wall (Figure 6-13). *It never forms a horizontal fluid level unless there is also air present opening up the pleural space.*

Whenever you see an obscured diaphragm, you must wonder whether there is fluid above it and look closely for an upward curve of density against the lateral chest wall or for a fluid level. *Do not call a curved fluid line in simple effusion a "fluid level."* Whenever you do see a true horizontal fluid level, you must check carefully for the margin of the lung, which is certainly present with pneumothorax and always visible somewhere. You must not forget to wonder what may be going on in that part of the lung which is concealed by the fluid shadow and to plan its better visualization. Massive effusions are more likely to be malignant in origin (Figure 6-14).

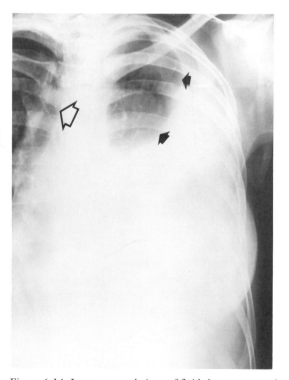

Figure 6-14. Large accumulations of fluid show a crescentic line ascending along the lateral chest wall in the PA view (*black arrows*). Remember that the same amount is sloping up the anterior and posterior chest wall. Note displacement of the trachea (*open arrow*) to the opposite side (mediastinal shift).

80

Pneumothorax

Although small amounts of pleural fluid collect far posteriorly against the diaphragm, small amounts of pleural air collect high over the cupola of the lung apex and against the upper lateral chest wall. They may be very difficult to see there because of the overlapping tangle of bones, and minimal pneumothorax is quite often missed unless you are looking carefully for it. It is more obvious when the lung is less well aerated, so that a film made *at full expiration* may show clearly the margin of slightly denser lung outlined by darker pleural air against the chest wall, or a film may be made PA with the patient lying on his good side. The air in the pleural space will then collect between lung and chest wall, where it is easy to see. This is called a *lateral decubitus film* (Figure 6-16).

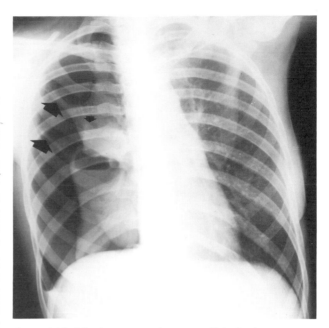

Figure 6-15. Massive pneumothorax, small hydrothorax. The right lung is only partly collapsed because of the dense pleural adhesions retaining it (*large arrows*). The *small arrow* points to the smaller of two cavities in the diseased lung. The larger cavity has a fluid level in it. You can see the three lobes collapsing separately in the pleural air. Note the small horizontal fluid-air interface in the right costophrenic angle, sure evidence that this is hydropneumothorax.

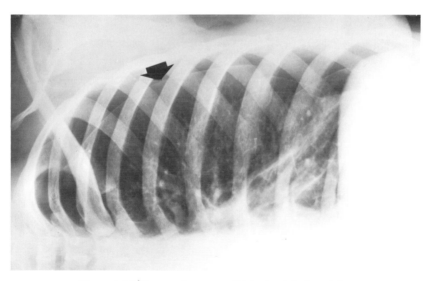

Figure 6-16. Pneumothorax seen PA in the right lateral decubitus position (patient lying on his right side, horizontal x-ray beam). The weight of the heart pulls the lung away from the chest wall, rendering a small pneumothorax easier to see. *Arrow* indicates lung margin.

81

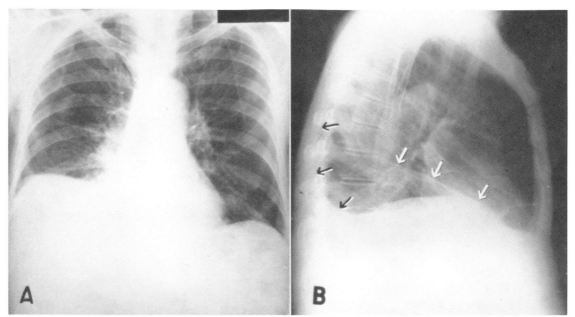

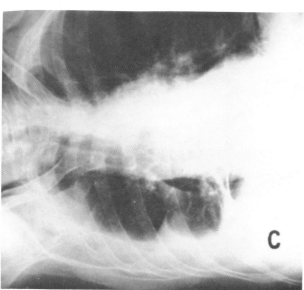

Figure 6-17. A: Subpulmonary collection of pleural fluid imitates a high right diaphragm in the PA view. B: Lateral film shows fluid curving up along the posterior chest wall (*black arrows*) and dipping into the major fissure (*white arrows*). C: Decubitus film shifts the fluid against the lateral chest wall, where it is seen to dip into the minor fissure.

The lateral decubitus chest film is useful in determining the presence of subpulmonic fluid. When the patient is placed on his affected side, fluid trapped beneath the base of the lung against the diaphragm can be dumped out into the pleural space against the lateral, now-dependent chest wall, as in Figure 6-17C. Without this maneuver the PA film might be interpreted as a "high right diaphragm." The lateral decubitus chest film is also useful for diagnosing small effusions in the patient who cannot be filmed upright.

Fluid may also be seen in the fissures. Remember that the planes of the two major fissures descend obliquely from high against the posterior chest wall to a point low against the anterior chest wall. Similarly, the plane of the minor fissure on the right is normally horizontal, extending forward and laterally from the middle of the major fissure at a level opposite the right hilum. Collections of fluid within these fissures will lie in the same planes, and you can look for them there. Frequently, when enough free fluid has accumulated, you can see it dipping into both major and minor fissures, as you do in Figure 6-17B and C.

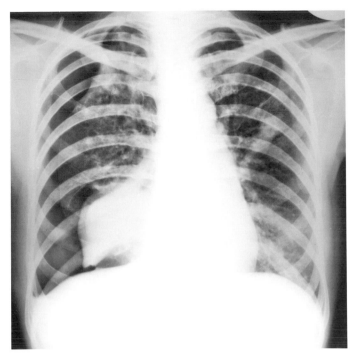

Figure 6-18 (*Unknown 6-2*). Clinically this patient had had fever and cough with hemoptysis for six months but had refused medical attention. Tuberculosis was the working diagnosis. Analyze the film.

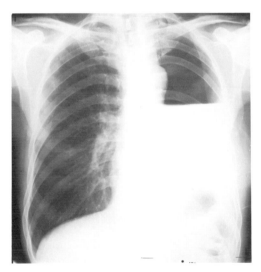

Figure 6-19A (*Unknown 6-3*). Locate the fluid level.

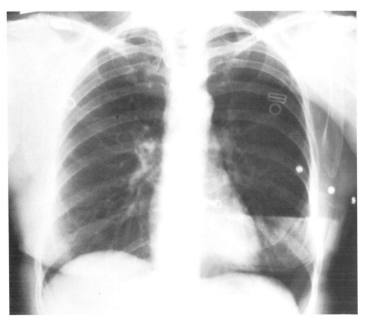

Figure 6-19B (*Unknown 6-4*). Locate the fluid level.

Pulmonary Embolism with and without Infarction

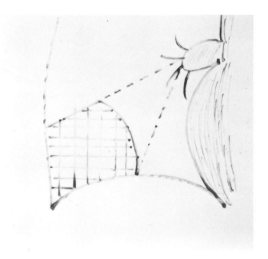

Figure 6-20. Diagram showing points in the development of the roentgen changes in pulmonary infarction (pruned-off vessels beyond the embolus near the hilum; a wedge of density in some part of the peripheral lung gradually increasing in density; elevated hemidiaphragm).

One cause of pleural effusion often overlooked by students is *pulmonary embolism,* which often requires isotope lung scans and pulmonary arteriography for diagnosis. At first the chest film is likely to be normal, but the roentgen changes which develop in pulmonary embolism are now well described and logically related to the pathology.

One could anticipate relatively underperfused lung tissue distal to the artery blocked by the embolus, just as one could predict that the hilar artery proximal to it would be dilated because of the presence of the embolus within it.

Pulmonary embolus may cause pulmonary infarction. Since infarction is always ischemia of pleura-based lung, one could also anticipate that a density would appear on the chest film, often at the lateral periphery of the lung, when intra-alveolar hemorrhage and, later, organization occur. Remember, though, that there is a good deal of pleura-based lung which abuts the fissures or even the mediastinum, so that infarcts do not always appear laterally on the chest film. They *are* more common there, and often present as rounded densities ("Hampton's hump") near the costophrenic sinus above an elevated diaphragm. This infarcted piece of lung, when it is close to the diaphragm, may have its shape obscured by the presence of some pleural effusion too, of course.

In early pulmonary embolism where infarction of the lung has not yet developed, one sees little or no change on the chest film. In patients who have sudden chest pain with dyspnea, one must entertain a high degree of suspicion that pulmonary embolism (often multiple) may have occurred even when the chest film is still normal. When the chest film is abnormal as a result of acute pulmonary embolism, the most common finding is that of diminished lung volume, usually manifested as elevation of a hemidiaphragm or atelectasis. Serial films may ultimately show one or more of the roentgen signs of lung infarction: pleural effusion and density in the lung (the infarct itself). The patient with clinically suspected pulmonary embolism *usually* requires a radioisotope lung scan and sometimes pulmonary arteriography.

84

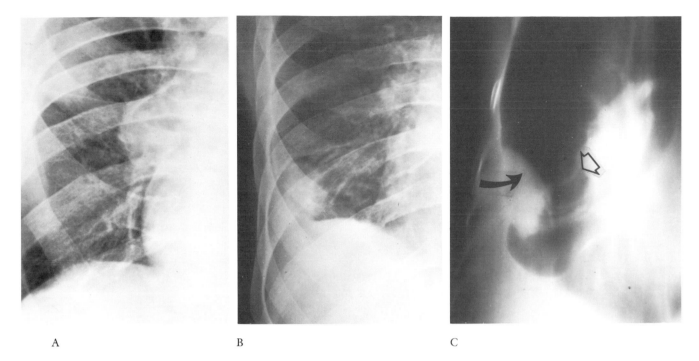

A   B   C

Figures 6-21A and B show the early and late development of characteristic roentgen findings in pulmonary infarction of the right base against the lateral chest wall in the right lower lobe. Remember that the middle lobe does not occupy the lateral sulcus. C is a tomogram. *Curved arrow:* wedge of infarcted lung (Hampton's hump). *Boxed arrow:* pruned hilar vessel. The small vessels seen below it are doubtless in the right middle lobe, which is still normally perfused.

Nuclear Medicine

The Use of Isotope Studies in Pulmonary Embolism

In order to comprehend the field of radiology in full, you must be familiar with all of the various imaging procedures by which visual information about the patient's body may be obtained. The field of nuclear medicine imaging is an immensely valuable aid in diagnostic work. It involves the use of *unstable isotopes (radionuclides) that disintegrate, predictably releasing gamma rays.* The emission of these rays may be "scanned" to produce an image on a screen and/or recorded photographically with the help of a *gamma camera.*

Lungs, bones, liver, spleen, kidney, heart, thyroid, and brain may all be evaluated with the help of such studies, and you must be prepared to learn their place in the workup of patients with various disease conditions. Currently used procedures will be discussed briefly for each area of the body as we go along. At this point it is the contribution of isotope scans to the diagnosis of pulmonary embolism with which we are concerned.

85

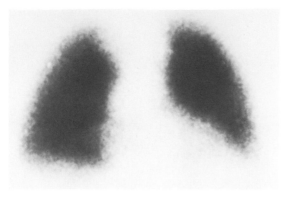

Figure 6-22. Normal perfusion scan, frontal projection.

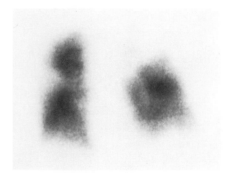

Figure 6-23. Perfusion scan in pulmonary embolism showing multiple defects.

Perfusion and Ventilation Lung Scans

In pulmonary nuclear imaging one substance used is "tagged" (radioactive) human serum albumin. Particles slightly larger than erythrocytes are injected intravenously. As they perfuse the lung, they are trapped in some of the capillary branches throughout the pulmonary arterial tree, where the emission of gamma rays continues until disintegration is complete. The particles become inactive in a matter of hours. Scanning techniques carried out during this interval produce an image of the lung (in terms of its arterial bed) which is photographically recorded. The distribution of the trapped emitting particles is normally uniform throughout the lungs, so the image produced should be that of two blackened lung-shaped shadows with the slightly asymmetrical heart shadow between them—white because it has no trapped particles (Figure 6-22).

This procedure is useful in the diagnosis of pulmonary embolism because the embolus has blocked a branch artery. The lung tissue peripheral to that block is *not* perfused with the isotope, therefore, so a "defect" (nonblackened area) is produced on the scan. This type of study is called a *perfusion scan*.

If a patient suspected of pulmonary embolism shows no perfusion defect on his scan, he can be presumed not to have an embolism.

When the perfusion scan is abnormal, a ventilation scan is performed. This procedure is carried out by the inhalation of a radioactive gas (xenon). In this way the degree of ventilation of all parts of the lung can be imaged. A number of disease conditions of the lung do cause alterations in ventilation (pneumonia, emphysema, tumors), but uncomplicated pulmonary embolism does not. Thus, a patient clinically suspected of having a pulmonary embolus who has a *perfusion scan defect* (as in Figure 6-24) *but a normal ventilation scan* (Figure 6-25) very probably *has* an embolus.

In older patients the presence of chronic obstructive pulmonary disease (COPD), often not apparent on the chest film, creates special problems in the diagnosis of pulmonary embolism. In these patients *matching scans* generally indicate a segment of abnormal lung causing defects on both scans and indicating both underperfusion and underventilation of that segment, probably not an infarct. But even patients with COPD can have pulmonary emboli. In such patients, when the clinical suspicion of embolus is high and life threatening, a diagnosis of embolism must be established with the help of angiography. The embolus itself can then be visualized radiographically as a lucent filling defect in a blocked artery (Figure 6-27) and the patient

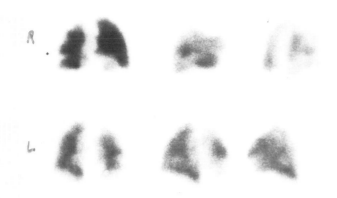

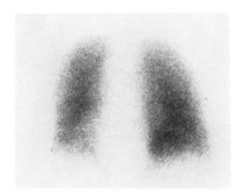

Figure 6-25. Ventilation scan (posterior view) in the patient in Figure 6-24 is normal. Q.E.D: VQ mismatch = pulmonary embolism.

Figure 6-24. Series of perfusion lung scans (anterior, posterior, two laterals, and two obliques) on a patient clinically suspected of pulmonary embolism. Note numerous defects in the perfusion of the peripheral lung.

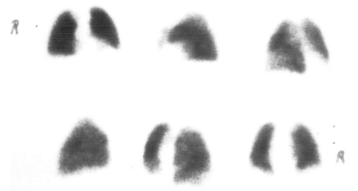

Figure 6-26. Same patient after sixteen days of therapy (anticoagulation). Perfusion scan is normal. Emboli have resolved.

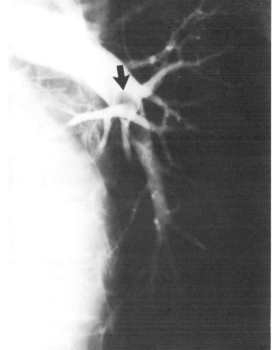

Figure 6-27. Pulmonary arteriogram in a patient with a large embolus (*arrow*) in the left lower lobe artery. Note good filling of the upper lobe vessels compared with that of the lower lobe vessels.

can be appropriately treated in order to prevent recurrent embolism, which may be fatal.

Pulmonary arteriography is a more accurate method than radioisotope lung scanning for diagnosing pulmonary embolism, but it is a more invasive and expensive procedure. It is usually indicated today when (1) the results of the lung scan are uncertain, (2) when the lung scan is interpreted as positive in a patient at risk for anticoagulation, or (3) when the lung scan is interpreted as negative in a patient with overwhelming clinical evidence for pulmonary embolism.

CHAPTER 7 Overexpansion and Collapse of the Lung; Causes of Mediastinal Shift

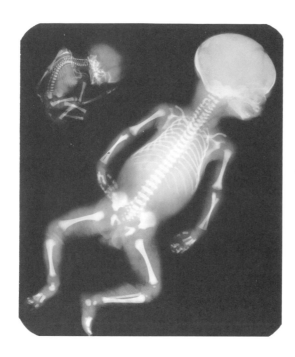

Figure 7-1. Stillborn twins, one dead at three months, one born dead at term. Note that lungs, heart, and abdominal structures blend into one uniform shadow.

When lung tissue is inflated with more than its normal content of air, it becomes more radiolucent than usual. No matter how clearly radiolucent the normal tissue on a chest film now looks to you, remember that it is quite logical that a cube of air should be more radiolucent than the same cube of air traversed by blood-filled capillaries. As you would expect, then, the roentgen appearance of overexpanded lung will be overall *increased radiolucency,* the affected lung appearing too dark with the exposures used for chest work. In addition, the lung markings will be spread apart as the vessels are separated farther and farther by the ballooned alveoli. In obstructive emphysema localized to one segment of lung this appearance may be so exaggerated as to be confused with pneumothorax. The true state of affairs may generally be determined by a careful fluoroscopic study or by inspiration and expiration films, for which you will need to consult your radiologist.

Atelectasis, on the other hand, causes the lung to appear less radiolucent than usual, and atelectasis of one lobe will be seen first as a difference in density between the two sides of the chest film. Thus you will be looking for an unaccountably dense area in the lung. You have already seen diffusely increased density due to the high position of the diaphragm in a film made at peak expiration, and you realize that that amount of decreased radiolucency at some phase of the respiratory cycle goes with every breath your patient takes.

You see in Figure 7-1 the film of a stillborn infant who has never breathed at all. His lungs and bony thorax are collapsed about the heart and mediastinal structures as one uniformly dense shadow within the rib cage, and they blend continuously with the shadows of the dense abdominal structures. The tracheobronchial tree is filled with amniotic fluid.

In Figure 7-2 the arterial tree of a segment of lung has been injected with opaque fluid and sealed off, inflation and deflation of the lung being carried out through a tube tied into the bronchus. In Figure 7-2A you see the lung collapsed around its arterial tree in just about the same degree of hypoaeration which would exist near the diaphragm at full expiration. In Figure 7-2B the specimen has been inflated to approximate the lung near the diaphragm at deep inspiration.

Below, in Figure 7-3, you see the lungs of a child at expiration and inspiration. (In childhood a range from posterior rib 7 to posterior rib 10 is normal for full respiratory excursion.) In this chapter you will learn the changes in the appearance of the chest film when both lungs are underexpanded and when both are overexpanded. Then we will consider the changes seen when the volume of one hemithorax is altered enough to produce shift of the mediastinum from its midline position.

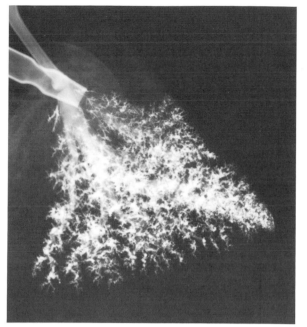 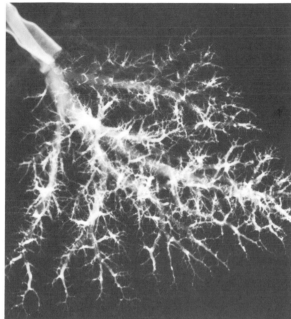

A: Expiration

B: Inspiration

Figure 7-2

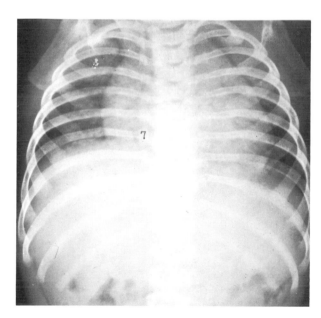 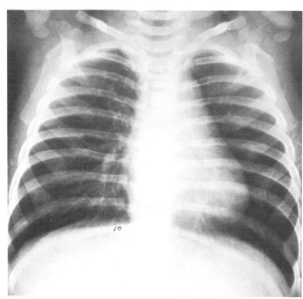

A: Expiration

B: Inspiration

Figure 7-3

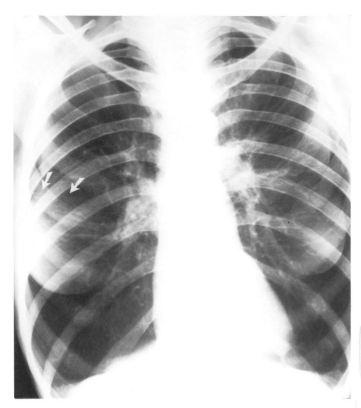

Figure 7-4. Emphysema in a heavy smoker, both lower lobes. The heart appears normal in size, but remember that right ventricular enlargement (cor pulmonale in this case) is difficult (or may be impossible) to recognize in the PA view alone. In the lateral view the lower half of the anterior clear space may be obliterated by forward extension of the massive right ventricle. Horizontal fissure (*arrows*) is slightly elevated and should be distinguished from the walls of the blebs seen in Figure 7-5.

Emphysema

With chronic emphysema the lungs usually are both overexpanded, the diaphragm low, flattened, and often serrated. Many cases will be obvious to you from the increased radiolucency you will see at the usual roentgen exposures for chest work. Lesser degrees of generalized emphysema may be much less obvious. In those patients the fluoroscopic finding of a diaphragm which moves down only slightly on inspiration and returns only very slowly on forced expiration will help to establish a diagnosis of emphysema. In many patients with emphysema the concomitant development of pulmonary fibrosis adds the shadow of a web of filamentous strands of increased density. These radiate outward from the hilum through the lung. Localized emphysematous bullae may be seen anywhere in the lung, like huge air cysts bordered by dense thin walls which enclose them. Rupture of such bullae, producing spontaneous pneumothorax, is not unusual.

Sometimes it is difficult to be certain from the PA chest film that the lungs are overinflated. When one looks at the lateral, however, the situation becomes much more convincing and shows hyperinflation with flattening of the diaphragm and increase in the AP diameter of the chest. Thin-section CT can beautifully delineate lung parenchyma and today may be used to confirm the chest films (as in Figure 7-6B), to identify bullae, and to classify the type of emphysema.

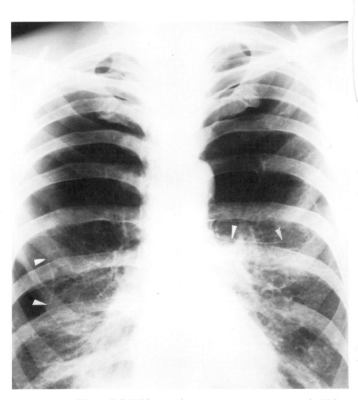

Figure 7-5. Widespread pan-acinar emphysema grade III in a patient with chronic bronchitis. *Arrows* mark walls of bullae.

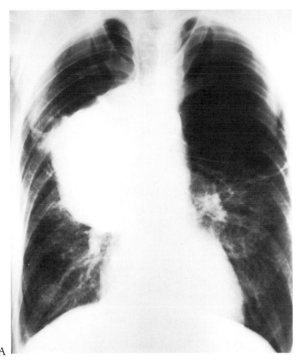

Figure 7-6

A: Bullous emphysema in a patient who smoked for years and now has also developed a lung cancer (the mass projecting to the right).
B: CT scan, same patient, with lung window technique. Note bullous destruction of left lung, which is useless. Imagine what perfusion and ventilation scans might show on this patient.

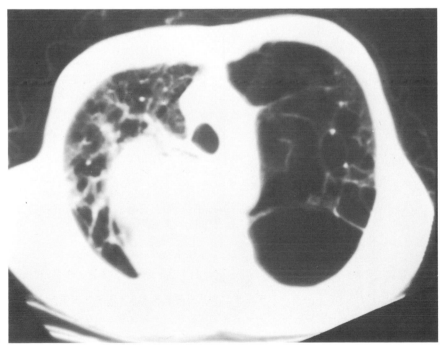

Normal Mediastinal Position

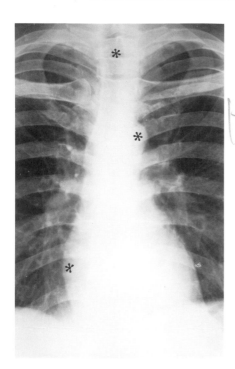

Figure 7-7. Well-exposed film showing the tracheobronchial tree. Markers indicate the three tag points by which one can determine the position of the mediastinum: the tracheal air column, the aortic arch, and the right heart border.

The first is the column of air in the trachea, visible as a dark vertical shadow on the PA chest film, normally a little to the right of the midline as it approaches the carina. The second is the white knob you see to the left of the spine at about the fifth rib posteriorly. This knob is the shadow margin created by the arch of the aorta as it swings posteriorly and turns downward to become the descending aorta. You see it, of course, only because there is radiolucent lung tissue abutted against it, and it will disappear if that lung tissue becomes airless or if a dense mass lies against the aortic arch.

Finding the trachea and the aortic arch in their usual locations, then, will tell you that the upper mediastinum is where it ought to be. When there is a marked decrease in the amount of air in the right upper lobe, for example, the trachea will be found shifted toward that side. The arch of the aorta will be pulled with it toward the midline, its shadow disappearing as it becomes superimposed upon that of the spine. In just the same way, the trachea and the aortic arch may be displaced to the left when there is a decrease in the air content of the left upper lobe. If you review the anatomic relations of the aortic arch, you will find that normally both upper and lower lobes adjoin it. For this reason if there is no air at all in the left upper lobe, it will lie, dense and much decreased in size, against the anterior mediastinum, and you may actually still see the aorta through it, illuminated by the overexpanded superior segment of the lower lobe. Check the position of the trachea and the aortic arch on some of the chest films you have seen so far.

The third tag point in determining the position of the mediastinum is the shadow of the right heart border. Major changes in the size of either *lower* lobe will swing the heart to one side, and it will look displaced. You may think that since we have not yet discussed the heart and cardiac enlargement, you will not be able to use the right heart border with much sense of security, but be reassured. Up to now we have

Some describe the mediastinum as a region. We prefer to think of it as a bundle of structures sandwiched between the two inflated lungs. With the exception of the air-filled trachea and main bronchi, all these structures have the same radiodensity and merge into a homogeneous shadow superimposed upon that of the spine in the PA projection. Thus, the shadows of the mediastinal structures cannot be separated from one another except by a variety of special procedures employing contrast substances, computed tomography, and magnetic-resonance imaging. On the routine chest film, only the lateral margins of the mediastinum outlined by air in the lungs on either side can be identified.

With changes in the air content of either lung, or with large accumulations of pleural air or fluid, the mediastinum will bow to one side like an elastic diaphragm. You will need to identify a few anatomic points along the margins of the mediastinal shadow and know their normal locations if you are to be able to recognize mediastinal displacement on a routine PA chest film. There are three of these signal points which ought to be included in your systematic chest survey.

shown you very few abnormal hearts and a good many normal chest films. Look back over some of them at the right border of the heart as it curves down toward the diaphragm. By the time you have looked at a dozen or so, you should be convinced that the border of the normal right heart shadow is about a fingerbreadth beyond the right border of the spine on a full chest film of 14×17 inches (and proportionately less on these reductions). Of course, this is a very rough working rule; you will learn how to modify it as you look at more and more films and appraise more and more enlarged hearts.

Obviously, elevation of the diaphragm compressing the liquid-filled heart from below will exaggerate the lateral projection of both heart borders. Accuracy about mediastinal position, therefore, will depend on your having counted the ribs so that you are sure the diaphragm is drawn down well. Obviously too, if the right

middle lobe lying against the right heart is consolidated, that border will disappear and cannot be used in tagging the position of the lower mediastinum. Also, the tag points will appear displaced in a patient with even minor degrees of scoliosis.

If, however, you are satisfied that the diaphragms are well down, that the clavicles and ribs are symmetrical and show no rotation, and that the right heart border appears to be in about its usual position, you can say then that the lower mediastinum is not appreciably displaced.

If the *whole lung* on one side collapses, then all three tag points will show a shift in position, since the whole mediastinum swings to that side. If *only an upper lobe* is involved, you may find that the trachea and the aortic arch are shifted, while the right heart border is not.

Figures 7-8 and 7-9. CT sections which illustrate shift of the mediastinum. Figure 7-8 (*left below*) is normal. Both scans have been made just below the level of the aortic arch. You can identify the ascending (*AA*) and descending (*DA*) aorta. The superior vena cava (*SVC*) lies against the ascending aorta on the right and is receiving blood from the azygous vein, via the forward-swinging azygous arch (*arrows*) encircling the air-containing radiolucent trachea (*T*). The trachea and lungs are much more radiolucent than the fat-containing triangle of anterior mediastinum extending forward to the sternum in the midline. The vascular structures have all been enhanced by intravenous contrast medium.

Now note in Figure 7-9 (*right below*) how the ascending aorta and superior vena cava (unenhanced in this scan) have swung to the left in this patient, who has a bronchogenic carcinoma which has obstructed the left upper lobe bronchus causing atelectasis of the left upper lobe. The collapse of the upper lobe has greatly diminished the volume of the left lung, so that the mediastinal structures are pulled to the left, the right lung expanding to fill the space. You can see the rounded mass of the tumor (*arrows*) and the concave margin of the major fissure beyond it.

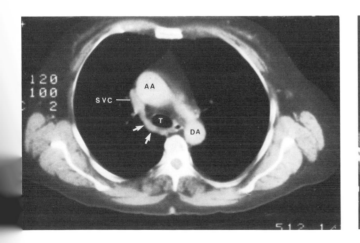
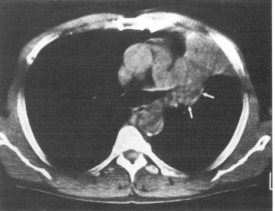

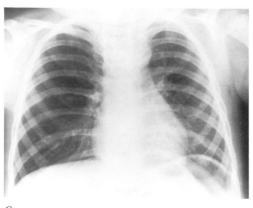

A

B

C

Mediastinal Shift

The mediastinum may be displaced *permanently* (as by surgical removal of the whole lung); *temporarily* (as when a large pleural effusion develops); or *transiently* (as when a foreign body in one major bronchus interferes with the inflation or deflation of that part of the lung during each inspiration). Permanent and temporary displacements of the mediastinum will usually be appreciable from the PA chest film, and you will be looking for them every time you check the three tag points in your systematic chest survey.

Because any single chest film only represents the state of affairs in your patient's chest at one particular fraction of a second in time, it is quite possible to expose the film when the mediastinum is in midposition, even though there is a definite mediastinal shift during some other phase of respiration. The single PA film made routinely at inspiration, which you hold in your hand later that day, may give no indication at all that there was a *transient shift of the mediastinum* at expiration. If you suspect there may be one, you ought to ask for *films made at inspiration and expiration*, a commonly used device for documenting transient mediastinal shift.

The mediastinum may be *pushed* to one side by pressure from an overexpanded lung, as in obstructive emphysema when air is drawn into that part of the lung with every breath but incompletely expelled. A check-valve foreign body may do this (see Figures 7-10B and C).

Obstructive emphysema probably also exists at some point in the natural history of any endobronchial tumor, although the obstruction is

Figure 7-10. A: Major collapse of the left lung. Note the pronounced mediastinal shift and high diaphragm (indicated by air in the gut under it, as well as crowded ribs on the left). A late postpneumonectomy film would look much the same. B and C: Transient mediastinal shift with a radiolucent endobronchial foreign body in the right main bronchus. At inspiration (B) the tracheal air shadow lies normally over the spine to the right of midline. The aorta and right heart border are in normal position. At expiration (C) it is the left lung which *can* deflate so that the trachea, aortic shadow, and right heart border all shift to the left as the mediastinum moves away from the side where there is air trapping (greater relative radiolucency of the right lung). A piece of chewing gum was recovered from the right main bronchus.

soon completed as the tumor grows, and the lung beyond it collapses as its air is absorbed or escapes to other segments. On serial films one would be able to observe the mediastinum at first displaced *away* from the side of the lesion by the overexpanded lung and, a week or so later, displaced *toward* the side of the lesion as the affected lobe collapses—another illustration of the value of serial films, of the proper evaluation of changing roentgen signs, and of constant discussion with the radiologist.

If you make a practice of thinking of the mediastinum as a flexible disc held in the midline *whenever the volumes of the two hemithoraces are equal,* you will not find it difficult to understand and remember how mediastinal shift occurs. The mediastinum *must* shift whenever there is a significant change in the volume on one side. Massive pleural effusion shifts the mediastinum to the opposite side. After pneumonectomy, or in massive collapse of one whole lung, pronounced mediastinal shift also occurs (Figure 7-10A). (Unilateral bullous emphysema may shift the mediastinum, compressing the good lung as in Figure 7-12.)

The mediastinum may *not* shift, on the other hand, if the various additions and subtractions in volume on one side cancel each other out, so that the volume of the abnormal hemithorax remains equal to that of the normal side. For example, in Figure 7-11 you see a patient with a large pneumothorax. Air trapped in the pleural space has added to the volume of the left hemithorax, but at the same time the left lung has collapsed to one-third its normal volume. Note that the mediastinum remains in the midline. Of course, with tension pneumothorax the mediastinum will shift away from that side.

The mediastinum *may* not shift if it has become fixed as a result of adhesions subsequent to inflammation, or because of tumor invasion. Furthermore, it may be checked in its displacement by pleural adhesions which prevent the full collapse of one lung.

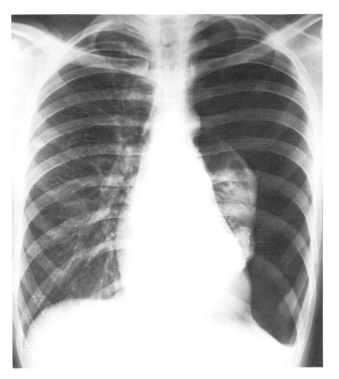

Figure 7-11. Pneumothorax with the mediastinum in the midline. The volume of pleural air is compensated for here by the degree of collapse of the left lung.

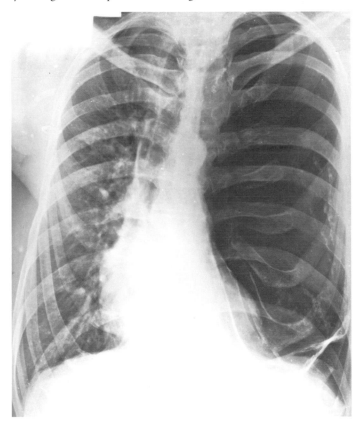

Figure 7-12. Obstructive bullous emphysema of part of the left lung, causing shift of the mediastinum to the right. No pneumothorax was present. Note that you do not see the outer surface of the lung, as you did in Figure 7-11.

95

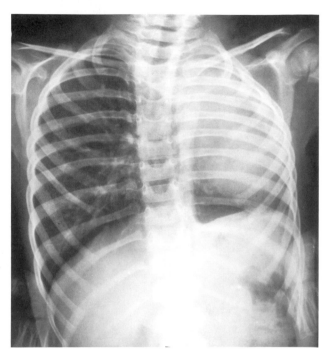

A

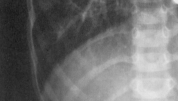

B

Figure 7-13. Permanently displaced mediastinum in a four-year-old who had agenesis of the left lung and compensatory overexpansion of the right lung coming across the midline anteriorly. A: The dense mass in the left hemithorax is the heart. B: Angiography delineates its structure. Note absence of the left pulmonary artery.

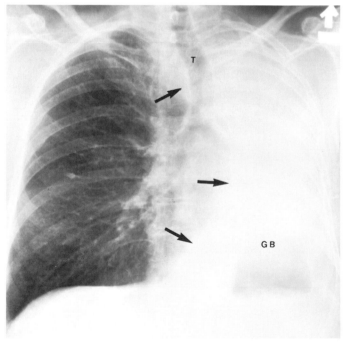

A

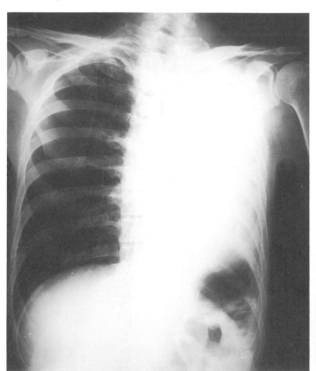

B

Figure 7-14A and B. Two patients with collapse of the entire left lung with compensatory overexpansion of the right lung. Note elevation of the gastric bubble (*GB*), implying a high (possibly paralyzed) left hemidiaphragm. There is pronounced displacement of all mediastinal structures to the left with herniation to the left of the right lung (*arrows*). Bronchoscopy: carcinoma obstructing the left main bronchus in both patients. *T* is the trachea.

Mediastinal Shift due to Collapse of One Lobe on the Right

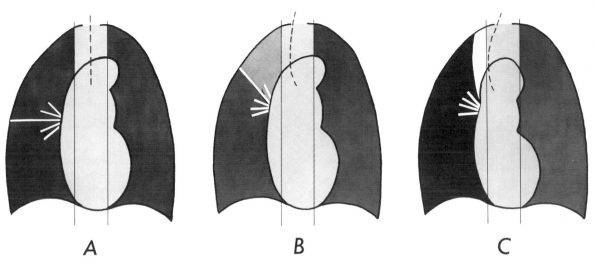

Figure 7-15. Collapse of the right upper lobe. A: Normal chest with normal position of the minor (horizontal) fissure, right hilum, trachea, aortic arch, and right heart border with equal aeration of all lobes. B: Right upper lobe collapsed 50 percent. Minor fissure deflected upward, trachea pulled slightly to the right. No change in right heart border. C: Major collapse of the right upper lobe, which is now a flat wedge of density against the superior mediastinum, trachea, and aortic arch tilted to the right. Right hilum drawn upward. Overaeration in the lower and middle lobes is compensatory. Note upward displacement of the hilum.

A collapsing lobe tends to fold up fanwise against the mediastinum in a characteristic manner, and a dynamic concept of these collapse patterns and the roentgen signs by which they are to be recognized is, again, nothing more than an exercise in the logic of radiodensities applied anatomically. You would anticipate, for example, that with atelectasis of the *right upper lobe* the location of the minor horizontal fissure separating it from the middle lobe could be seen increasingly well as the contrast increased between the poorly aerated lung tissue above it and the well-aerated lung tissue below it. Moreover, since the fissure is fixed at the hilum, it is natural that it would be seen to tilt upward from that fixed point as the upper lobe collapsed. When completely collapsed, the pancake-flat upper lobe would apply itself against the upper mediastinum and merge its shadow with that of other mediastinal structures. The shadow of the trachea would be drawn to the right, and the aortic arch would be drawn with it. The right hilum would be drawn slightly upward.

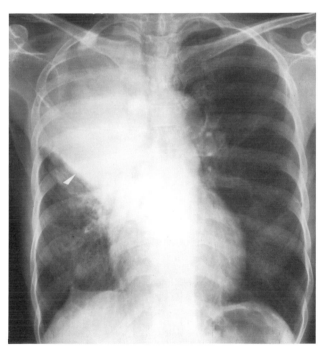

Figure 7-16. Patient with right upper lobe atelectasis distal to a bronchogenic carcinoma. *Arrow* indicates elevated minor fissure.

97

Collapsed Lobes on the Right

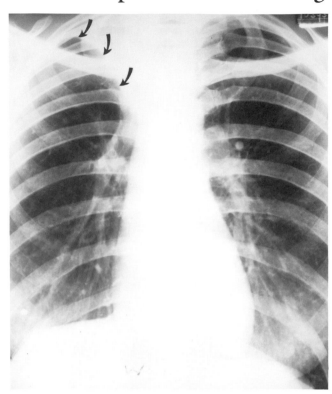

Figure 7-17 (*left*). Nearly complete collapse of the right upper lobe in a patient with a ten-year history of symptoms of cough and occasional hemoptysis. *Arrows* indicate the curving margin of an elevated minor fissure. At surgery obstruction of the right upper lobe bronchus by a bronchial adenoma was discovered and lobectomy performed. Note high right takeoff of vessels to the lower lobe.

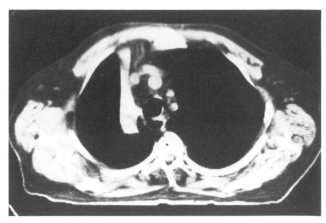

Figure 7-18. CT scan of another patient with collapse of the right upper lobe. The section is just above the aortic arch. You can identify the small flat upper lobe lying against the mediastinal structures, all of which are displaced to the right. Identify the left and right brachiocephalic veins (farthest anterior), then the trachea, and, between it and the brachiocephalic veins, the brachiocephalic artery. To the left of the trachea lie the left common carotid and left subclavian arteries. Compare with Figure 2-23.

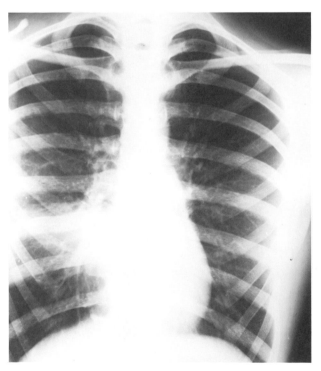

A

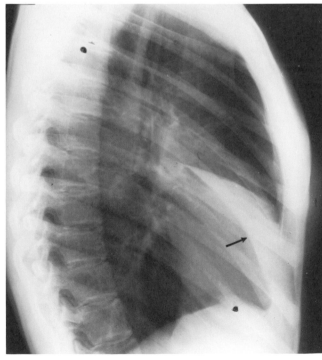

B

Figure 7-19. Collapse of the right middle lobe. A line drawn between the two black dots in the lateral view (B) would indicate the normal location of the major (oblique) fissure. Hence the lower part must be bowed forward. The minor fissure is depressed. The mediastinum is not displaced, as the volume of the right middle lobe is too small. Even if it totally collapses, there is not sufficient change in right lung volume to alter the position of the mediastinum.

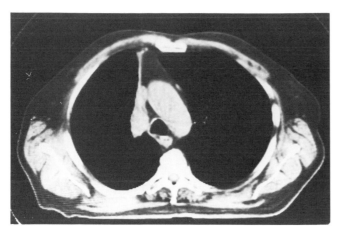

Figure 7-20. CT section showing right upper lobe collapse. This scan is made at the level of the aortic arch, lower than Figure 7-18. The aorta and the fatty anterior mediastinal triangle are displaced to the right.

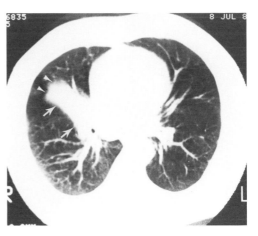

Figure 7-21. Collapsing right middle lobe. CT section with lung window technique. Section is much lower and through the heart. Compare with Figures 7-18 and 7-20. The right heart profile would be lost on the PA film in Figure 7-21.

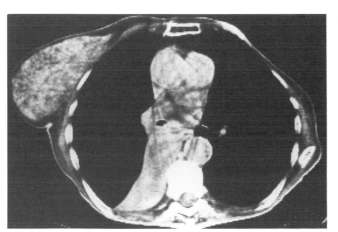

Figure 7-22. Right lower lobe collapsed posteriorly against the vertebral column and posterior ribs. This patient had had a left mastectomy. Note mass of metastatic nodes between the vertebral body and the flattened, anteriorly displaced bronchus intermedius.

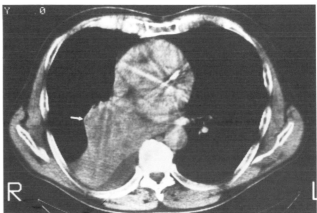

Figure 7-23. Right lower lobe collapse in obstructing bronchogenic carcinoma. Note the rounded tumor mass (*arrow*) bulging to the right, anterior to the collapsed lobe. Note too the pleural fluid collection (less dense) posterior to the collapsed lobe.

99

Mediastinal Shift due to
Collapse of One Lobe on the Left

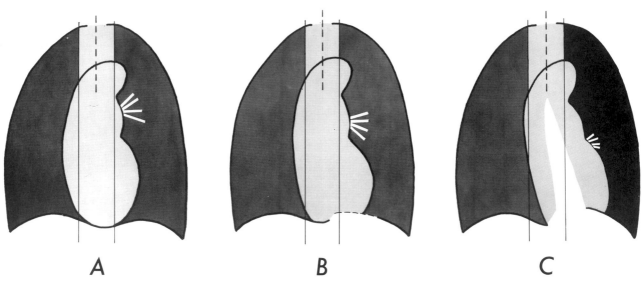

A   B   C

Figure 7-24. Collapse of the left lower lobe. A: Normal profiles and mediastinal tag points. B: Early signs of left lower lobe collapse—less heart shadow to the right of the spine, vague decrease in the lucency of the lower left lung field with preservation of left hemidiaphragm which, however, becomes slightly elevated medially. C: Massive collapse of the left lower lobe. Little or no heart shadow seen to the right of the spine. Medial half of the profile of the left diaphragm missing. Left lower lobe now a wedge of density seen through the heart and against the spine. Left hilum depressed.

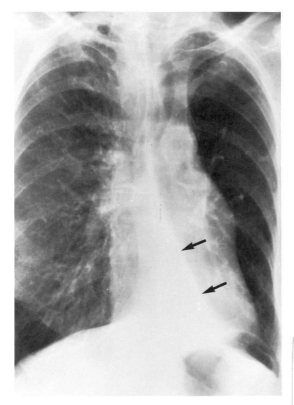

Now put together the signs of *left lower lobe* collapse in just the same deliberately logical way. Since the major fissure lines up with the beam of x-rays only in the lateral view and is always quite oblique to the ray in the PA view, no clear-cut margin between normal and atelectatic lung tissue is to be seen on the PA film as the left lower lobe begins to collapse. The heart gradually shifts to the left, however, so that you see less and less of the heart border to the right of the spine. You watch the left diaphragm become slightly more elevated and less and less clearly seen medially as the left lower lobe collapses against it, although the *lateral* half of the shadow profile of the diaphragm remains clear because of the compensatory expansion of the lingula of the left upper lobe, now touching it. The left

Figure 7-25. Left lower lobe collapse, seen as wedge of density through the heart. *Arrows* indicate margin of collapsed lobe. Overinflated left upper lobe. Medial part of left hemidiaphragm lost. Spine revealed and low left hilum obscured by displacement of heart to the left.

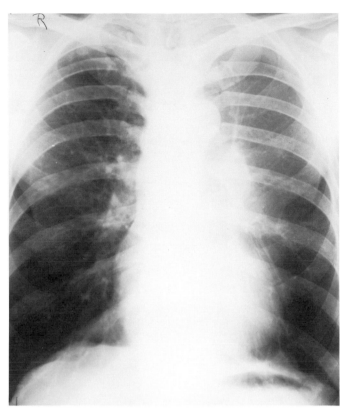

A

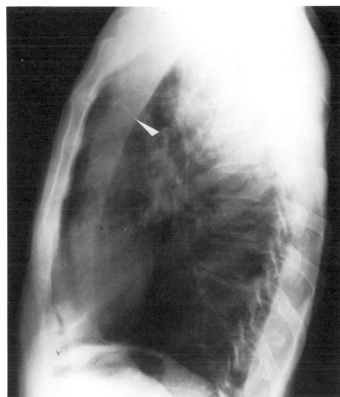

B

Figure 7-26. Collapsing left upper lobe due to obstructing carcinoma. Note veil-like density of left upper lung field and obscured left heart profile. The trachea is pulled to the midline and the aorta is too prominent, implying upper mediastinal shift. Lateral film (B): *arrow* indicates main fissure bowed forward as left upper lobe collapses. It is seen here as a slender wedge of density along the anterior part of the chest.

hilum is depressed, gradually disappearing behind the left border of the heart, an important and often missed roentgen sign of left lower lobe collapse. The lung markings of the left upper lobe appear spread apart and the lung tissue more lucent than that in comparable interspaces on the right. The totally collapsed lower lobe appears, finally, as a wedge-shaped shadow against the mediastinum posteriorly. Its outer margin is visible through the heart shadow, thrown into contrast by air in the normal lung tissue against it laterally, that is, in the overexpanded upper lobe (Figure 7-25). On the next page you will find CT scans to help you remember how the left upper and lower lobes collapse.

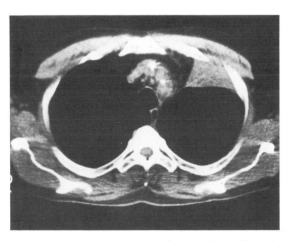

Figure 7-27. CT scan showing left upper lobe collapse in another patient, who had chest films similar to those in Figure 7-26. Note that the aortic arch is drawn forward and to the left, shortening the fatty wedge of the anterior mediastinum. The left upper lobe is seen as a wedge of density against the left anterior chest wall, with the hyperexpanded left lower lobe bulging into its posteroinferior surface.

101

CT Scans in Three Patients with Lobar Collapse on the Left

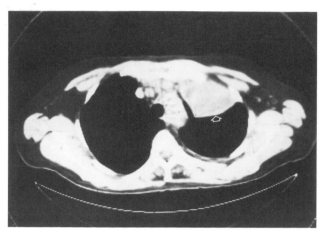

Figure 7-28. CT scan showing left upper lobe collapse. The section is at the level of the top of the aortic arch. The overexpanded superior segment of the lower lobe is pinched as a sliver of black between the atelectatic left upper lobe and the mediastinum. Here the posterior surface of the left upper lobe bulges backward because of a tumor mass within it. Open arrow indicates major fissure interface between left upper and left lower lobes.

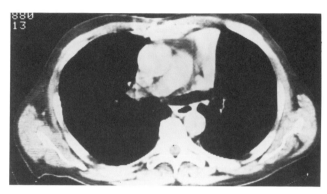

Figure 7-29. Left upper lobe collapse. Same patient as in Figure 7-28 but scanned lower down, at the level of the tracheal bifurcation. Here the lingula is seen flattened against the pulmonary trunk. The upper left cardiac profile would be lost in the PA film.

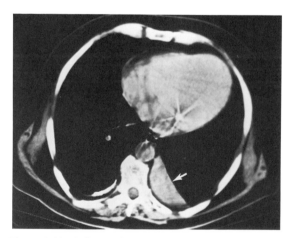

Figure 7-30. Collapse of the left lower lobe. Note mediastinal shift to the left (section level is through the heart). The left lower lobe always collapses posteromedially against the spine and posterior ribs. Arrow: displaced major fissure between upper and lower lobes.

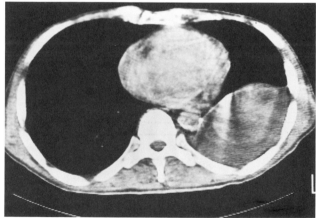

Figure 7-31. Collapse of the left lower lobe in another patient. Here mediastinal shift is much less pronounced because part of the lost volume is compensated for by a collection of pleural fluid engulfing the lobe. If you discount the motion-generated streak artifacts, you will see the crescent of less dense pleural fluid between the collapsing denser left lower lobe and the posterior chest wall. (Figure out the CT scan for a patient with collapse of the whole left lung.)

102

Tallying Roentgen Findings with Clinical Data

Roentgen observations which imply the presence of extensive emphysema or massive atelectasis will serve to remind you of distortions in architecture and aberrations of function which you might otherwise forget to consider in a particular patient. The old man with chronic emphysema is most concerned with his respiratory difficulties, but you will not be able to look at those overexpanded lungs and fibrous traceries of shadow on his radiograph without thinking of the increased work being done by the right side of his heart.

You must not forget, in looking at chest films, that changes in volume within the thorax may compensate for other changes and obscure them. If the mediastinum seems in its normal midline position despite the fact that one entire lung field is dense, you know only that the volumes of the two hemithoraces *are* equal. Underneath that white density there may be just enough collapse to compensate for the added volume of tumor or pleural effusion, and the radiologist will remind you that ultrasound or CT can differentiate fluid in the pleural space from tumor or atelectatic lung.

Remember that the radiograph is a shadowgram. Although you know that inflammation and tumor both render the lung dense, you must anticipate, for example, that in either condition some atelectasis is likely to be present as well, adding to the density of the already involved lung. Either tumor or inflammation may cause collapse of a lobe even though the entire lobe is not actually involved in the primary process.

The consolidated lobe in pneumonia often remains normal in size, as you saw it in Chapter 5; but equally often such a lobe will be distinctly decreased in size. In a good many patients with the clinical signs of pneumonia you may see some additional roentgen indications of atelectasis, resulting from poor aeration due to sticky endobronchial secretions. As you increase your knowledge of medicine, you will learn to evaluate the roentgen signs of lobar collapse according to whether, for example, your patient was admitted with clear-cut pneumonia or has only a minor degree of fever and cough the day following surgery. In the former instance you must think in terms of pneumonia-plus-atelectasis and treat accordingly. In the latter you must think in terms of atelectasis primarily, and consider the possibility of infection developing in the collapsed lobe. That they may look the same on the films should not disturb you, since you are using the radiographic findings as part of the entire clinical analysis rather than as oracular information. A respectable percentage of lung cancers are at first thought to be pneumonia with atelectasis, and only the unaccountable failure of the lungs to reexpand fully with proper treatment eventually raises the question of tumor.

It is immensely important for you to realize that the type of analysis of roentgen findings you have been learning offers you an improved understanding of the dynamic pathological changes within the thoracic cage of your patient. It is much more useful to you than any collection of diagnostic tags and labels. When you see mediastinal shift on a chest film or appreciate exaggerated radiolucency or the disappearance of normal profiles, you are recognizing roentgen findings rather than diagnoses. Such findings are heavy with implication about what is going on inside your patient. Their presence will often go a long way toward confirming, expanding, or exploding an original working diagnosis based on the history and physical examination.

CHAPTER 8 Study of the Mediastinal Structures

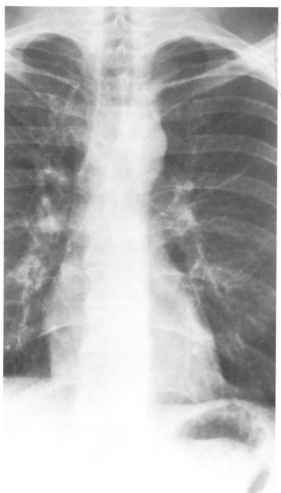

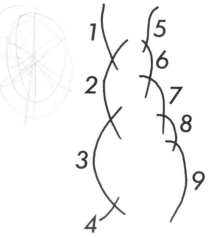

Figure 8-1 (*left*). The normal mediastinal profiles are all vascular and resolve into a series of nine intersecting arcs, as shown in Figure 8-2 (*above*): (*1*) right brachiocephalic vessels; (*2*) ascending aorta and superimposed superior vena cava; (*3*) right atrium; (*4*) inferior vena cava; (*5*) left brachiocephalic vessels; (*6*) aortic arch; (*7*) pulmonary trunk; (*8*) left atrial appendage; (*9*) left ventricle.

The heart is the largest of the mediastinal structures, and all of the profiles that bulge beyond the shadow of the spine on both sides in the PA chest film represent parts of the heart or of its great vessels. You can think of these profiles as nine intersecting arcs (Figure 8-2). Justify their identity on the basis of the angiocardiograms on the opposite page. Remember that some of the structures producing these shadows are more posterior in the chest (6) and others far anterior (2,7).

Remember too that when contrast medium mixed with blood fills a particular chamber of the heart, its shadow may seem to you quite different in shape from what you have learned about that chamber based on a gross examination of the heart and its surface markings. Where

a chamber is thickest its shadow will be most dense in the angiogram, and where it tapers off and becomes very thin a much less dense shadow is produced. Look at the shadow of the right ventricle, for example, in Figure 8-3. The slender, flattened part of the chamber, which extends far to the left against the interventricular septum in the PA view, hardly seems to belong to the dense massive shadow of the rest of the ventricle. Note also that you appreciate only vaguely the location of the tricuspid valve in this view, because the right atrium and right ventricle are partly superimposed. In the levogram notice that you see the dense upper margin of the crab-shaped left atrium through the shadow of the ascending aorta, in spite of the fact that you know the left atrium is on the posterior sur-

104

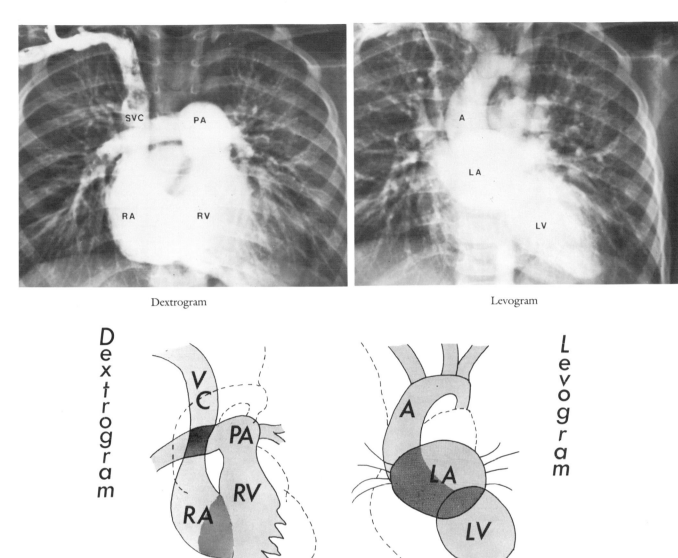

Dextrogram

Levogram

Figure 8-3 (*left above, with diagram below*). *Dextrogram*, taken from a series of films made as an opaque-loaded bolus of blood passed through the heart. You see the right chambers and pulmonary arteries.

Figure 8-4 (*right above, with diagram below*). *Levogram*, taken 3 seconds later when the right side of the heart had been cleared of opaque-containing blood. You see the left chambers and aorta. Note the pulmonary veins draining into the left atrium on either side. It is easy to see that the *venous* hilum is lower than the arterial hilum. This child had coarctation of the aorta; note indentation below the arch.

face of the heart and that the ascending aorta arises anteriorly. Their opaque-filled cavities have cast separate shadows outlining them for you, and the two shadows overlap in this view.

The plain film of the chest made PA, then, shows you a number of mediastinal bulges seen in profile against the radiolucent lung on either side of the spine, all of them vascular shadows. In addition, you can usually see air in the trachea, but all other mediastinal structures merge with one another and their shadows are superimposed upon those of the spine, the heart, and the sternum. You cannot account for the shadow of the esophagus or distinguish lymph nodes, thymus, or nerves; the thoracic duct merges with the shadows of other soft tissues and fluid-carrying vessels. Except for their marginal profiles and their branches entering the lucent lungs, even the great vessels are merged with other shadows.

105

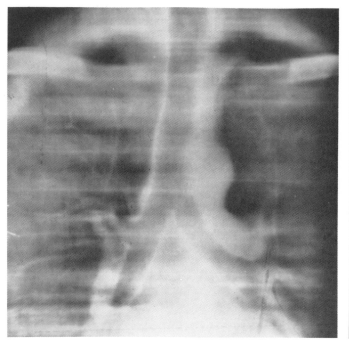

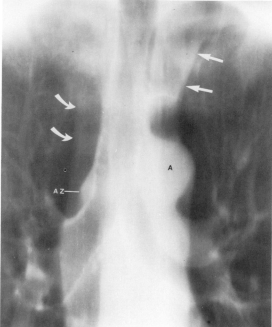

Figure 8-6. This coronal conventional tomogram visualizes many of the structures you have just identified in Figure 8-5. Note the bulge in the right paratracheal stripe, the azygos arch (*AZ*) about to empty into the superior vena cava, whose shadow is seen lateral and posterior to it (*curved arrows*). The left subclavian artery (*straight arrows*) is seen arising from the aortic arch (*A*).

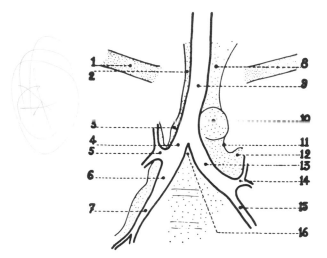

Figure 8-5 (*above, with diagram below*). Coronal tomographic study of the normal tracheobronchial tree.

- (1) Clavicle
- (2) Normal opacity of great vessels and tracheal wall
- (3) Azygos vein
- (4) Right main stem bronchus
- (5) Right upper lobe bronchus
- (6) Site of origin of right middle lobe bronchus
- (7) Right lower lobe bronchus
- (8) Normal opacity of vessels and tracheal wall
- (9) Trachea
- (10) Aortic arch
- (11) Concave profile between aortic arch and left pulmonary artery
- (12) Left pulmonary artery
- (13) Left main stem bronchus
- (14) Left upper lobe bronchus
- (15) Left lower lobe bronchus
- (16) Carina

On this page spread you are using the normal dark air column in the trachea and bronchi as a contrast medium—which you can do, of course, up to a point in any well-exposed chest film. In Figures 8-5 and 8-6 you have tomograms to study. These eliminate the superimposed images of other structures and afford you a more precise view of the tracheobronchial anatomy. Identify all the parts of the upper mediastinal structures visible in these plain tomograms and apply what you have now learned to recognize to the well-exposed chest films you will be seeing in your own patients. Upper mediastinal shift will be appreciable, as you learned in the last chapter, from displacement of the trachea in the PA film. The trachea is normally located slightly to the right of the midline because it is closely applied against the mass of the arch of the aorta. In older patients in whom the mass of the aortic arch becomes larger (ectatic) as a result of aging, the trachea may often be seen a little farther to the right without indicating mediastinal shift.

The esophagus, which lies just behind the trachea, is often deflected with the trachea by masses like the aortic aneurysm in Figure 8-7, in which the esophagus is visualized because the patient has swallowed barium. Here too, note that the entire upper mediastinum has not shifted but only certain of its structures (esophagus and trachea), whereas the mass of the aneurysm extends to the left. Aeration of the two upper lobes of the right and left lungs is equal.

The trachea may be visualized also with radiopaque contrast material, instilled under local anesthesia to suppress the cough reflex. This is called *bronchography* and is a special procedure little used today except in the staging of bronchiectasis. In questions of compression or invasion of the trachea plain tomography is more useful, as you see in the man in Figure 8-8 who was admitted with dyspnea and weight loss and soon developed stridor and great difficulty in breathing. Tumor is seen invading and narrowing the right main bronchus in this unfortunate patient, for whom radiotherapy would be only palliative. Both the mass of metastatic nodes and the narrowing of the trachea would be well visualized at CT.

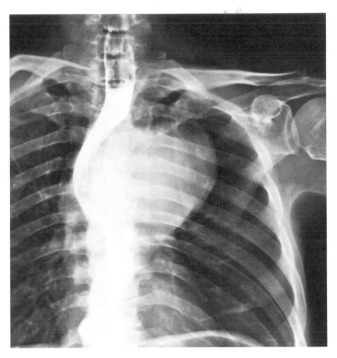

Figure 8-7. A patient with an aortic arch aneurysm causing deflection of the trachea and the barium-filled esophagus.

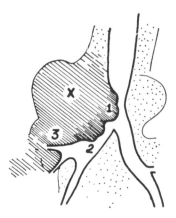

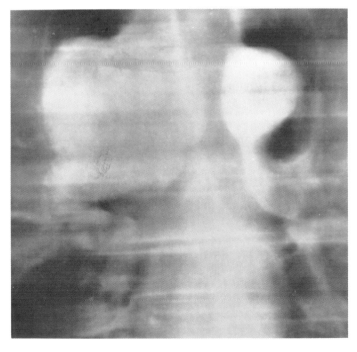

Figure 8-8 (*at right, with diagram above left*). Coronal midthoracic conventional tomographic study of a man aged 65 with dyspnea and weight loss. Note irregular narrowing of the trachea (*1*) and main stem bronchus (*2*). The mass (*X*) would appear on the regular chest film as an abnormal bulge on the right opposite the aortic arch. Note the downward deflection of a branch of the right upper lobe bronchus (*3*). Final diagnosis: bronchogenic carcinoma with spread to mediastinal lymph nodes.

107

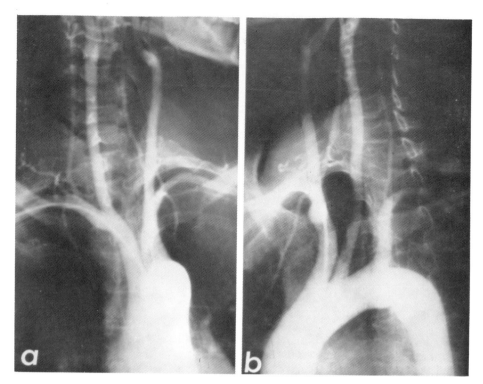

Figure 8-9. The normal aortic arch and the brachiocephalic artery. Opaque fluid was injected at the arch through a catheter placed into the right brachial artery. The patient in *a* is almost AP (very slightly rotated to the left). In *b* he has been sharply rotated to his right, unrolling the aortic arch so that its branches no longer overlap. Remember that both arterial and venous structures account for arcs 1 and 5 in Figure 8-2, but that here only the arteries are contrast filled.

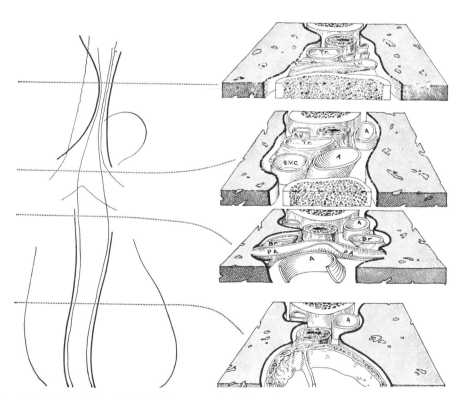

Figure 8-10. Mediastinal relationships in cross section. *Tr*, trachea; *IV*, innominate (brachiocephalic) vein; *AV*, azygos vein; *A*, aorta; *SVC*, superior vena cava; *Br*, bronchus; *PA*, pulmonary artery. Heavy lines are pleural reflections. Remember that in this diagram you are looking at the *top* of the section from front to back, whereas on all CT scans you are looking up at the scan from the patient's feet, with the spine toward you.

108

CT Sections:
4 Levels, 4 Patients

For decades *angiography* has been able to document alterations in the heart and brachiocephalic vessels. What you see in Figure 8-9 is a thoracic aortogram. Here the bolus of contrast material has been injected via a catheter threaded into the brachial artery. In *a* the patient is lying flat and in *b* he has been turned to his right. Imagine the superior vena cava lying against the arch on the right. Note that in *b* you can identify the brachiocephalic artery arising first and then dividing into the right subclavian and right common carotid arteries. Next, the left common carotid artery and the left subclavian artery arise in turn from the arch of the aorta.

Study of the mediastinum in the living patient has been revolutionized by computed tomography. You will be able to appreciate the precision of this new development in radiology when you study the serial CT scans (in different patients) at the right. In Figure 8-11, made just above the arch of the aorta through the brachiocephalic vessels, you can easily identify the anteriorly placed right and left brachiocephalic veins, which in the scan just below have joined to form the superior vena cava.

Figures 8-9a and 8-10 to your left afford you a *frontal* view with the vertebrae away from you, whereas the CT scans are conventionally displayed so that you are looking *up from the patient's feet* with the vertebrae down.

Now look back from Figure 8-12, in which you see the sectioned arch of the aorta, to Figure 8-11, in which you can identify the vessels it gives off: the brachiocephalic (or innominate) artery, and then in turn the left common carotid and left subclavian arteries. Note the trachea to the right of the arch of the aorta in 8-12 and its bifurcation (*B*) just posterior to the arch in 8-13, as well as the branching major bronchi in 8-14. The ascending and descending limbs of the aorta and the pulmonary trunk branching into left and right pulmonary arteries are all clearly seen in 8-14. The density of the anterior mediastinum in Figure 8-12 is normal thymus in an adolescent (*arrow*).

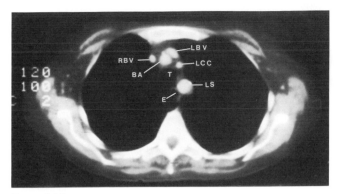

Figure 8-11

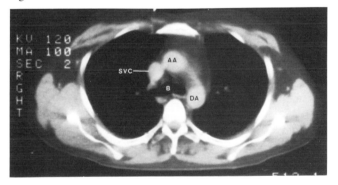

Figure 8-12

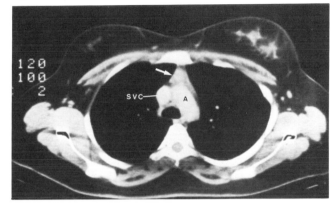

Figure 8-13

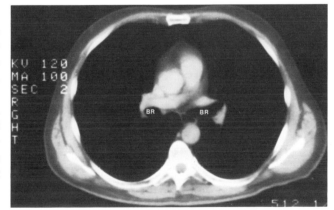

Figure 8-14

109

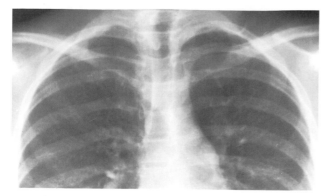

Figure 8-15. The normal superior mediastinum flattened between the two inflated upper lobes.

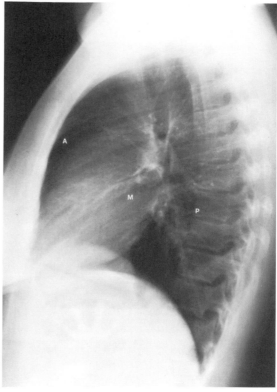

Figure 8-16. The mediastinal zones: *A,* anterior mediastinum; *M,* middle mediastinum; *P,* posterior mediastinum and paraspinal area.

Mediastinal Compartments and Masses Arising from Them

The mediastinum, considered as a disc of structures compressed between the two inflated lungs in the PA chest film, is seen en face in the lateral chest film instead of in tangent. One can divide it into anterior, middle, and posterior sections and discuss the structures and masses in each. Unfortunately, there is some difference of opinion in labeling the various compartments of the mediastinum. Some writers place the heart in the anterior mediastinum; some place it in the middle mediastinum. For our purposes one need not put too fine a point on it, since *anterior mediastinal masses* generally arise from the region anterior to the heart and are seen, in the lateral chest film, to fill in the radiolucent anterior clear space in front of the heart. Such masses include goiter extending down from the thoracic inlet, thymoma, teratoma, and lymphoma. The last often extends back to occupy also the middle compartment and of course may involve any part of the mediastinum, because lymph nodes are located in all compartments.

Middle mediastinal masses generally arise from structures posterior to the heart: the esophagus (carcinoma as well as dilatation of the esophagus itself in achalasia and scleroderma), the tracheobronchial tree (bronchogenic carcinoma and cysts), and lymph nodes located there. *Posterior mediastinal masses* are often neural in origin (ganglioneuromas, neurofibromas) and, of course, aneurysms of the posterior part of the arch and the descending aorta are posterior mediastinal masses.

Near the diaphragm one also sees masses related to the herniation of abdominal structures through the diaphragm (hernias of Morgagni and Bochdalek, and those paraesophageal hernias we call hiatus hernias, which are often symptomatic). Pericardial cysts occur most often in the right paracardiac angle. They are seen on the frontal chest film to ablate part of the right heart shadow, and on the lateral film to superimpose on the heart shadow.

110

Masses in the superior part of the mediastinum or thoracic inlet are often (but not always) *goiters* in which the thyroid mass extends down into the mediastinum. Compare Figure 8-17 with the appearance of the normal thoracic inlet in the frontal view in Figure 8-15. Note how the trachea in Figure 8-17 is deflected.

Now analyze Figure 8-18. Does this CT section belong to the patient in 8-17? Note that the trachea is deflected by a large mass in the anterior mediastinum. Compare with Figure 8-11 on the last page spread by tipping the page so that you can look at 8-18 and 8-11 together. Yes, Figure 8-18 proved to be a goiter, but it is not the same patient as in Figure 8-17: the trachea is deflected to the left, not to the right. Note also that it is compressed.

Analyze Figure 8-19. There is a mass in the superior mediastinum, extending to both sides, but it proved to be a mass of tumor-invaded lymph nodes metastatic from a distant primary site. The metastatic nodes were located so high in the sternal notch that they were easy to biopsy.

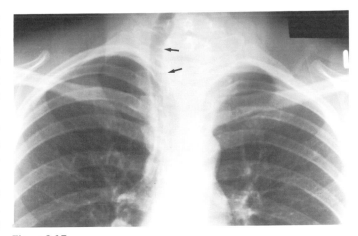

Figure 8-17

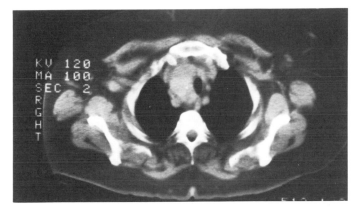

Figure 8-18

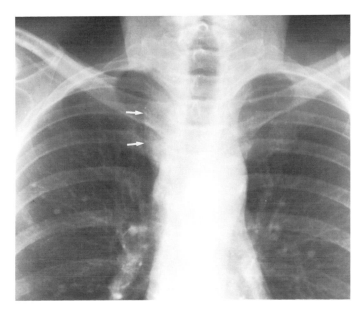

Figure 8-19

111

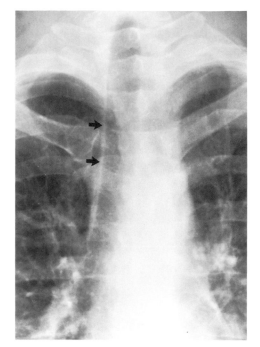

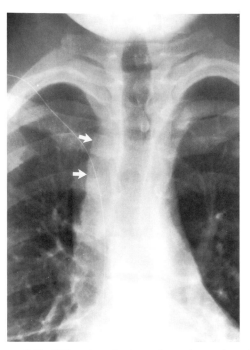

Figure 8-20. Normal mediastinum for comparison with Figures 8-21 and 8-22. *Arrows* indicate the right paratracheal stripe.

Figure 8-21. Widened mediastinum due to hemorrhage following trauma (see text).

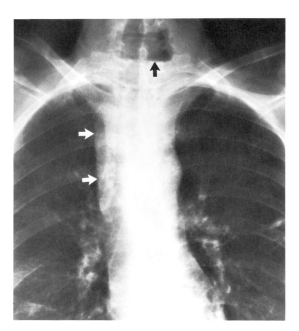

Figure 8-22. Mediastinitis widening the shadow of the superior mediastinum (see text).

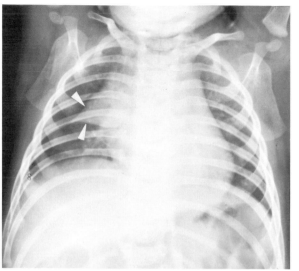 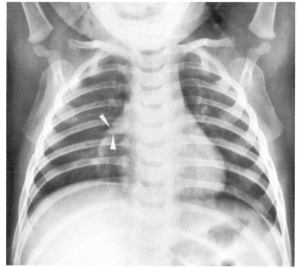

A   B

Figure 8-23. The normally enlarged thymus of an infant seen as a triangular, sail-shaped shadow overlapping the hilum as it projects laterally from the anterior mediastinum. It will be better visualized at expiration (A) than at inspiration (B) a moment or so later.

By no means all obvious thickening or widening of the upper mediastinum is caused by tumor mass of one kind or another. Compare the three illustrations on the page to your left. Figure 8-20 is normal and shows normal thickness of the right paratracheal stripe and the slightly-to-the-right-of-midline location of the trachea that you have learned to expect.

Figures 8-21 and 22, however, show definite widening of this region. The patient in 8-21 had a mediastinal hematoma (*arrows*) following traumatic insertion of a subclavian venous catheter. The catheter was removed and replaced with a right arm central venous pressure line, which you can see in this illustration. The patient in Figure 8-22 had difficulty in swallowing and high fever before admission; she has a retropharyngeal abscess (air-fluid level indicated by *black arrow*) and extension downward into the mediastinum with development of mediastinitis (*white arrows*). Note the mottled appearance and indenting of the upper mediastinum. This case serves as a reminder that the mediastinum is a continuation of the soft tissues of the neck. Infection and other processes may extend from one region to the other in either direction.

The *thymus* is normally large in infancy and gradually regresses as it is replaced with fat in the adult. You have in Figure 8-23 the appearance on the chest film of the normal infant thymus, a sail-shaped shadow extending from the mediastinal border and seen somewhat better at expiration than at inspiration. In Figure 8-12 you have already seen the normal, rather dense thymus extending from the arch of the aorta anteriorly to the sternum as a triangular wedge at CT. Look back at that figure and compare it with the less dense anterior mediastinal region of the somewhat older patient in Figure 8-13, in whom the usual fatty decreased density of the anterior mediastinum is well seen.

Anterior Mediastinal Masses

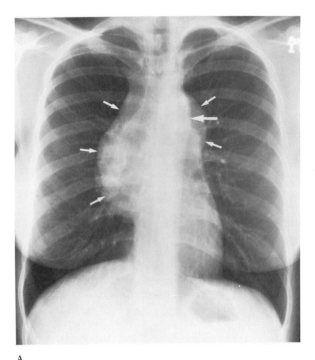

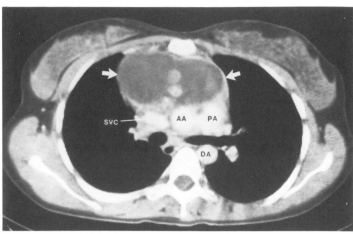

B

A

Figure 8-24
A: Teratoma in the anterior mediastinum (see text).
B: Same patient at CT.

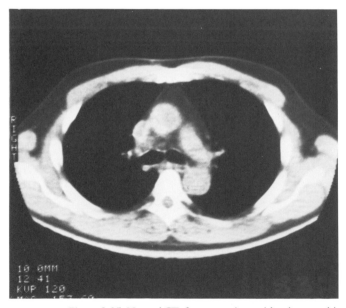

Figure 8-25. Normal CT, for comparison with others on this page spread.

114

Masses in the mediastinum anterior to the heart are generally one of four kinds: ectopic thyroid (goiters extending substernally), teratomas (benign or malignant), thymomas, or lymphoma. The mass in the chest film of the patient you see in Figure 8-24A was asymptomatic. Note that it is plastered against the right side of the heart and ablates the right heart shadow just as pneumonia or large segments of collapsed lung do. This mass, however, lies across the location of the horizontal fissure and bulges outward so that it does not conform anatomically to either of those diagnoses. You know even from the PA view alone that it must be located anteriorly against the heart, since the upper part of the heart border is lost. You can also see its left margin as distinct from the far-posterior arch and descending aorta (*long arrow*). It is, therefore, most likely to be one of the four masses we have listed above.

Now look at the CT scan in Figure 8-24B and decide what the tissue composition of the mass is likely to be. The density of the vascular structures tells you that intravenous enhancement has been used, and this throws into contrast the lucency of the well-encapsulated mass, which must

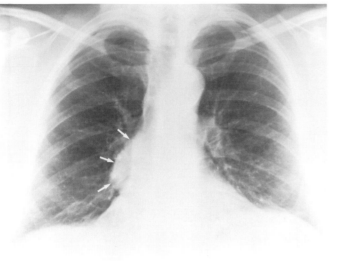

A

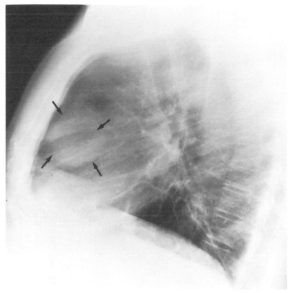

B

Figure 8-26. Anterior mediastinal thymoma in PA and lateral chest films (A and B) and at CT (C).

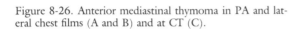

C

be largely composed of fat. It has within it, however, several round calcific densities, so it is not entirely fatty. It must logically be a teratoma, therefore, as indeed it proved to be on resection. The dense areas were cartilage partly calcified.

Notice the posterior displacement of the superior vena cava, the ascending aorta, and the pulmonary artery (compare with Figure 8-25, a normal scan made very slightly higher, as you can tell from the tracheal bifurcation). The descending aorta is normally located against the vertebra.

Thymomas also appear as anterior mediastinal masses, often asymptomatic, sometimes occurring in conjunction with symptoms and signs of myasthenia gravis. The mass (*arrows*) in Figure 8-26A was asymptomatic and might therefore have been any of the four entities, although it is low in the chest for thyroid.

Note that with the two views the plain films tell you that the mass is smaller than the one you have just been studying in Figure 8-24. For this reason it does not completely ablate the heart margin; small masses seldom do. Compare the matching CT scan, Figure 8-26C, with the other two on this page spread. Again the anteriorly placed mass deflects the aorta and superior vena cava posteriorly. At surgery it proved to be a thymoma.

Note that while Figure 8-25 was made at the level of the tracheal bifurcation, both 8-24 and 8-26 must be a bit lower, since the air-filled structures representing the major bronchi are now widely separated.

115

Anterior and Middle Mediastinal Masses

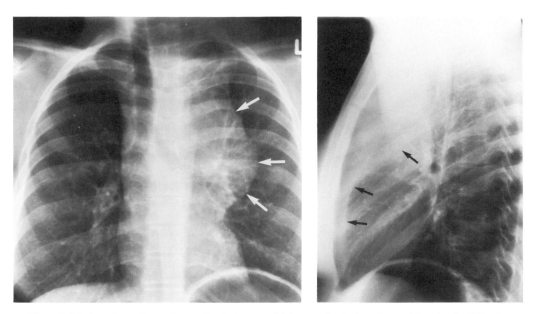

Figure 8-27. Anterior and superior mediastinal mass, which proved to be lymphoma. Note density filling in the anterior clear space in the lateral view.

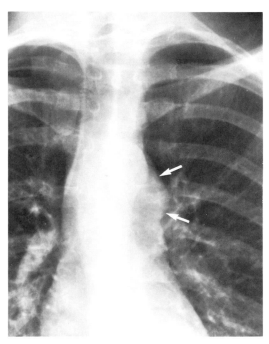

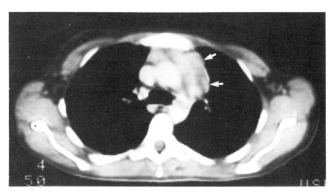

B

Figure 8-28. Hodgkin's lymphoma. Posteroanterior radiograph (A) and CT (B) of chest. The findings are in effect those of anterior mediastinal lymphadenopathy.

A

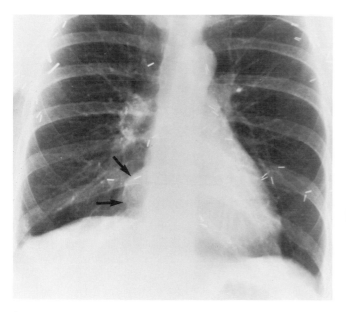

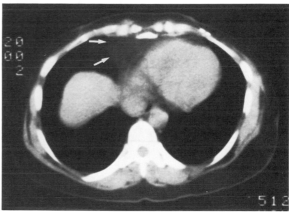

B

A

Figure 8-29. This patient had a history of bilateral mastectomies for carcinoma. At her annual checkup, although she was asymptomatic, her physician was concerned about the right paracardiac mass seen in A. However, on CT (B) made low in the chest, the anteriorly placed mass is seen to be low in density (Hounsfield units, −136) and therefore is typical of a paracardiac fat pad or lipoma rather than recurrent tumor.

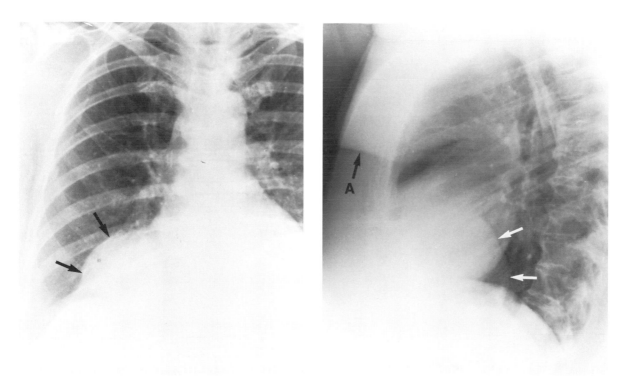

Figure 8-30. Pericardial cyst. The PA and lateral films demonstrate a round mass in the right cardiophrenic angle (*arrows*). CT would indicate its cystic character. The patient was asymptomatic. *A* indicates air against the undersurface of the patient's arm.

117

Posterior Mediastinal Masses

Masses occurring in the paraspinal or posterior mediastinal areas are usually neural masses arising in nerves as they issue from the spinal cord. Because they apply themselves snugly against the ribs and spinal column, they often cause erosion of bone and back pain. In Figure 8-31 an oval mass is seen extending to the right of the spine across four rib spaces. Note that there is erosion of the fourth and fifth ribs inferiorly (*white arrows*) with dense reactive bone along the inferior medial margin of each. The spaces between the fourth and fifth and the fifth and sixth ribs are wider than the contralateral spaces on the other side of the spine. The margin of the mass can also be seen extending down behind the heart and displacing the barium-filled esophagus to the left (*black arrows*). You know that this is not an anterior mediastinal mass because it does not obliterate the heart border. It proved to be a ganglioneuroma.

The CT scan on another patient, seen in Figure 8-32, shows a partly calcified mass lying against the posterior ribs on the left. This too proved to be a ganglioneuroma. Benign posterior mediastinal masses are more common than malignant ones.

Other posterior mediastinal masses include aneurysms of the descending aorta. They can generally be seen through the heart on the PA chest film.

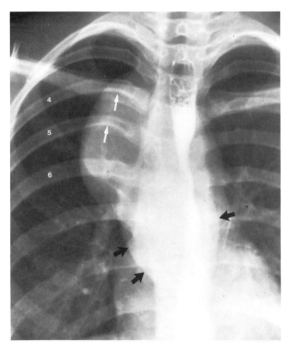

Figure 8-31. Posterior mediastinal ganglioneuroma. How would the CT scan look?

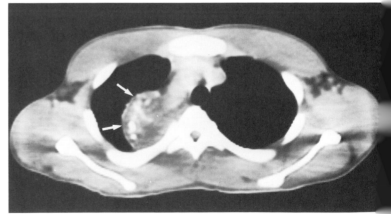

Figure 8-32. Posterior mediastinal mass in another patient. How would the PA chest film look?

Problems

Unknown 8-1 (Figure 8-33)
Analyze the film and decide whether the lesion in the right upper lobe (*single arrow*) could be related to the mediastinal mass (*two arrows*). The patient was admitted with superior vena caval syndrome.

Unknown 8-2 (Figure 8-35, bottom of page)
Analyze this CT scan taken at the level of the claviculomanubrial junction. Decide what you might find on physical examination.

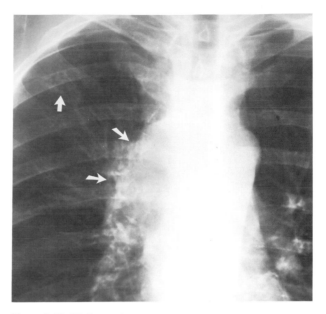

Figure 8-33 (*Unknown 8-1*)

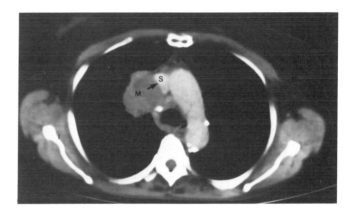

Figure 8-34

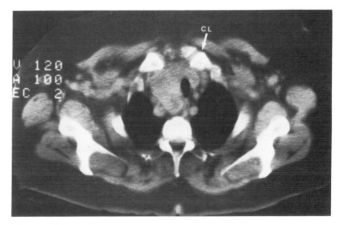

Figure 8-35 (*Unknown 8-2*)

119

CHAPTER 9 How to Gather and Use Imaging Data (Example: Tuberculosis)

You already realize that this book is not at all intended as a reference book in which you can look up classic and pathognomonic radiologic "patterns." There are very few of those, for radiology is not pattern recognition but a system of pathologic deductions made in the light of the patient's clinical story.

Radiographs of very thin parts of the body like the hand can be compared to a low-power study of the gross pathology which has altered the morphology of the bony and soft-tissue structures there. Radiographs of thicker parts of the body are also records of morphologic changes, but must be viewed and interpreted as summation shadowgrams of the changed morphology of many superimposed layers of tissue. CT returns us to the more simplified record of the altered morphology of one slice of the patient, and we can build a three-dimensional concept of the change in form of any structure with successive scans.

Radiologists are thus morphologists who have at their command a wonderful range of imaging data which they can combine in various ways to produce the information you need about your patient's organs and tissues. It is certain that once you have graduated from medical school you will see little or no gross pathology. You will not find time to attend autopsies, and you will miss many clinical pathologic conferences you mean to attend. Unless you are a surgeon you will probably see few gross specimens to help refresh your knowledge of pathologic change, and as time goes on your memory of what you learned in school about morphologic change in disease states will become dimmed. In fact, you will find that your daily contact with radiographs and other imaging data is the only practical means you have for reviewing clinical pathology as you continue in practice. For this reason it is essential, as you study this book looking at images, to think of the changes in morphology produced by various diseases, and to get into the habit of looking at radiologic imaging studies of all kinds as pathology documented through newer imaging modalities rather than through classic gross and microscopic study. In this way you will use imaging data to review pathology and the spectrum of disease.

It is vital to remember that several different disease states *can* produce similar morphologic changes in a given organ. You already know that this may mean that *morphologic change can be deduced from a radiograph but that the agent causing it cannot always be identified*. Bilateral disseminated interstitial changes in the lung are a good example and one we have already discussed.

If you are feeling insecure about "radiologic diagnosis" at this point, therefore, you need some direction about how to continue to learn useful information without attempting to make of radiology a card-sorting device that it cannot be. Suppose you say to yourself, "I have learned how to look at the bony thorax, the soft tissues, lungs, diaphragm, and mediastinum . . . but I don't feel I know anything about diagnosing tuberculosis. Of what use is it just to be able to recognize a pleural effusion, for example?" There, indeed, you can begin.

Stop and list for yourself the *morphologic changes* produced by the tubercle bacillus in the lung alone, changes with which you are familiar and whose images you *do* know how to recognize on radiographs. You will see that you already do have a pretty good idea about the radiographic recognition of tuberculous change.

To start with, of course, you know that identification of the etiologic agent in tuberculosis is never settled by x-ray. Tuberculosis is a laboratory diagnosis, not a radiologic one, for all the morphologic changes it produces can be closely mimicked by fungus, among other agents. Once you accept this fact, however, you will list a number of roentgen changes you *would* know how to recognize in a patient with proven pulmonary tuberculosis.

120

Pleural effusion is one easily recognized manifestation, the organism being recovered from the tapped fluid even in the absence of visible changes in the lung. Shadowy infiltration of the parenchyma may be visible when you compare the interspaces with those on the opposite side in the asymptomatic patient who recently had a positive skin test. More extensive infiltration with or without cavitation may be documented and followed on serial films, as well as healing under therapy. You have seen enlarged hilar and paratracheal lymph nodes which although not at all specific for tuberculosis may be a part of the roentgenographic documentation, and you know that those nodes may calcify as they heal.

Tuberculosis may produce pneumothorax, and you know how to look for air in the pleural space. Miliary tuberculosis will be recognizable on the chest film once the minute interstitial granulomas reach 2 millimeters in diameter, although you know they cannot be differentiated radiographically from miliary carcinomatosis, disseminated in the same fashion to the interstitium via the capillary bed.

Remember, these are roentgen findings documenting pathologic change both for you and for the radiologist, and while they do not inform you about the etiologic agent they do inform you about the extent of the disease in your patient. Some disease conditions produce no roentgen change because they produce no gross morphologic change, or because they kill or are cured before any such changes can develop. The common cold, for example, is not accompanied by any useful radiologic findings in most cases.

You must realize too that there may not have been time as yet for the disease process you suspect to produce the imaging changes you have learned to associate with that disease. The radiologist needs to be a good clinician and to remind you of this fact from time to time, to be able to anticipate for you how soon you may expect those changes to develop and how they may alter in the course of the disease.

You need now to become a collector in tallying disease processes with imaging changes. As you collect visual images and relate them to the implied pathophysiology, you will be reviewing and adding to your overall knowledge of medicine and weaving the tight fabric of information necessary for you to become an accomplished clinician. Start your image collection with the cases of proven pulmonary tuberculosis on the following pages.

The Spectrum of Radiologic Data in Bacteriologically Proven Pulmonary Tuberculosis

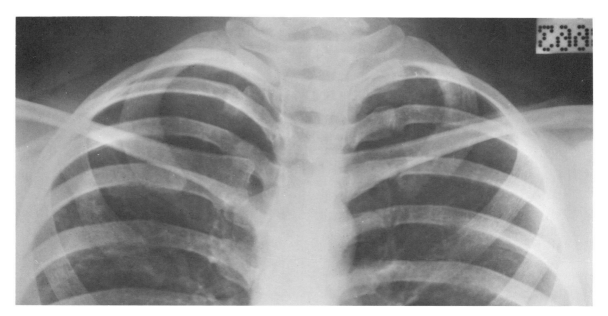

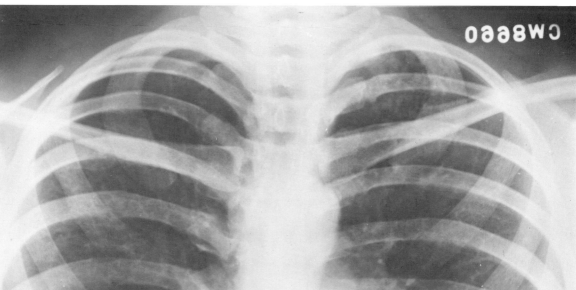

Figures 9-1 and 9-2. An example of *minimal apical tuberculosis* in details from two chest films made on the same patient. Figure 9-1 (*above*), a routine film made in September, is normal. Figure 9-2 (*below*), made five months later, shows numerous small, fluffy shadows in the lung tissue at the left apex, in the second and third interspaces, and superimposed on the first three ribs. Compare the interspaces. Up to this point in the book you have seen a number of instances of the roentgen shadows which may be produced in the chest film by tuberculosis. Add to them now the cases of tuberculosis which follow, and you will have a nucleus of images to start your collection.

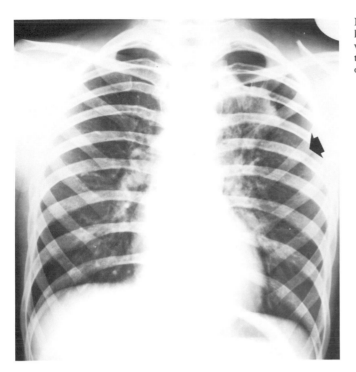

Figure 9-3. *More extensive tuberculosis,* left upper lobe, with small pneumothorax (**arrow** indicates visible margin of lung). Strands of shadow extending to the chest wall are pleural adhesions over the apex, restricting the degree of collapse.

Figure 9-4. Silicosis in a miner with sputum positive for acid-fast bacilli. Most of these myriad lesions must be silicotic nodules, but at least a few represent infiltrative granulomas. No diagnosis of "tuberculosis" is to be made from this film, of course.

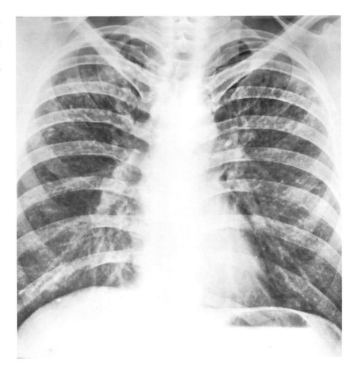

123

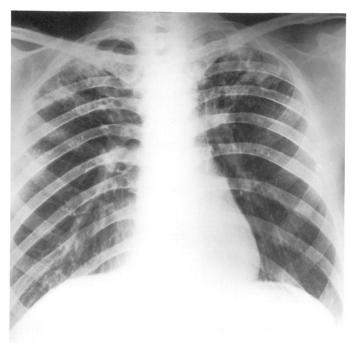

Figure 9-5. *Bilateral chronic upper lobe tuberculosis.* Note that in addition to the obvious infiltrative parenchymal streaks in both upper lobes, ringlike cavities are present. The one on the right can be seen rising above the medial end of the right clavicle, and the one on the left overlies the fourth rib near the lateral chest wall. Note also the very characteristic vascular lung markings extending down into the lower lung fields from the hila. These are longer, straighter, and more vertical than the normal lower lung markings and may be likened to the taut guy ropes of a tent. Their appearance is easy to remember when you realize that in this type of upper lobe tuberculosis there is so much scarring and retraction that the upper lobes are markedly reduced in size and both hila are drawn upward, stretching the vessels to the lower lobes.

Figure 9-6. *Cavitation in a relatively new tuberculous lesion.* Considering the size of the cavity here, there is less extensive parenchymal density than might be expected in chronic involvement. When you compare carefully the lung seen in the seventh, eighth, and ninth interspaces on the two sides, those on the left appear normal, while those on the right show scattered soft shadows. Think now of the pathologic process which is going on, rather than of the roentgen shadows. Consider that the balance between the resistance of the patient and the virulence of the disease must determine the rate of tissue breakdown. This being so, it must follow that the relation of the size of the cavity to the type of inflammatory density in the involved lung around it, as you see them in the x-ray, provides an index to the state of the host-disease balance. In a portion of lung showing many soft, fluffy shadows, the sudden appearance of a large, thin-walled cavity probably means rapid tissue breakdown in poorly resisting lung. A similar cavity in a segment of lung known to have been diseased for a long time, and showing instead the dense, discrete, and stringy shadows of healing fibrotic lesions, would not carry the same implications. Just so, the progress of changes in a series of films made at intervals provides a useful index to the patient-disease relationship and all the factors which may influence it, as well as the success or failure of therapy.

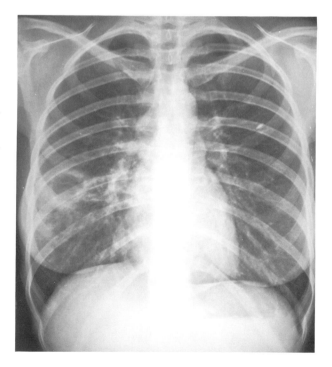

124

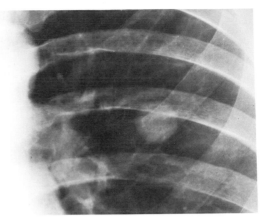

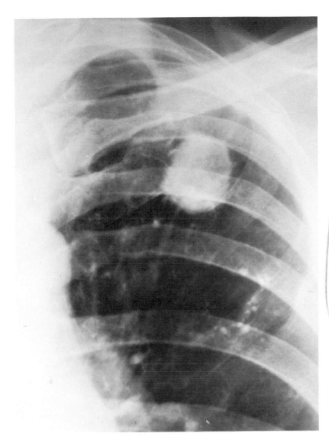

Figures 9-7 (*left*) and 9-8 (*above*). *Tuberculous granulomas* in the lung may closely simulate solitary tumors, either primary or metastatic. Some granulomas contain no calcium, others calcify centrally (or expand around and engulf an earlier calcific focus). Still others calcify peripherally and appear to have a shell.

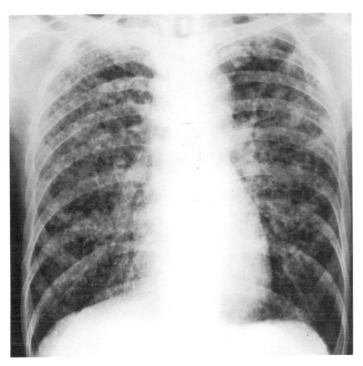

Figure 9-9. *Miliary tuberculosis*. The innumerable lesions scattered throughout the parenchyma here, and probably resulting from hematogenous spread, have been engrafted upon a lung field in which there was already some tuberculous infiltration in the upper lobes. In looking at any film, you have to consider that the shadows you see may represent acute changes superimposed on chronic ones.

The progress of tuberculosis documented over three years, before the advent of antituberculous drug therapy . . .

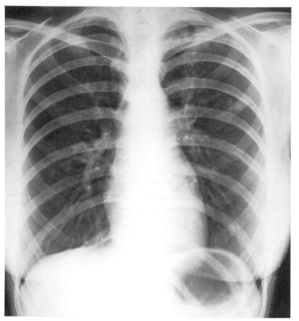

A. December 1943

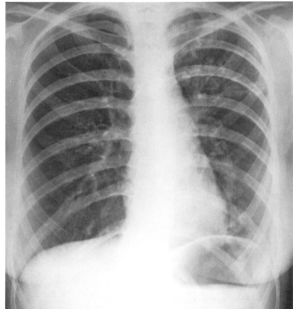

B. August 1944

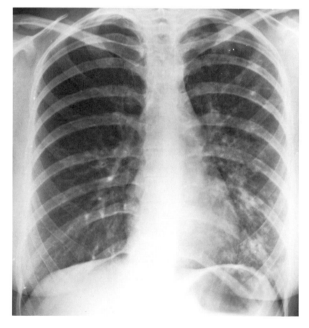

C. February 1945

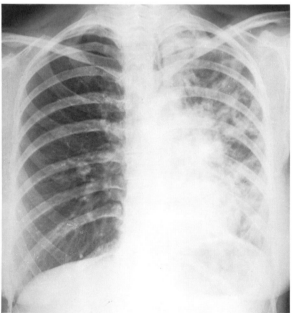

D. February 1946

Figure 9-10. *Serial films over a period of three years in a patient with tuberculosis.* In A she has a soft infiltrative lesion extending upward from the left hilum to the apex. In B, made eight months later, there is progressive involvement of the left upper lobe and new areas of density extending down toward the left diaphragm, which may be either in the lingular segment of the upper lobe or in the lower lobe. In C, made six months later, there is involvement throughout the left lung, but with the development of scar tissue the patches of shadow have taken on a harder, denser, and more discrete appearance. D, a year later, gives you radiographic indications that there is much more scar tissue retraction than on the earlier films. Note that the trachea and the heart have been drawn over to the left. Cavitation is obvious in the upper lobe. You see the profile of the diaphragm still. In E, there appears to be an immense cavitation replacing the upper lobe (absence of lung markings). The left diaphragmatic profile and that of the left heart border have disappeared, indicating consolidation, and there is new spread of the disease to the right lung. Some pleural effusion on the left cannot be excluded. F is a radiograph of the postmortem specimen of the two air-inflated lungs, the vessels of which have been injected with an opaque substance.

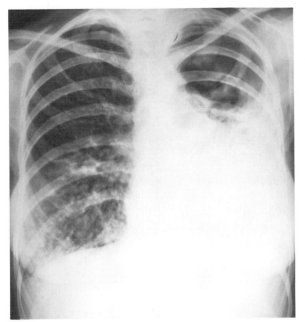

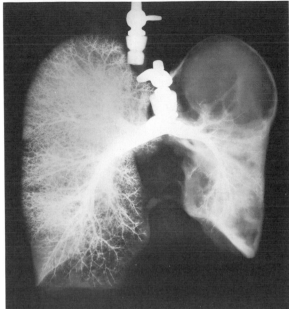

E. August 1946   F. October 1946

. . . and in a recent patient, healing.

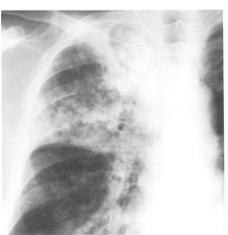

A

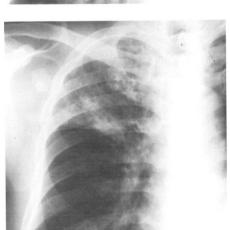

B

Figure 9-11 (*at left*). *Healing of tuberculosis*. A patient with proven right upper lobe tuberculosis (A, *above*), which is seen in B (*below*) to be resolving on drug therapy. Note the upward retraction of the horizontal fissure as the process heals. Ultimately this patient became symptom free and sputum negative and was considered cured.

Unknown 9-1

As an unknown for this chapter try listing all the roentgen changes you can think of which could be produced by bronchogenic carcinoma. You have seen a number of them in the preceding chapters and you will be able to imagine others. As an embellishment for this exercise, think of each one as belonging to a patient who presents himself for the first time in your office this afternoon. In that way you will be tallying roentgen-pathologic changes with signs and symptoms and preparing yourself for the modes in which patients with the disease may first be encountered. If you make the effort of writing down your list, you will be able to tick it off against the answer at the back of the book (which is admittedly incomplete).

127

CHAPTER **10** The Heart

Today a variety of simple and sophisticated imaging procedures is available to provide detailed information about the structure and function of the heart. These include chest films, fluoroscopy, echocardiography, computed tomography, cine-computed tomography, radioisotope examinations, angiography, and magnetic-resonance imaging.

Generally the *plain-film* diagnosis of heart disease is limited to the determination of cardiac enlargement (overall size and specific chamber enlargement), pulmonary vascular abnormalities, and congestive failure. The other imaging techniques can give detailed information about myocardial thickness, precise chamber size, and the presence of valvular disease, coronary artery disease, or pericardial disease. Several of these techniques also provide information about cardiac function.

In this chapter we propose to discuss, first, the plain-film findings in heart disease, and then to give you examples of help provided by more complex studies.

Measurement of Heart Size

We are a race of measurers, partly because it is easier to measure than to think. Both accurate measurement and an analysis of the significance of the findings form the basis of good science. Before angiocardiography was developed, making possible the study of the individual cardiac chambers, the overall size of the heart was measured in its every dimension and some of these measurements proved useful. Since the development of specialized cardiac imaging, however, much less reliance is placed on plain-film measurements in a cardiac patient. Nevertheless, in day-to-day routine patient problems, evaluation of the shadow of the heart on the plain film of the chest will prove useful to you. You can develop for your own daily use a *rough* estimate of the size of the heart, using only the measurement you make on a PA film (which enlarges the heart by projection less than 5 percent). If you know one easy-to-carry-out measuring system and employ it on every PA chest film you study, you will soon develop an ability to *estimate* heart size. A left lateral film, now a routine part of the chest film study, will enhance the accuracy of plain-film assay of heart size.

You must add to this mode of assaying the status of the heart an awareness of *the ways in which cardiac enlargement may be (1) simulated (as on a poor inspiration film) or (2) masked (as in a large left pleural effusion)*. Even more important, you must have some familiarity with changes in the *shape* of the heart due to specific chamber enlargements, since a change in shape either with or without enlargement may sometimes indicate the type of heart disease which is present.

In sum, then, you must be able to estimate overall cardiac size while accepting the important limitations of that estimate, to discount conditions which may simulate enlargement, and to be aware of the changes produced in the shape of the cardiac profile by various disease processes. These things every physician ought to know comfortably.

The simplest method of measuring the heart is to determine its relation to the width of the chest at its widest part near the level of the diaphragm. This is called the *cardiothoracic ratio,* and it is calculated from the PA chest film only. Measure between two vertical lines drawn tangential to the most prominent point on the right and the left cardiac profiles. The prominence of the bulge on the right is usually a little higher than the apex of the left profile. In adults the width of the heart should be less than half the greatest thoracic diameter, measured from inside the rib cage at its widest point.

128

No ruler is necessary for this measurement, nor do you need to remember anything more than the 50-percent figure. Using any handy piece of paper with a straight edge (the handiest will often be the margin of the patient's own film envelope), determine the width of the heart. Then decide whether this width exceeds the distance from the midpoint (spine) to the inside of the rib cage (half the transthoracic diameter). Still more simply, you can measure from the midline to the *right* heart border and see whether that distance will fit into the piece of lung field to the *left* of the heart, something you can do from the back row at ward rounds! For example, in Figure 10-1 is the distance from *A* to the midline less than or greater than from *B* to *D*?

The left lateral film is an excellent check on the PA appearance of the heart. When apparent enlargement to the left in the PA view is checked on the left lateral chest film, any increase in the *mass* of the left ventricle will extend the border of the heart posteriorly and low against the diaphragm. Conversely, increase in the mass of the right ventricle will be seen in the lateral film to fill in the lower part of the anterior clear space behind the sternum but will not extend the heart posteriorly.

No doubt you measured the heart in Figure 10-1 and found it normal in size; but compare it now with almost any of the chest films in the preceding chapters and you will certainly be struck by the flat, almost absent aortic arch. This young patient had been discovered to have hypertension. The possibility of coarctation of the aorta was suggested in view of unobtainable pressure in his legs. Reinspection of his chest film revealed the saucered erosions of the undersurface of his ribs, where the dilated intercostal arteries had developed as collateral pathways. His coarctation was successfully revised surgically, restoring him to normal health and life expectancy. Figure 10-3 (next page) is a detail of the chest film in Figure 10-1. The radiologic manifestations of coarctation are seldom present in children younger than 10. You must remember too that a number of other conditions *can* cause rib notching. Neurofibromatosis is one.

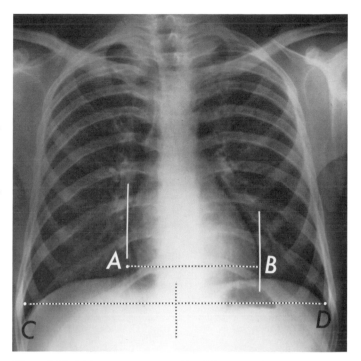

Figure 10-1. This young man was filmed because a heart murmur was detected on routine physical examination. Is his heart enlarged?

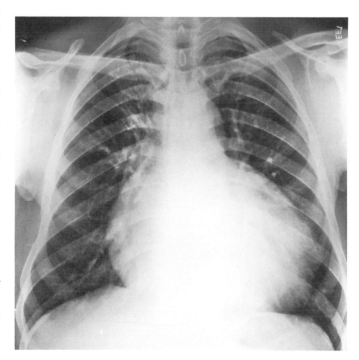

Figure 10-2. Measure this patient's heart for enlargement.

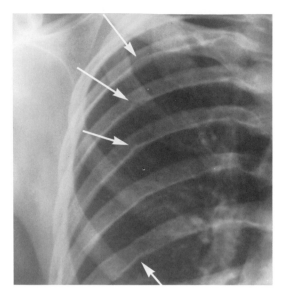

Figure 10-3. Detail from Figure 10-1. *Arrows* indicate rib notching.

Factors Limiting Information Obtained by Measurement

It is valuable to realize that heart shadows may be abnormal in shape even though normal in size. They may also be enlarged with or without a distinctive change in shape; hearts which decompensate may be enlarged and shapeless.

Hearts may also be only *apparently enlarged* for a variety of reasons which you must be able to discount. You already know some of the ways in which cardiac enlargement may be simulated. You have seen it in chest films made at *expiration* (Figure 10-4A) and it is logical to expect that a high diaphragm will tilt the heart upward, bringing its apex closer to the lateral chest wall. In addition, the flare of the ribs is greater at inspiration and decreases at expiration, further altering the apparent cardiothoracic ratio. In any patient in whom you would have reason to expect the diaphragm to be high, you will be anticipating an *apparently* enlarged heart shadow. In the presence of *any kind of abdominal distension* (late pregnancy, ascites, intestinal obstruction) you may not be able to estimate heart size for this reason.

Remember too that portable chest films are usually made AP and result in an appreciable enlargement of the heart shadow by projection, since the heart is farther away from the film. If the patient is filmed supine, then the diaphragm is likely to be higher. Valuable data may be obtained from bedside chest films on the very sick patient, but an estimate of heart size is not among them.

The next point to be checked is that there is *no rotation* of the patient. You have already seen in an earlier chapter the degree to which rotation may produce an appearance of widening of the heart and mediastinal shadows, and you know that symmetry of the clavicles and ribs gives you assurance that no rotation is present. We will be discussing intentionally rotated oblique films in more detail, at which time you will be able to study more closely the precise effect of rotation on the cardiac shadow.

Deformity of the thoracic cage will, of course, often render impossible any attempt to measure the size of the heart, and you would not expect to be able to do so in severe scoliosis, for example. The solitary (but symmetrical) deformity of a depressed sternum usually displaces the heart to the left, and your suspicions will be aroused when you find no right heart border from which to measure. A lateral film will settle the matter.

You might wonder whether the size of the heart shadow would be increased if the film happened to be taken at full diastole, and decreased if it were made at the end of systole. The shadow *is* slightly different at the extremes of the cardiac cycle, but the difference is not usually enough to matter in a rough estimate such as the cardiothoracic ratio, at least in adults.

It is vital that you develop an immense degree of caution with regard to making pronouncements about apparent enlargement of the *infant* heart as you see it on chest films. This is particularly true in the infant under 1 year of age. Because an infant cannot be requested to "take a deep breath" and because of the basic difference in proportion of abdominal size to thoracic size, the normal diaphragmatic level in the infant is higher than in the adult. He is usually filmed AP

130

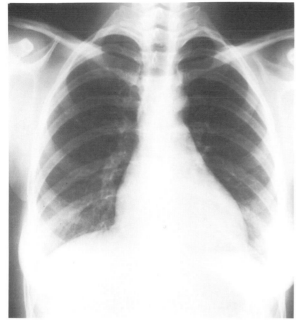

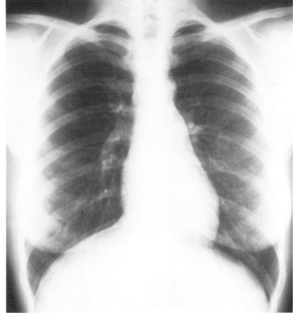

Figure 10-4A. This appears to be cardiomegaly but it is only a normal heart at expiration.

Figure 10-4B. The same heart at inspiration.

and supine. He wriggles and is hard to immobilize, which produces rotation. He has not yet developed the proportion of lung size to heart size characteristic of the adult and present already in the older child. Remember that the thymus overlying the heart may also mimic cardiomegaly. Beware of x-ray appearances suggesting cardiac enlargement under 1 year, therefore, without supporting clinical evidence.

On the other hand, always remember that *overdistension of the lungs* for any reason compresses the heart and mediastinal structures from both sides and narrows their PA shadow. In the dyspneic patient with low diaphragms and in the emphysematous patient, therefore, the heart size as measured on the PA chest film may be *deceptively small* and not inform you at all reliably about the cardiac status. In patients with chronic emphysema the heart is often found at autopsy to be enlarged by weight as a result of right ventricular hypertrophy (cor pulmonale), although no cardiac enlargement had ever been noted radiologically.

Noncardiac disease may mask true cardiac enlargement. If you think back through the earlier chapters, you will have no difficulty appreciating the degree to which mediastinal or pulmonary disease may render the dimensions of the heart unobtainable. Any density which obscures one cardiac profile makes it futile to try to estimate heart size. Thus, neither the size nor the shape of the heart can be studied from plain chest films in the patient who has a massive pleural effusion, consolidation in the anterior part of either lung, or a large anterior mediastinal mass.

True mediastinal shift is usually the result of some important change in intrathoracic dynamics and may so alter the position of the heart that measurements are meaningless (collapse of one entire lung, for example).

Examples of Apparent Abnormality in Heart Size and Difficulties in Measuring

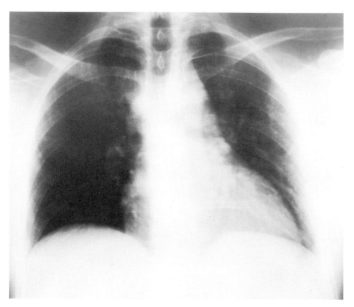

Figure 10-5. This chest film made AP recumbent simulates cardiac enlargement.

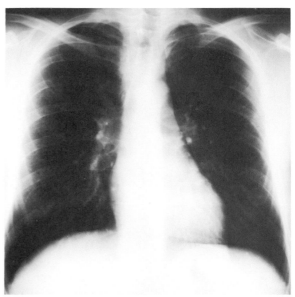

Figure 10-6. PA film of same patient standing.

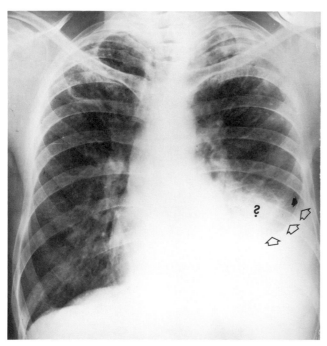

Figure 10-7. Here, because of a combination of pleural and pulmonary pathology, heart size cannot be estimated. (*Boxed arrows* mark a fluid line crossing a rib margin, *black arrow*. *Question mark* indicates probable lingular consolidation further obscuring the left heart border in this patient with known upper-lobe tuberculosis.)

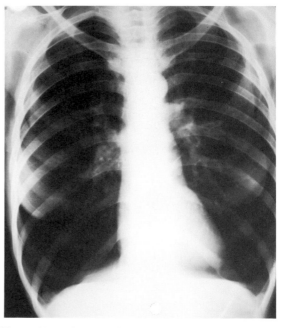

Figure 10-8. The heart does not appear enlarged, but cor pulmonale is present in this patient with emphysema and overdistended lungs.

132

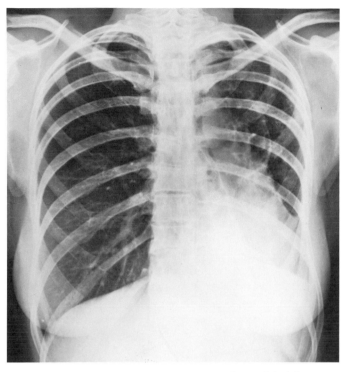

Figure 10-9. The heart is not well seen in collapse of the left lower lobe (or of the whole left lung).

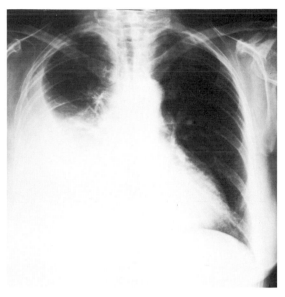

Figure 10-10. The heart size cannot be estimated in massive pleural effusion.

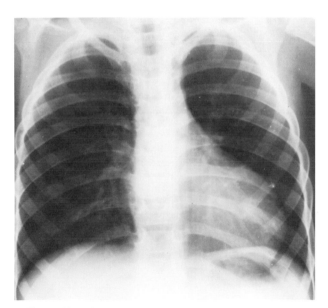

Figure 10-11A. Pectus excavatum. The heart is displaced slightly to the left.

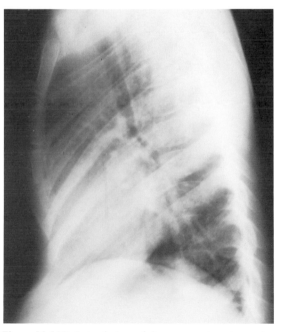

Figure 10-11B. Lateral view of the same patient shows depressed sternum and decrease in AP midline dimension.

133

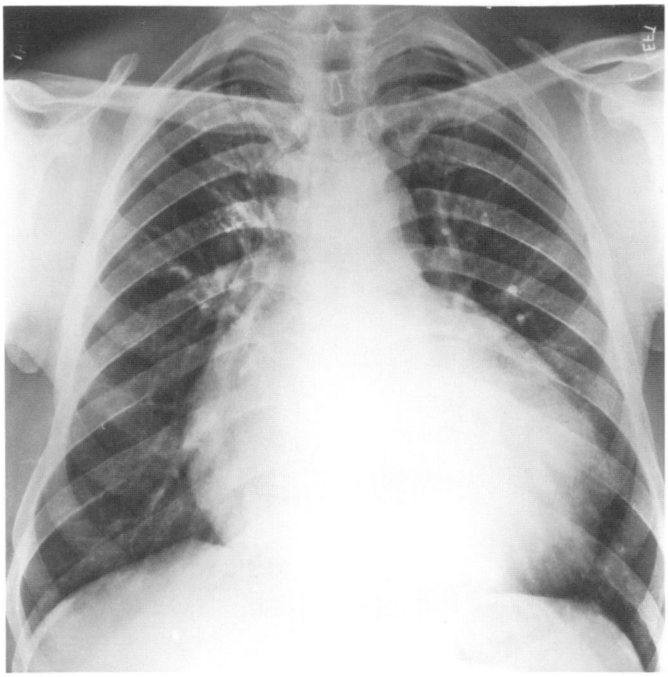

Figure 10-12 (see text).

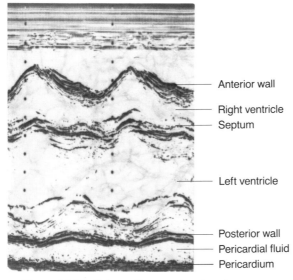

Figure 10-13. Echocardiogram showing the presence of pericardial fluid between the posterior wall of the heart and the pericardium, normally in contact.

Labels on figure:
Anterior wall
Right ventricle
Septum
Left ventricle
Posterior wall
Pericardial fluid
Pericardium

Interpretation of the Measurably Enlarged Heart Shadow

Consider now a chest film in which, after checking out all potentially misleading factors, you find that the measured heart shadow exceeds its allowed 50 percent of the transthoracic diameter. How can you distinguish between the shadow cast by cardiac hypertrophy, cardiac dilatation, and pericardial effusion around the heart?

Figure 10-12 gives you an example. A patient with acute rheumatic fever and pancarditis shows obvious enlargement of the heart shadow. You know from your study of pathology that there may well be valvular involvement, myocardial damage, and pericarditis with effusion. The heart disease is properly termed pancarditis, and dilatation of the chambers due to poorly functioning valves and an inflamed, inefficient myocardium, as well as the presence of pericardial fluid, could all be contributing to the production of such a large shadow. In fact, all were present at autopsy.

As you look at PA and lateral chest films on any patient having an enlarged heart, there are a number of findings that will help you. You may be able to recognize a predominantly enlarged *left* ventricle from the extension to the left in the PA view and posteriorly in the lateral. *Right* ventricular enlargement will show no posterior extension on the lateral film but anterior fullness filling in the lower part of the anterior clear space. Remember that plain chest films may show ventricular enlargement but do not differentiate hypertrophy from dilatation.

If the heart is decompensating, it will tend to shapelessness and extend to both right and left in the PA view, suggesting either failure or pericardial effusion. Effusion is usually documented currently by *echocardiography,* a sonographic record of the reflection of sound waves from the wall of the heart and from the pericardium, separated by a layer of fluid (Figure 10-13). In clinical practice a review of the patient's old films is probably the best way to assess the development of cardiac enlargement, in and out of failure. Sudden shapeless increase in size should suggest pericardial effusion to you.

Enlargement of Left or Right Ventricle— Help from the Lateral Film

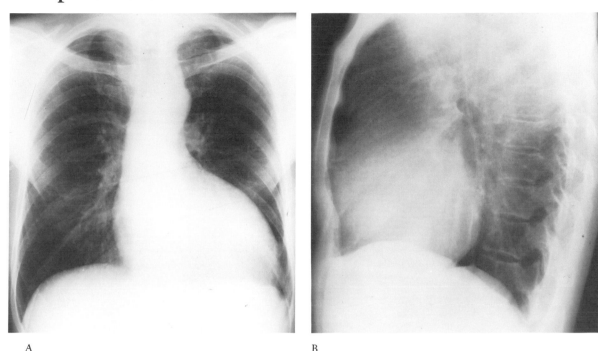

A

B

Figure 10-14. A: Left ventricular enlargement with characteristic shape. B: Lateral view, same patient. Note extension posteriorly of the left ventricle.

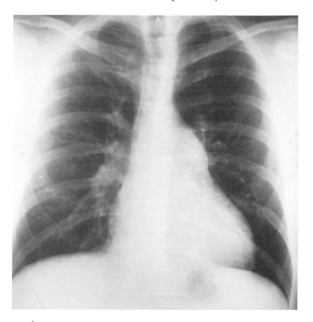

A

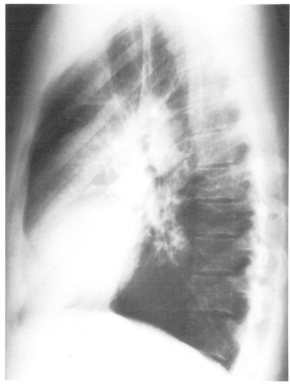

B

Figure 10-15. A: PA in patient with right ventricular enlargement. Note that this view shows only generalized cardiac enlargement. There is a straightened left heart border and enlargement of the pulmonary trunk. B: The lateral film shows the enlarged right ventricle filling in the anterior clear space. Note that the heart is flat posteriorly.

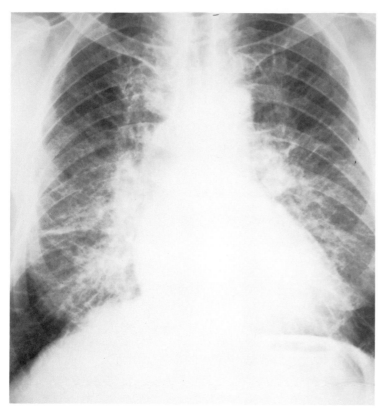

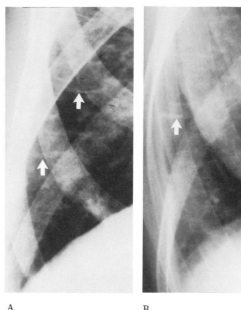

Figure 10-17. A: Kerley's B-lines (*arrows*) represent thickened interlobular septa seen tangentially close to the chest wall. This patient had lymphatic spread of carcinoma, not cardiac failure. B: Kerley's B-lines (*arrow*) in a patient with mitral valvular disease and a history of repeated episodes of congestive failure.

Figure 10-16. Moderate congestive failure. Note the general increase in vascular markings, engorged hila, Kerley's B-lines, and fluid in the horizontal fissure.

The Heart in Failure

Important indications of the physiological state of the failing heart will be found on studying the hilar and pulmonary vessels carefully. In addition to the increasing size and shapelessness of the cardiac shadow, you should look for evidence of pulmonary venous engorgement. The vessels are seen to extend farther than normal into the lung field. The normally thin-walled and hence indistinguishable bronchi become "framed" in interstitial fluid accumulating around them. When seen end-on they appear as white rings (Figure 10-18A). This is often called peribronchial cuffing and can be observed to decrease as the patient improves under therapy and the lung interstitium is cleared of water (Figure 10-18B). Pleural effusion in cardiac failure may be bilateral or unilateral, and is more frequent on the right.

The lungs appear hazy and less radiolucent than normal because of retained water, and soon Kerley's B-lines appear. These are short, horizontal white linear densities very close to the peripheral margin of the lung. They have been proven to represent the thickened interlobular septa with their engorged lymphatics, and may ultimately remain present in the patient who has been repeatedly in and out of failure.

Often rapid accumulation of interstitial fluid spills over into the alveoli and one sees the development of alveolar *pulmonary edema* as in Figure 10-19, a patient with a massive myocardial infarction whose left ventricle failed very rapidly. Pulmonary edema occurs in noncardiac conditions (water overload, renal failure, heroin overdose, and inhalation injury or burns).

Pulmonary edema may be unilateral or unequal bilaterally, but in general produces the so-called bat-wing appearance you are familiar with, symmetrical about both hila. It may appear

136

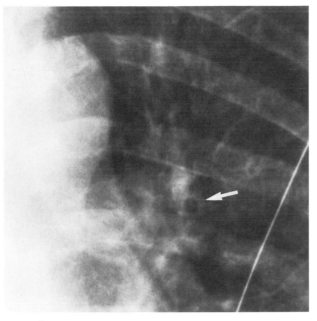

A

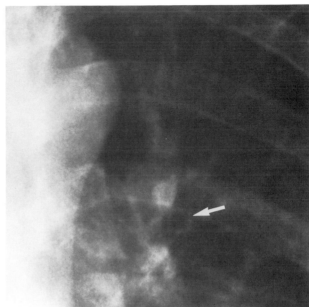

B

Figure 10-18. A: Detail of area around the left hilum in a patient with congestive failure. Note the increased vascularity with interstitial fluid accumulating about all hilar structures, blurring the outline of the vascular trunks and producing "peribronchial cuffing" (*arrow*). B: Clearing after therapy.

rapidly after sudden left ventricular failure or be superimposed on the more gradual roentgen findings of cardiac failure. Note how the vessels of the hilum, bathed in interstitial fluid as they are, disappear in Figure 10-19 together with the superimposed shadows of innumerable fluid-filled alveoli. Compare the hilar vessels in Figure 10-16, in which they are becoming indistinct. Similar early loss of the interface outlines of the hilar vessels is seen in the patient in Figure 10-18A; in the B film, after good response to therapy, they are seen again emerging from their fluid bed.

Serial chest films provide an excellent means of following the progress of a cardiac patient through an episode of failure, and you will find that they tally well with other clinical signs available to you. The patient should generally be sent to x-ray for the better-quality films available there.

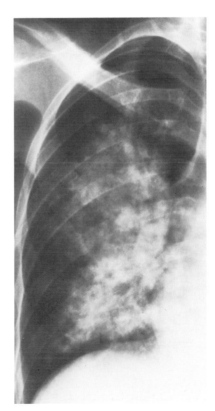

Figure 10-19. Alveolar pulmonary edema in a perihilar distribution.

137

Variations in Pulmonary Blood Flow

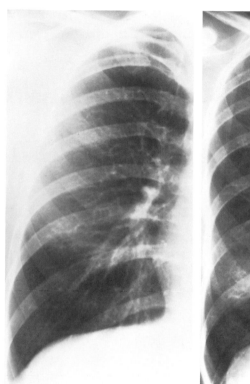 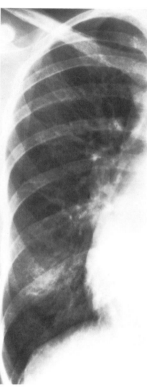 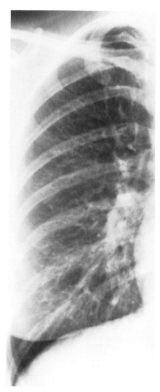 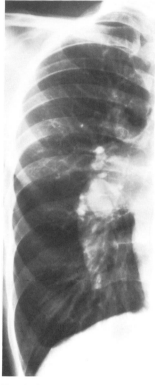

A. Normal pulmonary vasculature.

B. Pulmonary venous hypertension.

C. Increased pulmonary vasculature (left-to-right shunt).

D. Pulmonary arterial hypertension.

Figure 10-20

(1) Normal Pulmonary Vasculature

Pulmonary blood flow in the upright patient is much greater at the bases of the lung than it is at the apex. This is apparent on normal chest films and is partly due to the fact that the lung is pyramidal in shape with more lung tissue and more vessels superimposed at the base nearer the diaphragm (Figure 10-20A).

(2) Pulmonary Venous Hypertension

The pattern of pulmonary venous hypertension is seen in patients with elevated pulmonary venous pressure, usually caused by left ventricular failure or by obstruction of left atrial outflow, as in mitral stenosis. This pattern is identified on chest films by increased prominence of the upper lobe vessels, decreased prominence of the lower lobe vessels, and haziness of the hilar vessels (Figure 10-20B). In congestive failure the pulmonary venous hypertension pattern is seen *underlying* varying degrees of interstitial and alveolar pulmonary edema.

138

(3) Increased Pulmonary Vasculature

Increased pulmonary blood flow may be seen in both cardiac and noncardiac conditions. In patients with congenital heart disease and a left-to-right shunt, the lesser (pulmonary) circulation is constantly being overloaded with blood returned to the right chambers from the left chambers. This is commonly seen in interatrial or interventricular septal defect, and, to a lesser degree, in patent ductus arteriosus. An example of a noncardiac cause of increased blood flow would be an arteriovenous fistula or malformation elsewhere in the body.

(4) Pulmonary Arterial Hypertension

Pulmonary arterial hypertension is caused by conditions which *decrease* the flow of blood through the pulmonary capillary bed. Some are uncommon (such as tricuspid atresia); others are common (emphysema). Decrease in the volume of the peripheral vascular bed may result from showers of pulmonary emboli, vasoconstrictive states, and long-standing shunts. You have seen an example of the "pruned-tree" appearance of such a constricted arterial bed in Figure 4-17, a wedge arteriogram. As you would expect, the lung field in such patients shows the decreased vasculature you see exemplified in Figure 10-20D above. Note that the hilar trunks are enormously dilated in response to the constricted arterial bed.

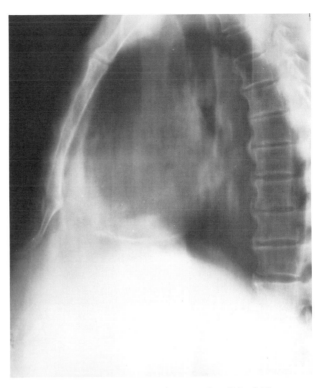

Figure 10-21. Lateral tomogram shows pericardial calcification in a patient with constrictive pericarditis.

Cardiac Calcification

Various parts of the heart may calcify. These include valve leaflets, valve rings, coronary arteries, ventricular wall aneurysms, and the pericardium itself. Thrombi in the left atrium and cardiac neoplasms also calcify. Large areas of calcification can often be seen on plain films, but most calcifications are small and may be identified in the moving heart only by fluoroscopy or some other technique. Figure 10-21 shows a shell of calcification around the heart in a patient with constrictive pericarditis. Cardiac fluoroscopy has been superseded today by echocardiography, which can offer more detailed information about the interior of the moving heart without using ionizing radiation.

139

The Anatomy of the Heart Surface

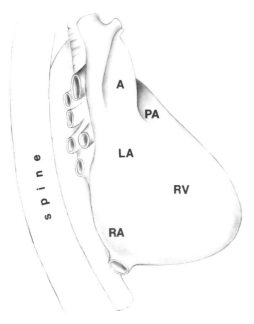

Right and Left Anterior Obliques

The right and left anterior oblique films of the chest are still used, so you will want to understand them. Justify these two projections with the help of the diagrams and drawings on this page spread and the next two. Turn to the angiocardiograms (next page spread) in order to realize how the opaque-filled masses of the various chambers project in the frontal view, first during the period when the opaque bolus is passing through the right chambers and then after it returns from the lungs and opacifies the left chambers.

Figure 10-22A. Orientation of the heart for a right anterior oblique view. Figures 10-23 and 10-24 (*below*) show you how the patient is oriented with the right anterolateral surface of the chest closest to the cassette.

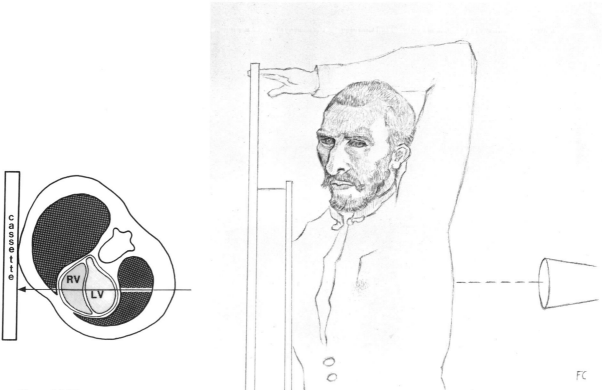

Figure 10-23

Figure 10-24

140

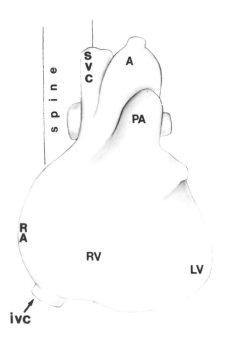

Figure 10-22B. Surface of the heart as it would appear on a routine frontal chest film.

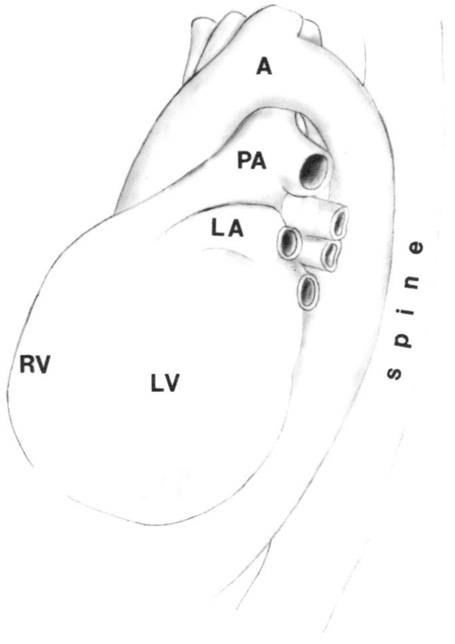

Figure 10-22C. Orientation of the heart for a left anterior oblique view. Figures 10-25 and 10-26 (*below*) show you how the patient is oriented with the left anterolateral surface of the chest closest to the cassette.

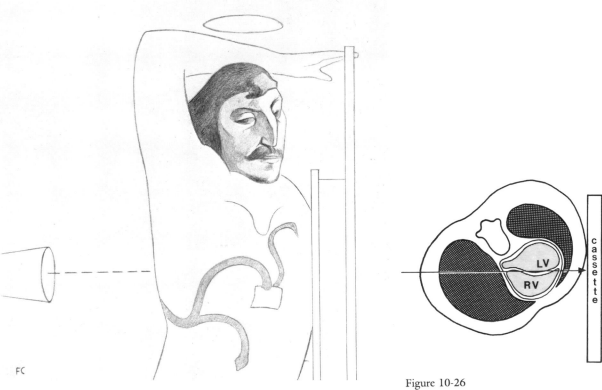

FC

Figure 10-25

Figure 10-26

Identifying Right and Left Anterior Oblique Views

On the normal right anterior oblique film, the heart is to the right of the spine (your right) and looks triangular with a flat posterior surface.

On the left anterior oblique film, the heart lies to the left of the spine and is much more bulbous in shape, with a rounded posterior surface.

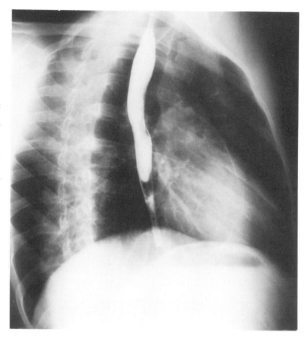

Figure 10-27A. RIGHT ANTERIOR OBLIQUE.

Angiocardiograms Show the Interior of the Heart

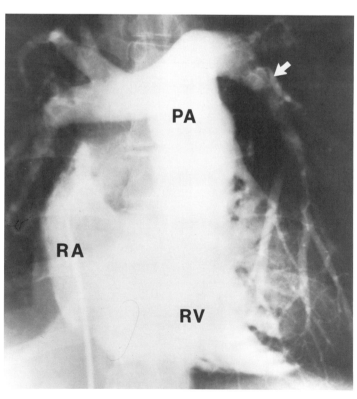

The interior of the four heart chambers can be visualized radiographically by angiocardiography. For this procedure a percutaneously inserted venous catheter from either a femoral or a brachial vein is advanced until its tip is in the right atrium. A bolus of contrast material is then injected, during which rapid serial films are made, usually in the frontal projection. When contrast medium opacifies the right side of the heart, this is called the dextrophase and an image obtained at that time is called a dextrocardiogram (Figure 10-28A). The *arrow* indicates the pulmonary artery supplying the left lower lobe. Note that the right atrium is thin walled and makes up most of the right heart border. The

Figure 10-28A. DEXTROCARDIOGRAM.

142

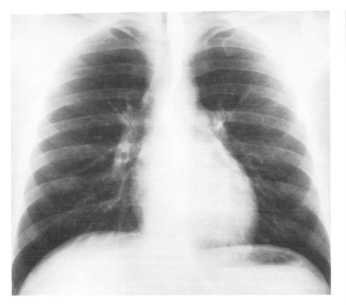

Figure 10-27B. POSTEROANTERIOR VIEW.

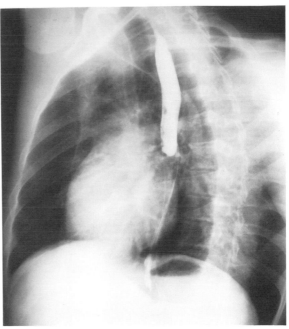

Figure 10-27C. LEFT ANTERIOR OBLIQUE.

Three Views, Same Patient

indentations in the outline of the right ventricle are muscle trabeculae. Did you remember that the right ventricle is more trabeculated than the left? Compare the two on these images. If you look carefully, you can locate the site of the pulmonic valve.

The levocardiogram was filmed after the bolus of contrast medium had passed through the pulmonary circulation and returned to the heart, where it opacified the left chambers. The *arrow* points to the vein draining the left lower lobe. Note that it enters directly into the left atrium. At this point in the cycle the ascending aorta is only faintly opacified. Notice how the left ventricle makes up the left heart border.

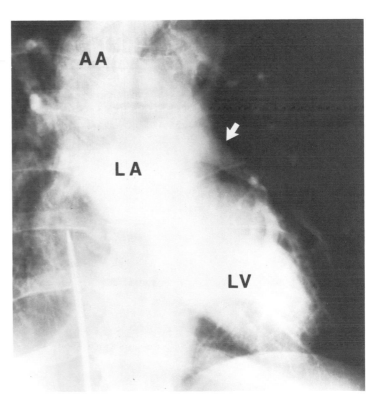

Figure 10-28B. LEVOCARDIOGRAM.

143

Coronary Arteriography

Coronary arteriography is carried out commonly in patients having symptoms of cardiac muscle ischemia. Contrast material is injected via a catheter inserted into the femoral or brachial artery and, under fluoroscopic guidance, hooked into the orifice of the right or left main coronary artery. Films are made in standard projections and varied as required to best show the course of the artery. Stenoses and occlusions caused by atherosclerotic disease are identified precisely by this method.

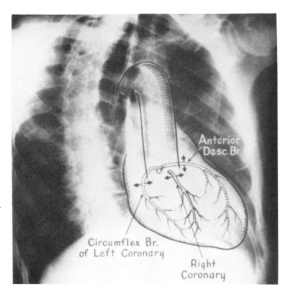

Figure 10-29A. Coronary artery anatomy, right anterior oblique projection.

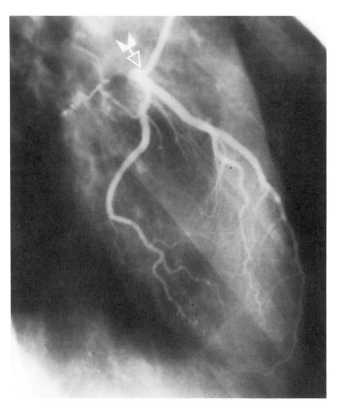

Figure 10-30. Normal left coronary arteriogram (right anterior oblique view). In these photos *open arrow* indicates catheter tip in origin of artery.

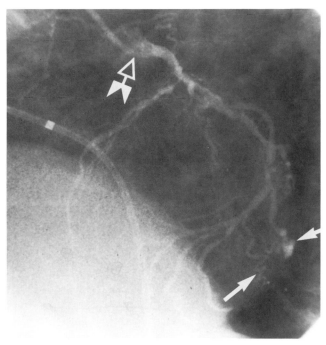

Figure 10-31. Diffusely atherosclerotic left coronary artery. Note the luminal narrowing of the entire vascular tree, multiple sites of stenosis, and formation of collateral branches (*arrows* to tortuous branches).

144

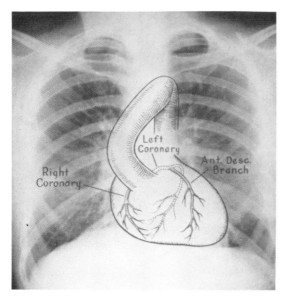

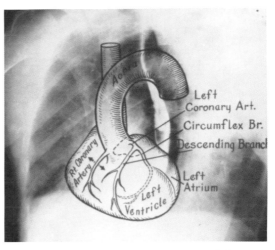

Figure 10-29C. Coronary artery anatomy, left anterior oblique projection.

Figure 10-29B. Coronary artery anatomy, frontal projection.

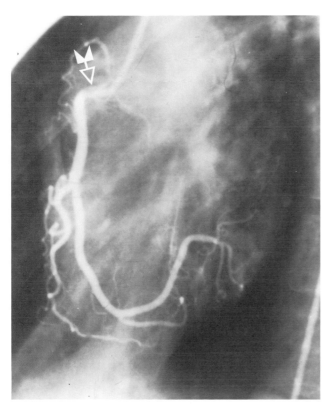

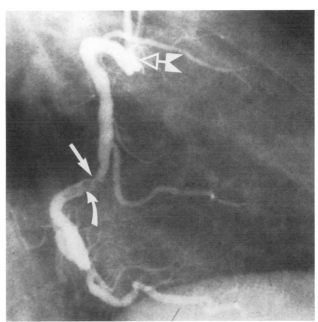

Figure 10-33. Atherosclerotic right coronary artery in a patient with an acute myocardial infarction. Note the tight stenosis (*straight arrow*) with intraluminal thrombus (*curved arrow*) just distal to the stenosis.

Figure 10-32. Normal right coronary arteriogram (left anterior oblique view).

145

Classic Changes in Shape with Chamber Enlargement

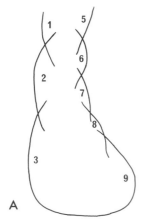

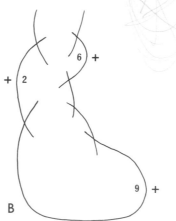

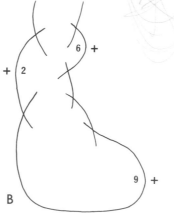

Figure 10-34. Changes in the shape of the heart with specific chamber enlargements, expressed in terms of alteration of the nine intersecting arcs responsible for the PA profile of the heart and great vessels (compare Figure 8-2). Note: the normally concave slope between arcs 6 and 9 is often called the cardiac waistline.

As you looked at the shadows of the heart in Figure 10-29 on the preceding page spread, you were accepting the fact that the heart size was normal and also the fact that the *shape* of the heart was normal.

Try now to imagine what would happen to the size and shape of the heart with increasing degrees of *left ventricular enlargement*. Predict the change in shape of the heart that one might expect in long-standing resistance to outflow through the aortic valve—as in aortic stenosis, coarctation of the aorta, or systemic hypertension. You can appreciate that the shadow of the left ventricle will project farther to the left on the PA view (Figure 10-34B) and that it will extend farther posteriorly in the lateral view. The posterior surface of the heart (as seen in the lateral view) should normally clear the anterior surface of the vertebral column, but in advanced cardiac disease with left ventricular enlargement, especially in decompensation, the posterior surface of the heart is often seen to overlap the spine to some extent. Left ventricular enlargement is often associated with aortic stenosis and chronic hypertension, both of which may cause enlargement of the aorta (Figure 10-34B, 2 and 6). With aortic stenosis this may be due to post-stenotic dilatation.

Now imagine that the *left atrium* enlarges as it would in a patient with mitral valvular disease with stenosis and insufficiency. What would you expect that to do to the heart shadow on the PA view? Remember that the left atrium lies posteriorly just underneath the carina, higher than the major chambers. When it enlarges it will produce fullness across the heart at about the level of the "waistline" (arc 8), producing the shape you see in Figure 10-34C. In the left oblique view the normally open aortic window between the ascending and descending aorta will be filled in by the enlarging atrium. A well-penetrated PA film will show the air-containing carina to be splayed, and usually the widening of the subcarinal angle will be due primarily to elevation of the left main bronchus as it rides over the expanding left atrium.

In the right anterior oblique view, the displacement of the esophagus posteriorly will be evident too, as you see in Figure 10-35B. The patient was given barium paste to swallow, outlining the esophagus as it lies against the poste-

146

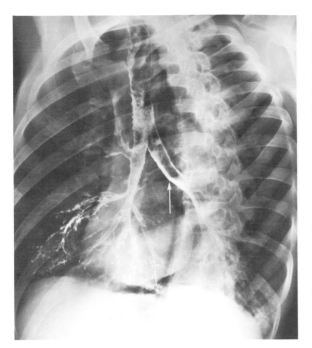

Figure 10-35A. Left anterior oblique showing normal subcarinal angle during a bronchogram. The carina sits atop the left atrium; when that chamber dilates, the left main bronchus (*arrow*) will be lifted, so that the subcarinal angle is increased.

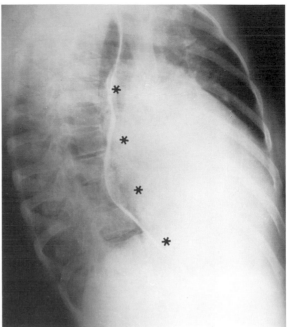

Figure 10-35B. Right anterior oblique in a patient with mitral valvular disease and insufficiency, showing posterior displacement of the barium-filled esophagus by the dilated left atrium. *Asterisks* indicate normal course of the esophagus.

rior surface of the heart. Normally the esophagus lies just anterior to the spine in the midline, bisecting the chest in the lateral view.

In the PA view, as the left atrium enlarges in mitral disease, it first fills in the left cardiac waistline so that the left heart border becomes convex instead of concave, and then the atrium extends to the right so that its margin is visible along the *right* heart border, above the profile of the right atrium and overlapping it—the "double shadow" so frequently referred to as a classic sign in left atrial enlargement (Figure 10-35C).

Observe in this figure that in addition to the enlargement of the left atrium there is also extension of the left ventricle to the left, as in Figure 10-34D, left ventricular enlargement in mitral disease of long standing. This may result from work overload on the left ventricle, which has to overcome the inefficient backward flow of some blood into the left atrium through the poorly closing mitral valve. Enlargement of the left ventricle may also be seen in patients with combined aortic and mitral valvular disease in whom the resistance and insufficiency of a deformed aortic valve adds to the work the left ventricle must do.

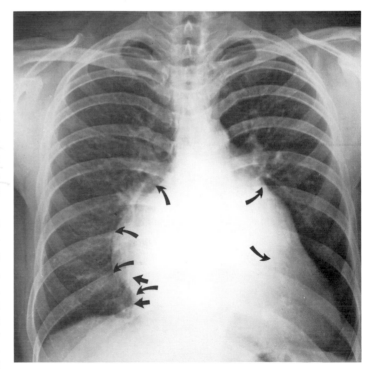

Figure 10-35C. Frontal view of a patient with mitral insufficiency and a huge left atrium (outlined by *curved arrows*), which projects both to the left and to the right. Profile of right atrium is indicated by two *straight arrows*. This creates the double shadow along the right heart border seen in advanced mitral insufficiency.

Problems

Try analyzing the four hearts on these pages before reading the text.

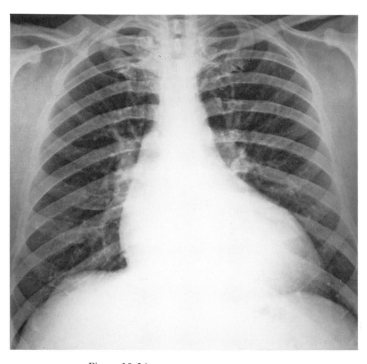

Figure 10-36

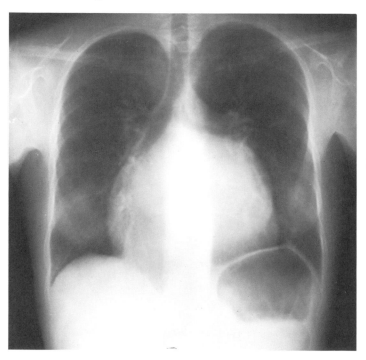

You begin now to have a feeling for the basic differences in shape between the heart shadow with predominantly left ventricular enlargement and the heart in which the left atrium is dilated. They are the most important specific chamber enlargements for you to be able to recognize. When, from the PA view, you suspect either, you will try to confirm your impression by examining the obliques and the lateral views.

The patient in Figure 10-36 has measurable cardiac enlargement and a shape which must have suggested to you left ventricular enlargement. You have noted the concave left waistline and extension of the apex to the left, which would be confirmed in the lateral view with posterior projection of the left ventricle. This patient had classic murmurs of aortic stenosis and insufficiency, probably of rheumatic origin. Note the flat shadow of the aortic arch.

Change in the shape of the heart resulting from enlargement of the *right* chambers is much more difficult to recognize. The right atrium will be immensely dilated in tricuspid atresia, as you could anticipate. We do not reproduce an example here, because that entity is exceedingly rare. The right ventricle enlarges in cor pulmonale and in pulmonic stenosis. When it does (as you have already seen in Figure 10-15), the PA may show the heart to be deceptively normal or have the normal left ventricle displaced to the left. (Since the right ventricle is located anteriorly, no part of it is seen in profile in the PA view.) When you examine the lateral film, however, you will be struck by the filling in of the lower part of the anterior clear space and by the flat posterior surface of the heart, unlike the rounded posterior projection of left ventricular enlargement. Of course, in today's practice of medicine and radiology one is not limited by the data available from plain chest films. CT and magnetic-resonance imaging have added new dimensions of accuracy in appraising the relative

Figure 10-37

size of the chambers of the heart, of the thickness of the cardiac wall, and of abnormality of function and structure of the valves, as you will see in the next few pages.

The patient in Figure 10-37 is seen to have clearly measurable enlargement of the heart in this PA film, made with supervoltage technique so that you can see the air in the carina and the marked increase of the subcarinal angle with elevation of the left main bronchus. The patient had the murmurs of mitral stenosis and mitral insufficiency and a markedly dilated left atrium. This is a classic example of a mitral heart.

The left border of the heart may exhibit the convex waistline sometimes found in young people, so that you will be cautious in proclaiming that straightening of the left heart border always signifies increased left atrial size. Remember too that filling in of the normally concave waistline may be due to fullness which is either posterior (as in left atrial dilatation) or anterior (as in any condition causing dilatation of the main pulmonary artery, such as poststenotic dilatation in pulmonic stenosis, or dilatation due to patent ductus arteriosus).

The patient in Figure 10-38 had mitral stenosis and insufficiency. She has measurable cardiac enlargement in this single view, elevation of the left main bronchus seen just above the left eighth rib, and a double shadow along the right heart border, all classic signs of left atrial enlargement in mitral disease. She was dyspneic because she was going into failure. The patient in Figure 10-39, on the other hand, was short of breath because of an incipient attack of asthma—of which she had a long history. She has slight straightening of the left border, to be sure, but has no cardiac enlargement and no clinical signs of cardiac disease. The straightened left heart border here is probably due to slight fullness of the main pulmonary artery, resulting from increased pulmonary bed resistance during asthmatic attacks. Patients with emphysema from any cause may show this.

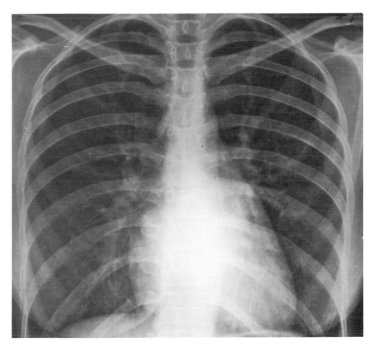

Figure 10-38

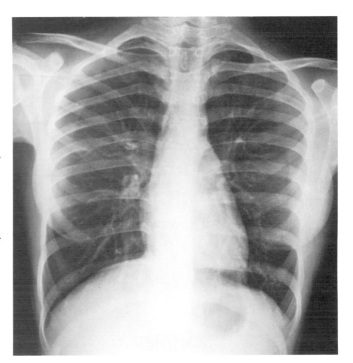

Figure 10-39

Nuclear Medicine and the Heart

You will have noted that we have not used the terms "hypertrophy" and "dilatation," but rather "enlargement" of a particular cardiac chamber. It is difficult if not impossible to differentiate between hypertrophy and dilatation of the heart from plain films. Of course, the two conditions can be distinguished by imaging techniques that depict ventricular wall thickness, such as angiocardiography, CT, and magnetic-resonance imaging. As you will learn from this section, the past decade has seen an explosion of techniques for imaging the heart. Only coronary arteriography, as you have seen in Figures 10-31 and 10-33, can document precisely and visually the location of atherosclerotic plaques in the coronary circulation which produce stenoses and occlusions. It is an invasive procedure, however, requiring arterial catheterization and injection of contrast material.

There are three noninvasive radioisotope techniques currently being used for the diagnosis of cardiac disease.

The first is a method for imaging myocardial infarction with *technetium pyrophosphate* and other bone seekers. These concentrate in necrotic and dying tissue, and can be identified within the involved portions of the heart from one to five days after myocardial infarction has taken place.

The second technique involves the use of *radioactive thallium* to evaluate coronary artery perfusion. Thallium, like potassium, accumulates in well-perfused, well-oxygenated muscle cells within a few minutes after intravenous injection. A normal heart shows a uniform distribution of radioactive thallium throughout the myocardium, whereas an ischemic heart will show areas of decreased thallium activity.

The third technique, *radionuclide ventriculography,* tests ventricular function with radioactive agents that label a patient's blood pool, such as technetium-labeled red blood cells or human serum albumin. Following injection of the isotope the patient's heart is imaged under a gamma camera that is coupled with a computer. The image information can be manipulated and analyzed to determine the stroke volume and ejection fraction. Blood within the chambers of the heart can be imaged either with a complex of computed frames or by cine technique, to show size and shape of the cardiac chambers, position of the great vessels, thickness of the ventricular walls, filling defects in the chambers, wall motion, and identification of dyskinetic segments.

In Figure 10-40 you see an illustration of the first method, myocardial infarction imaging. Here the isotope, technetium pyrophosphate, injected three hours earlier, has been picked up by the ribs and sternum but not by any part of the myocardium. This is a normal study in a patient whose chest pain was found later to result from a different cause. In Figure 10-41 (another patient with chest pain), in addition to the visible ribs, there is a spot of activity representing the damaged myocardium. This proved to be due to a new myocardial infarct, technetium pyrophosphate having gradually accumulated in the dying muscle over a period of two days.

In the overwhelming majority of patients the diagnosis of myocardial infarction is made without the use of technetium pyrophosphate imaging. This examination, however, is useful when the electrocardiogram and enzyme results are equivocal, or when they are unreliable because the patient's workup was delayed for several days, or when the infarct occurred after cardioversion or cardiac surgery. The disadvantages of this method include the fact that technetium will accumulate also in breast tumors, callus about fractured ribs, and aneurysms, for example. With transmural infarcts of the myocardium, however, the sensitivity of the method is high.

In Figures 10-42 and 10-43 you see an illustration of the second method, a thallium perfusion scan. When a patient is at rest, perfusion to the myocardium distal to a stenosis is generally normal or near-normal. Under stress, the increased demands placed on the myocardium are reflected by a demand for increased oxygen and increased perfusion. In this circumstance the decreased coronary vascular reserve distal to a stenosis is best demonstrated. Consequently thallium scanning is performed during exercise, usually on a treadmill. For both scans shown here thallium was injected at peak exercise; scanning with a gamma camera was performed shortly thereafter. In the normal patient (Figure 10-42) the ion is shown readily concentrated in well-functioning myocardium so that the image obtained in the left anterior oblique projection appears as a doughnut-shaped ring, the ventricular myocardium. In Figure 10-43, though, there is a defect (*arrow*) in the septum and the inferior wall where no thallium has yet entered the muscle cells, because that portion of myocardium is underperfused and poorly oxygenated. A later coronary arteriogram showed a tight stenosis in the left coronary artery.

Thallium stress imaging has proven to be a highly sensitive and specific test for the detection of coronary artery disease, in fact more sensitive than exercise electrocardiography. Nevertheless, the thallium test should not be considered as a replacement for stress ECG examinations in patients with suspected coronary disease; rather, it should be reserved for those patients in whom the ECG is nondiagnostic. Thallium stress imaging is considerably more expensive and is not always readily available.

Of course, this brief explanation only suggests the complexity of the whole subject, but it will serve at least to offer you a basic comprehension of the principles involved and to enlist your interest in the great potential aid available from isotope studies in the evaluation of some types of cardiac disease.

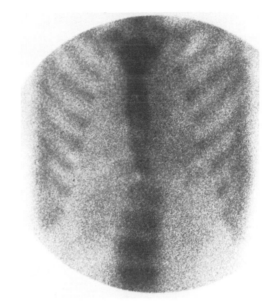

Figure 10-40. Normal technetium scan.

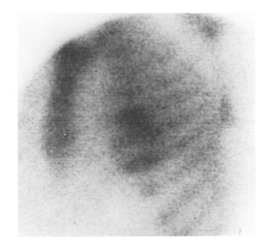

Figure 10-41. Technetium pyrophosphate scan in myocardial infarct.

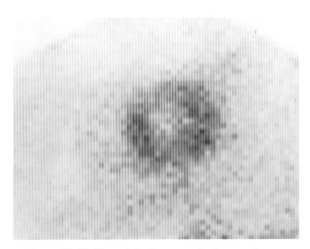

Figure 10-42. Normal thallium scan during exercise.

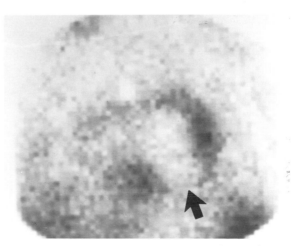

Figure 10-43. Thallium scan during exercise in a patient with coronary artery stenosis.

Magnetic-Resonance Images of the Heart— Coronal Plane

To help you understand the three-dimensional anatomy of the four cardiac chambers and their associated great vessels, we suggest that you review the labeled anatomic structures on this series of coronal magnetic-resonance (MR) chest scans of a young woman. Figure 10-44 is the most anterior section through the cardiac apex; Figure 10-48 is the most posterior section through the left atrium. (Compare the coronal frozen body-slice radiographs in Chapter 2.)

Remember that moving blood in cardiac chambers and blood vessels appears black at MR. Note the thick muscular wall of the left ventricle. Note also the carina and right pulmonary artery just above the left atrium in Figure 10-48.

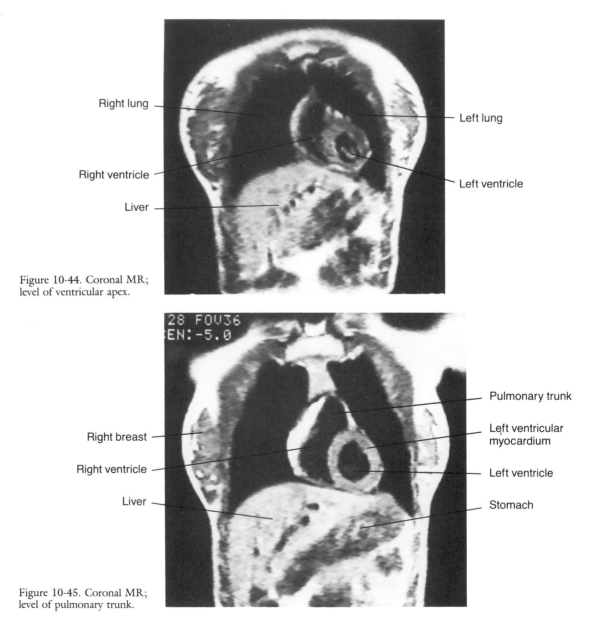

Figure 10-44. Coronal MR; level of ventricular apex.

Figure 10-45. Coronal MR; level of pulmonary trunk.

152

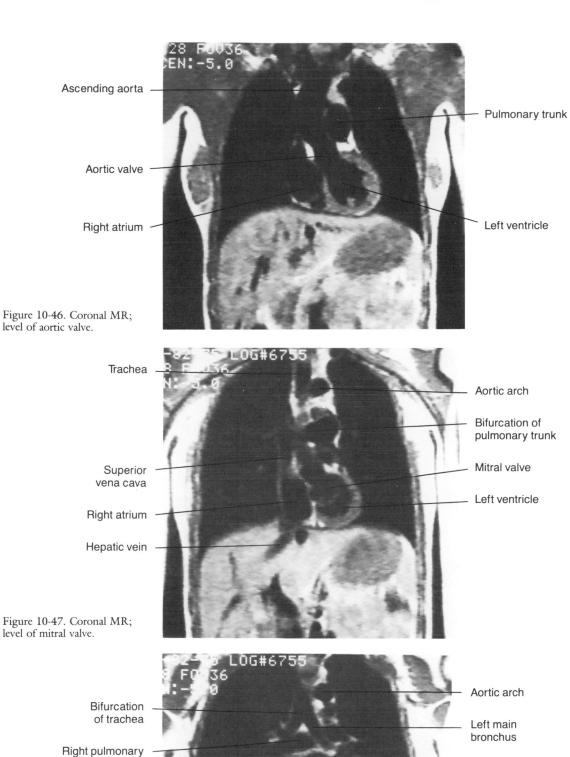

Ascending aorta

Pulmonary trunk

Aortic valve

Right atrium

Left ventricle

Figure 10-46. Coronal MR; level of aortic valve.

Trachea

Aortic arch

Bifurcation of pulmonary trunk

Superior vena cava

Mitral valve

Right atrium

Left ventricle

Hepatic vein

Figure 10-47. Coronal MR; level of mitral valve.

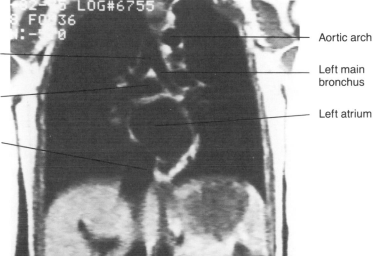

Aortic arch

Bifurcation of trachea

Left main bronchus

Right pulmonary artery

Left atrium

Inferior vena cava

153

Figure 10-48. Coronal MR; level of left atrium.

Computed Tomography of the Heart— Axial Plane

This series of axial CT scans shows the anatomy of the heart and great vessels from the division of the pulmonary trunk (main pulmonary artery) at level 1 down through the top of the right diaphragm. These images were obtained following an intravenous bolus of contrast material with an ultrafast CT scanner that eliminates artifacts caused by cardiac motion. The study was performed on a middle-aged man following coronary artery bypass graft (CABG) surgery to determine patency of the various grafts. As you probably know, this procedure involves placement of vein grafts from the root of the aorta down alongside the great vessels and heart into the ventricular myocardium to supply blood to ischemic areas.

In level 1 (Figure 10-49) note the anterior location of the ascending aorta and the posterior location of the descending aorta. Metallic clips can be identified in levels 1 and 2 at sites of by-pass graft surgery. The highest cardiac chamber, the left atrium, is seen in level 3. Note the patent grafts (opacified with contrast) in levels 4 through 8.

In level 5 the right atrium, right ventricle, and a portion of the left ventricle are first seen. This scan is located at the level of the aortic valve. The leaflets of the mitral valve are well shown in level 6 between the left atrium and the left ventricle. The tricuspid valve can be identified in level 7 between the right atrium and the right ventricle. Note the calcified atherosclerotic plaques in the descending aorta. The left atrium can no longer be identified, since level 7 is below it. Level 8 best shows the interventricular septum between the right and left ventricular cavities. Once again, note the thick wall of the left ventricular myocardium as compared to the right, and the bundles of papillary muscle extending into the left ventricular cavity.

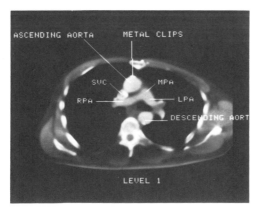

Figure 10-49. CT level 1. MPA, RPA, and LPA indicate the main, right, and left pulmonary arteries.

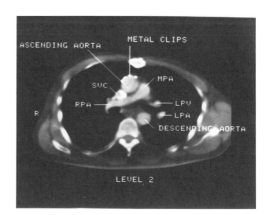

Figure 10-50. CT level 2.

154

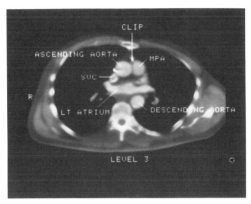

Figure 10-51. CT level 3.

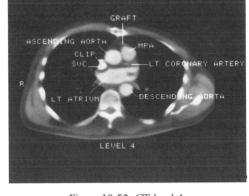

Figure 10-52. CT level 4.

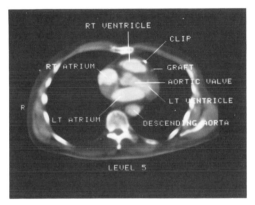

Figure 10-53. CT level 5.

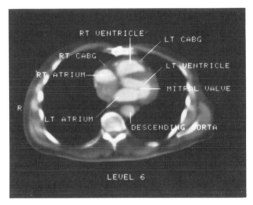

Figure 10-54. CT level 6.

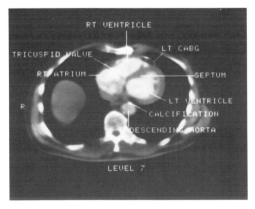

Figure 10-55. CT level 7.

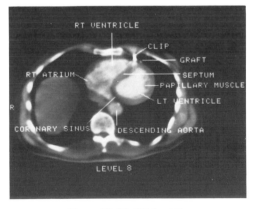

Figure 10-56. CT level 8.

155

CHAPTER 11 The Abdomen: How to Study the Plain Film; Abdominal CT; Sonography

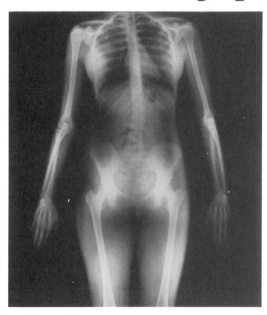

Figure 11-1. Abdomen, chest, and bones filmed together for comparison of radiodensities.

Radiographic study of the region of the abdomen is, in its way, perhaps a little more difficult and a little more subtle than that of the chest, but it is equally interesting from the standpoint of the opportunity it affords you to discover how much radiologic information can be obtained through reasoning. Material learned by appreciating the logic of its appearance is easily retained because it can be reasoned out again if it is forgotten. Radiographic study of the abdomen is largely reasoning. In this chapter we will address first the way in which you should examine plain-film radiographs of the abdomen. A section on normal CT of the abdomen follows, and, finally, one on sonography in this, its most richly useful region.

The Plain-Film Radiograph

The wide differences in radiodensity of the chest structures provide profiles and margins which are easy to see and to interpret as you first begin to look at x-ray films. In the abdomen, however,

organ masses and great vessels may merge into a confluent gray shadow so that their borders and profiles vanish. *Only when some structure of differing density lies against one you wish to know about can you see its boundary*—often only a small segment of that boundary—from which you may be able to deduce something about the size and shape of the organ in question.

The striking radiolucency of air within the bowel will occur to you at once as providing the sort of boundaries and outline segments you need. You will use this information constantly in assaying from plain films the size and shape of organs and masses within the abdomen.

Thus, for example, all air-containing structures may be swept into the left side of the abdomen by a grossly enlarged liver, whose mass is seen as a large gray shadow but whose *margin* is often only visible to you outlined by air in the colon (Figure 11-3). The stomach, when filled with fluid, lies against the spleen and blends with its shadow invisibly, giving no information about its size; but if the stomach is inflated with air, it may be seen to be clearly indented from the left and displaced medially by an enlarged spleen. All air-containing structures may be displaced upward out of the pelvis by a large ovarian cyst or a distended bladder. Individual large-bowel and small-bowel loops, like a circle of dark beads, will outline the upper surface.

Variable as the content of air in the gut certainly is, it will still prove extremely useful to you in tagging abnormalities in the size and shape of other organs, and you will soon form a visual baseline with regard to the amount and location of air-in-gut which you can expect to see. There is normally at least a little air in the stomach and a fair amount distributed throughout the colon. In the healthy, ambulatory adult the small bowel usually contains little or no air, but normal infants and bedridden adults frequently show considerable amounts of small-bowel air without any abdominal pathology to account for it.

By definition a "plain film" is a film made without any artificially introduced contrast sub-

156

stance. For this reason you should call it a *plain film* rather than a "flat plate," an obsolete term which derives from a time when images were made on large glass plates. The so-called KUB (kidney, ureter, bladder) is a plain film. Although we must in this chapter discuss first the plain film of the abdomen, you will find that you will better anticipate the location and appearance of the air-outlined gut *after* you have seen all parts of the gastrointestinal tract filled with barium. *In barium studies the lumen of the gastrointestinal tract is rendered visible, but in the plain film you will be depending on transient air content alone for information,* and you will realize that many parts of the gut are ordinarily invisible because they contain fluid, food, or feces, or are collapsed. Sometimes parts of the colon will be outlined by their content of semisolid feces with which bubbles of air have been mixed. This casts a distinctive speckled shadow and may be just as useful as air-filled gut in indicating the position of neighboring structures or in locating parts of the colon itself. Such speckled fecal shadows always identify colon and are not seen in the small bowel.

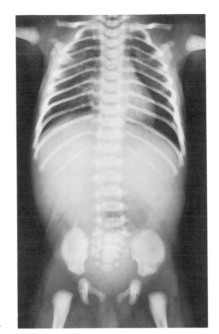

A

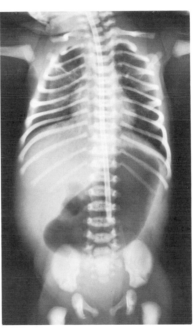

B

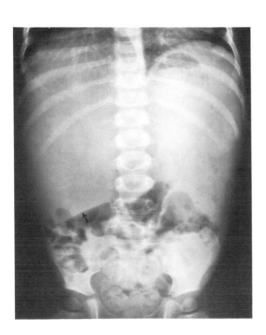

Figure 11-2. A: Airless abdomen in a four-day-old girl who had been vomiting since birth. All the organs blend together as one confluent gray shadow. B: Same patient, stomach inflated with air. Note density of catheter. The right side of the stomach lies against the liver.

Figure 11-3 (*left*). The margins of the liver (*arrow*) and spleen are outlined by air in the gut. You know the film was made standing because of the fluid level in the fundal stomach bubble. The liver and spleen in this small boy were immensely enlarged by lymphoma.

Identifying Parts of the Gastrointestinal Tract from Intraluminal Barium and Then from Air Content

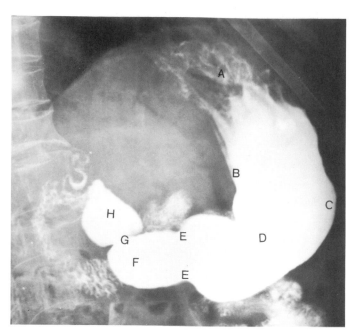

Figure 11-4. The stomach is visible here because it is filled with barium sulfate. *A*, fundus; *B*, lesser curvature; *C*, greater curvature; *D*, body; *E-E*, indentation of a peristaltic wave; *F*, pyloric antrum; *G*, pyloric canal; *H*, first portion of the duodenum (the duodenal cap or bulb).

Barium casts of various parts of the gut produce white shadows on the film, the margins of which distinctly reproduce the character of the mucosal pattern. The rugae of the stomach are quite different from the plicae of the small intestine and from the smoother, more widely spaced haustral indentations of the colon. To identify their barium-filled appearance is to anticipate differences in their dark air shadows on the plain film, as well.

The distribution through the abdomen of air in the gut is determined to some extent by the degree of fixation of the several structures. The stomach may vary considerably in size, but it *is* fixed to the diaphragm and to the duodenum, which is partly retroperitoneal. The small bowel enjoys the liberty of its ample mesentery, folded into the midabdomen. The transverse colon varies widely in position, hanging from its mesocolon; the ascending and descending portions of the large bowel are relatively fixed laterally in the anterior compartment of the retroperitoneum. Within this degree of latitude you will learn to identify different parts of the air-filled gut by their locations as well as by their distinctive mucosal patterns.

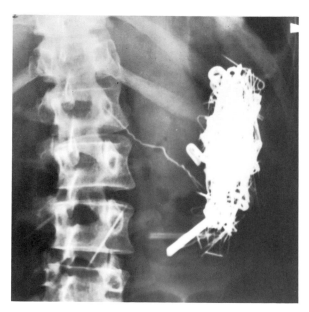

A

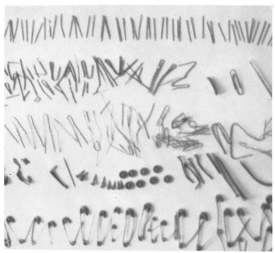

B

Figure 11-5. A psychiatric patient claimed to have "swallowed a pin" and complained of abdominal pain. The radiograph (A) shows an overlapping tangle of many metallic objects. At gastrotomy 287 metallic and glass objects were removed (B).

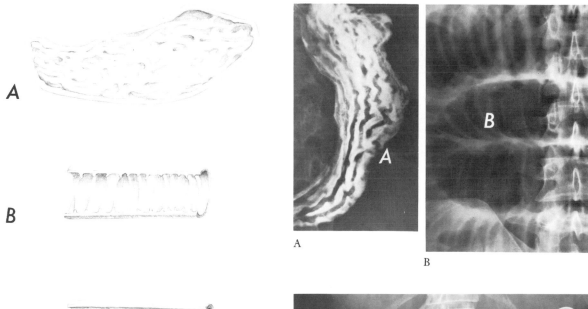

A

B

Figure 11-6. The mucosal lining of segments of the gastrointestinal tract differ enough anatomically to be identified from the appearance of their respective air shadows. Compare the pattern of the mucosal folds of the stomach (A), the valvulae conniventes of the jejunum (B), and ileum (C) with the haustral indentations of the colon (D). Remember that hollow organs *full of barium* (as in Figure 11-4) look quite different from the same organs *filled with air* or lightly coated with a smear of barium.

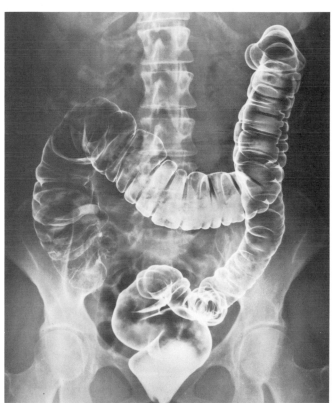

C

Figure 11-7. Examples to help you. A: The rugae of the stomach are seen as black wavy shadows, opaque barium filling the valleys between them. B: The distinctive plical folds inside the jejunum appear as transverse ridges with air between (here seen inside distended small bowel in a patient with intestinal obstruction). C: The normal colon coated inside with barium and distended with air.

159

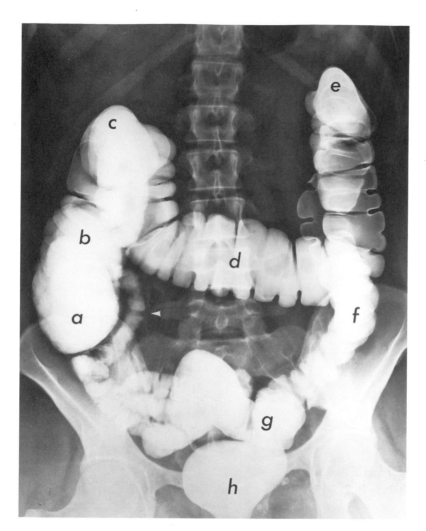

Figure 11-8. Normal distribution of the colon. *a*, cecum; *b*, ascending colon; *c*, hepatic (right) flexure; *d*, transverse colon; *e*, splenic (left) flexure; *f*, descending colon; *g*, sigmoid colon; and *h*, rectum. Note overlap at flexures in the frontal view. When the patient is turned, they are seen unrolled. *Small arrowhead* points to the terminal ileum, which often fills at barium enema.

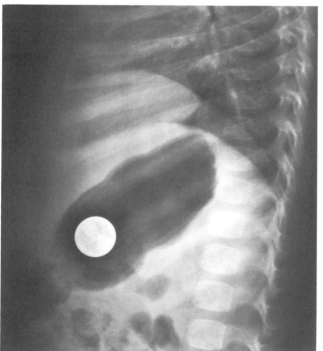

Figure 11-9. Lateral view of an air-filled stomach containing a penny. (Is it a Lincoln-head or an Indian-head penny?)

Identifying Fat Planes, Tangentially Viewed, as Normal Markers

Fat distributions within the abdomen also help you to make certain decisions about the structures they invest. The wide apron of the omentum will *not* help you, because it is distributed across the abdomen and never seen in tangent. The perirenal envelope of fat, however, provides a tangential radiolucent layer outlining the kidney mass with a dark line where more x-rays reach the film to blacken it.

In the same way precisely, the fatty layer next to the peritoneum in the abdominal wall is seen where the sagittally directed ray of a supine plain film strikes it and indicates the lateral limit of the peritoneal cavity. At each side where the fat layer turns posteriorly toward the patient's back, the beam catches it tangentially and the dark line produced on the film is called the flank stripe.

The flank stripe disappears when the flank itself becomes edematous. This is perfectly logical: fluid infiltrating the fat renders it as dense to the x-ray beam as the muscle which adjoins it. With inflammation near the flank (as in appendiceal abscess, for example) the flank stripe on that side may disappear, while the opposite one remains normal. In exactly the same fashion, perirenal inflammation may erase the perirenal fat line.

Concentrated accumulations of fat, such as may be present within a dermoid cyst, produce localized round radiolucent shadows on the film, visible because of their juxtaposition with surrounding structures of greater density.

As you will see in the next chapter, it is their surrounding radiolucent fat that renders abdominal organs and masses so readily identifiable in cross section by computed tomography. Obese patients are harder to examine clinically and often have suboptimal plain films, but they may be easily examined by CT.

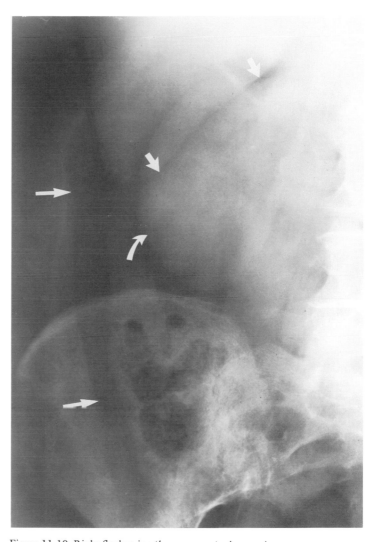

Figure 11-10. Right flank stripe (*longer arrows*), close against which lies the ascending colon—indicated, as it so often is on the plain film, by the characteristic speckled shadow of feces mixed with air. The margin of the liver is clear (*shorter arrows*) and the *curved arrow* indicates the tangentially viewed perirenal fat.

161

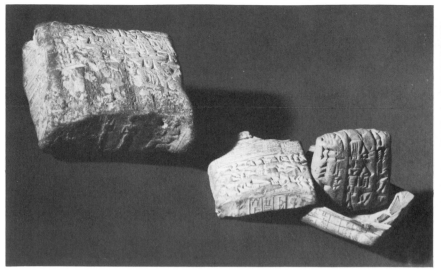

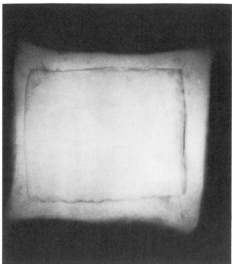

A   B

Figure 11-11. A: Clay tablets from the ancient Sumerian city of Ur. Business transactions were recorded in this way, and because the tablets were fragile and the records precious, an outer envelope of clay was added, bearing the same information in duplicate. B: The envelope of air between the inner and outer layers of baked clay is well shown in this radiograph of the intact clay tablet. The parallel between this and any fat-encased or gas-encased anatomic structure of greater density is obvious.

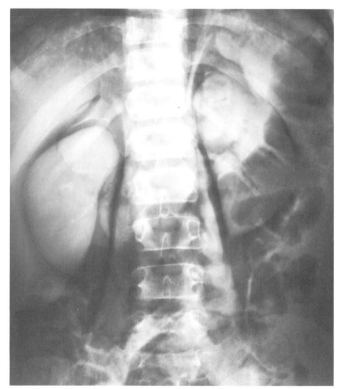

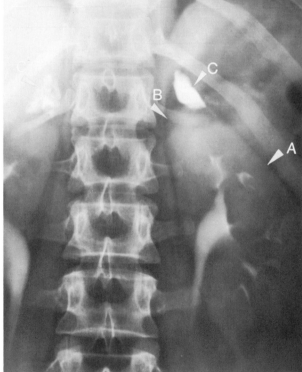

Figure 11-12 (*left*). A gas injected into the retroperitoneal space here has outlined the kidneys even more dramatically than does the fatty envelope you usually depend on to locate them on a plain film. Compare this with Figure 11-13 (*right*) where *A* is the margin of the parenchyma, *B* the upper pole, and *C* the calcified adrenal gland. (This patient had Addison's disease.) The renal calyces and pelvis are seen because a renally excreted contrast substance has been injected by vein (the intravenous urogram).

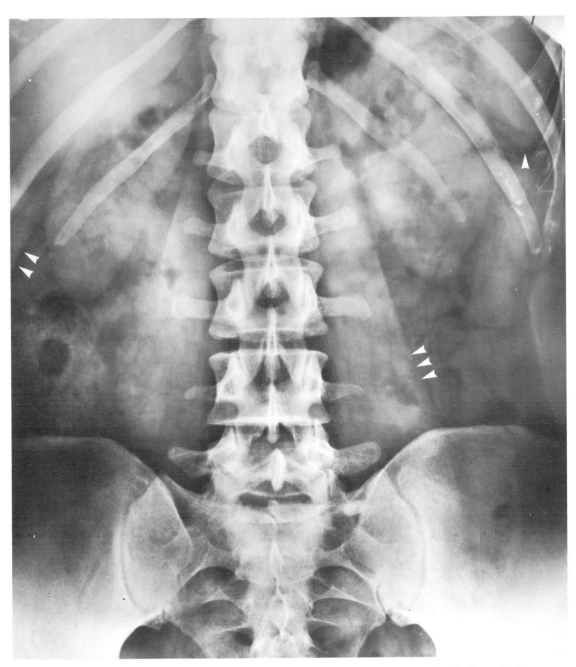

Figure 11-14. Soft tissues unusually well seen on the abdominal plain film. *Single arrowhead* indicates the tip of the spleen. *Double arrowhead* marks the lower margin of the liver, which you can follow obliquely upward across the shadow of the kidney. *Triple arrowhead* indicates the left psoas margin. The psoas shadows are generally symmetrical and are seen sharply because of fat in the psoas sheath. Here the lower part of the right psoas is obscured by something of equal density lying against it. Note dark air in the stomach overlying the upper pole of the left kidney, and the haustrated, air-filled transverse colon superimposed on the middle of the left kidney. The entire outline of the right kidney is well seen. Note the left flank stripe.

163

Identifying Various Kinds of Abnormal Densities in the Abdomen

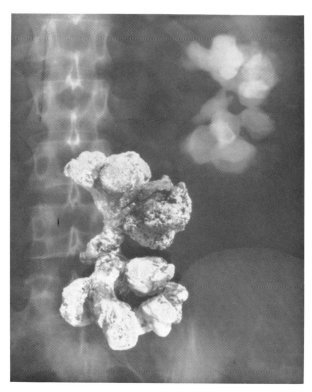

Figure 11-15. Stag-horn calculus in the left kidney. The photograph of the surgical specimen has been superimposed on the abdominal plain film and photographed with both transmitted and direct illumination.

Abnormal radiodensities can be provided by any area of calcification sufficiently large to absorb some of the beam. For example, phleboliths (calcified thrombi in the veins) will be seen as dense white nuggets. Gallstones calcify much less commonly than kidney stones, but both have a characteristic location and often show a distinctive radiographic structure in their shadows as well. Calcified gallstones are frequently laminated and faceted. Gallstones, more often than kidney stones, form over a long period of time in a pool of fluid of slowly changing metabolic composition—hence the lamination seen in the radiograph. They are also more often multiple and are made to rub against one another with the contractions of the gallbladder—hence the faceting. The very characteristic stag-horn renal calculi (Figure 11-15) fill up the entire renal pelvis and calyces, closely resembling the shadow of opaque fluid you see on a urogram.

Calcification of the capsule of any organ will resemble the radiograph of an eggshell, more dense peripherally where it is caught tangentially by the ray (Figure 11-18). Calcification in the wall of a hollow organ will look very similar, and you will often see this type of calcification in the aorta of older patients. Sometimes it will indicate the presence of an aneurysm of that great artery (Figure 11-20). Plaques of calcium caught by the ray in tangent will provide an interrupted white outline, as you would expect. An artery of smaller caliber, when its wall becomes calcified, will show linear white margins like the rose stem in the first chapter, and they will be serpiginous and parallel if the artery describes a tortuous course (Figure 11-19). You will recognize them as characteristic of a cylinder of dense material about a more radiolucent core, x-rayed from the side.

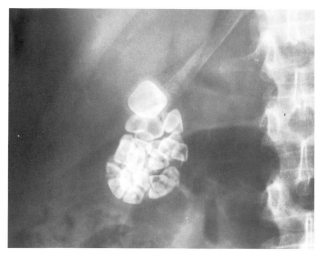

Figure 11-16. Cluster of faceted calculi in the gallbladder. Note that these have been formed in such a way that their outer surfaces contain more calcium. Now look closely. The large, square, uppermost calculus shows a new layer of lesser density. This illustrates the development of lamination in large gallstones which have been present for a long time.

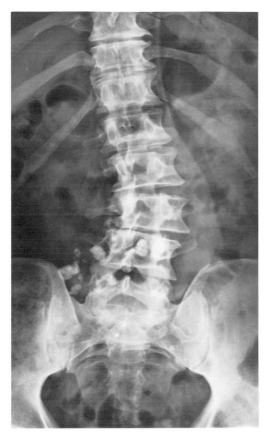

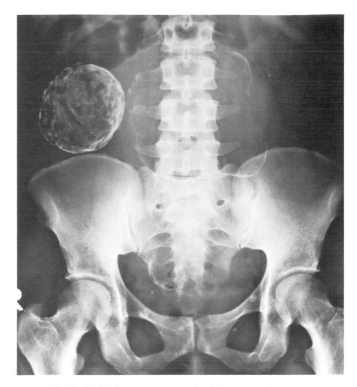

Figure 11-17. A cluster of calcified mesenteric lymph nodes overlie the course of the right ureter near the upper border of the right sacroiliac joint. This patient was positioned as straight as possible in the supine position. Note the obliquity produced in the midlumbar spine by his degree of scoliosis. Only the left psoas muscle can be seen.

Figure 11-18. Multiple enormous uterine leiomyomas in a 42-year-old woman complaining of constipation and dysuria. The patient had lived all her life in a remote rural area and had never consulted a physician before. The specimen removed at surgery showed many intramural, pedunculated, and submucous fibroids with varying degrees of calcification. The only visualized air-filled loops of bowel are displaced into the upper abdomen by the enormous uterine tumors.

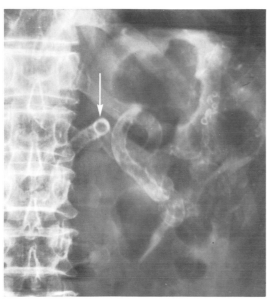

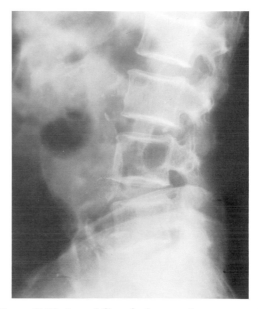

Figure 11-19. Calcified tortuous splenic artery. Note parallel winding white lines. *Arrow* indicates segment passing AP, hence filmed end-on and appearing as a white ring.

Figure 11-20. Lateral film of a large aortic aneurysm with calcified wall.

165

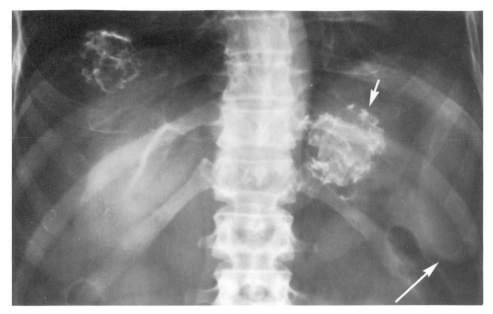

Figure 11-21. Calcified amebic abscesses in the liver. *Long arrow* indicates the tip of the spleen, which is not enlarged. *Short arrow* points to old abscess in the left lobe of the liver.

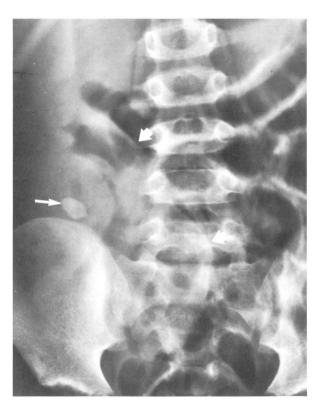

Figure 11-22. Abdomen of a 5-year-old boy. Air-filled gut is seen displaced away from the right flank by a large soft tissue mass (*wide arrows*) in which there is an oval dense shadow suggesting calcium (*thin arrow*). The calcification proved to be an appendolith within a large appendiceal abscess. Note scoliosis concave toward the abscess.

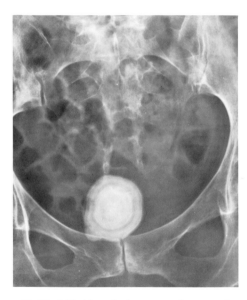

Figure 11-23. A bladder calculus present for some time was finally removed via the suprapubic route. Note lamination.

166

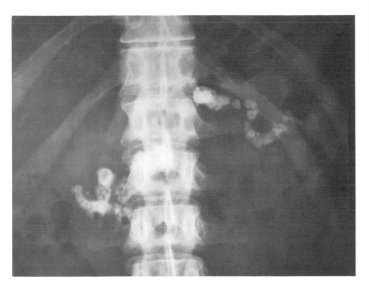

A

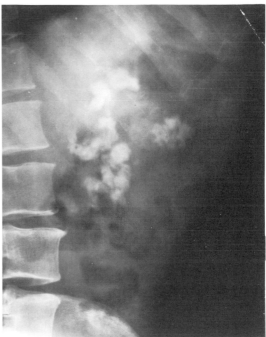

B

Figure 11-24A and B. AP and lateral films of an alcoholic patient with chronic pancreatitis. Note the irregular calcifications in the pancreas, seen overlying the gastric air shadow on the AP projection and anterior to a calcified atherosclerotic aorta on the lateral projection.

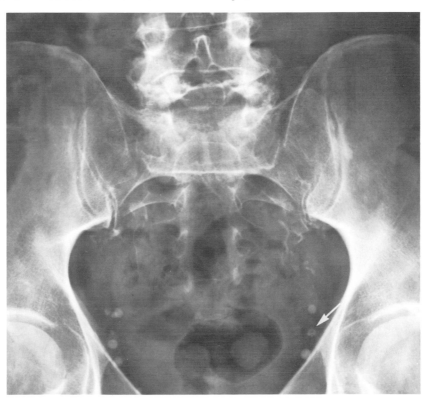

Figure 11-25. Plain film of the bowl of the pelvis showing clusters of phleboliths on both sides. The one indicated by the *arrow* shows a central lucency indicating the recanalization typical for a phlebolith. These are too round and smooth to be ureteral calculi.

167

Learn to Study the Plain Film Systematically

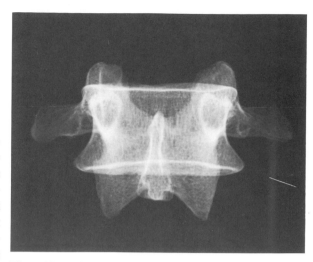

Figure 11-26. AP radiograph of a single disarticulated vertebra.

The plain film of the abdomen is important because it is so simple to obtain, involves no danger or discomfort for the patient, and can be immensely informative without complex procedures. So much can be learned, in fact, from plain films of the abdomen in so many different conditions that every physician should be familiar enough with them to study intelligently those on his own patients and to recognize some of the common aberrations.

There are many subtleties in the interpretation of abdominal plain films, to be sure, and it is easy to feel, when you first begin to look at them, that you are missing important and obvious changes. At your stage of learning, an orderly manner of approaching the analysis of an abdominal plain film is strongly recommended. We suggest that you make a practice of *looking first at the bones* on a plain film of the abdomen (vertebral column, lower ribs, pelvis), excluding from your mind's eye all other structures. (If you do not look at the bones first, you will almost certainly forget them later.)

Then examine carefully the *soft tissues* of a series of smaller areas, including the left upper quadrant, right upper quadrant, both flanks, midabdomen, and pelvis, in that order. In each soft-tissue zone you will be *checking border indicators, organ masses, and fat lines, looking for calcification and for any shift in position or change in shape of the structures you see and identify.*

Then check out the gastrointestinal (GI) tract, accounting for all parts of it in order, whether distended with gas or containing only a small amount, and recognizing some parts of the colon by their content of solid or semisolid feces.

Finally, decide whether there are any gray soft-tissue shadows or radiolucencies not yet accounted for in your survey, and if there are, try to reconcile them with the patient's history and physical examination.

Begin with the spine . . .

The shadows of the *lumbar vertebrae* may appear very confusing when you first look at them, but they will be easy to comprehend and remember once you have analyzed them part for part. To begin with, the boxlike body of a vertebra, extending anteriorly, would have a very simple radiologic structure if it could be seen by itself and not superimposed on the complex posterior articulating processes. Because it is literally a flat cylindrical box of dense compact bone filled with spongy bone, you would expect it to radiograph with a shell of tangentially seen—and therefore denser—bone outlining it, and an interior of many superimposed slender white trabeculae with dark marrow spaces between.

Add to this box outline, now in the AP projection, the two pedicles, cylinders of compact bone extending straight backward on either side of the spinal canal. Because they too are filled with spongy bone, they will radiograph as cylinders seen end-on and, as you can predict, will appear on the film as two white circles. Now as you look at the vertebrae on any plain film of the abdomen, you can account for the two "eyes" which you see superimposed on the upper part of each vertebral body.

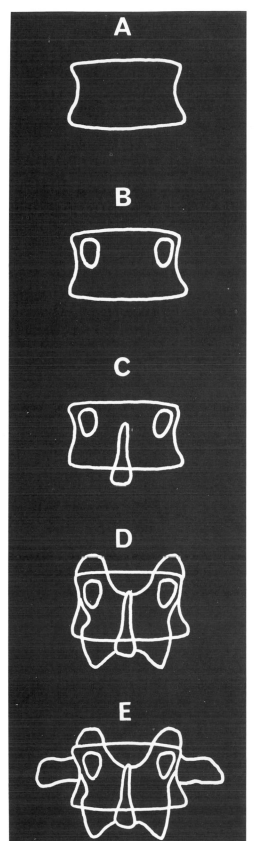

Figure 11-27

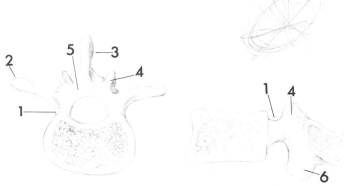

Figure 11-28. A single vertebra seen from above and from the side. *1*, pedicle; *2*, transverse process; *3*, spinous process; *4*, superior articulating process; *5*, lamina; *6*, inferior articulating process.

The centrally located white teardrop is the compact bone investing the spinous process, also filled with spongy bone. The pairs of superior and inferior articulating processes are also to be seen as wings of bone extending upward and downward from each vertebral body to create a butterflylike shadow behind the vertebral body. Finally, the transverse processes extend out to each side, varying slightly in shape from level to level.

If you always think first of the outline of the vertebral body as you look at the spine on an abdominal film, and then add the posterior structures one by one, you will not be confused by the jumble of overlapping bony parts. A pathologic process which destroys any part of these bony structures will cause the disappearance of a shadow you are now expecting to see and can usually trace because of its symmetry with the same structure on the other side, or above or below at a different level.

The bilateral symmetry of the posterior structures superimposed upon the vertebral body will be useful to you in another way, because it tells you that the ray passed sagittally through the patient. Routinely, plain films of the abdomen are made AP with the patient supine, but some barium studies are made PA with the patient prone. (Why?) Many types of special procedures are performed in conventional degrees of obliquity, and you will find that the appearance of the vertebrae indicates the obliquity of the ray.

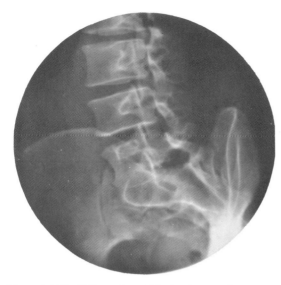

Thus, if you see the boxy bodies of the vertebrae cleanly separated from their posterior structures, you will know that you are looking at a *lateral* film; but if the bodies and posterior structures are precisely superimposed and bilaterally symmetrical, you are looking at a film made with a *sagittal* ray. *Obliques* will show you the vertebrae about as you see them in Figure 11-29, and note that now you can see through the obliquely directed posterior articulations.

Figure 11-29. Oblique view of the lumbar vertebrae.

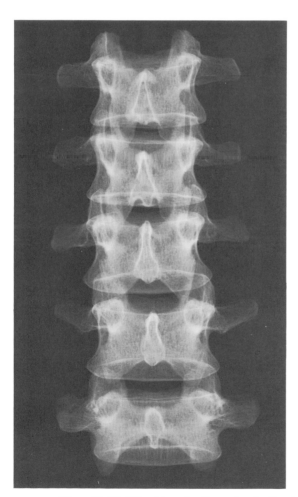
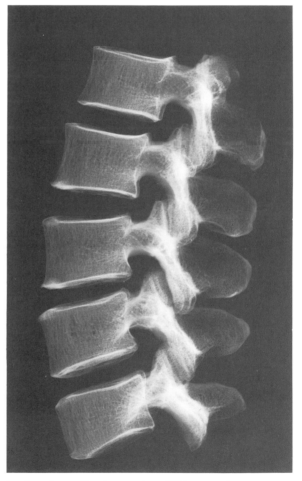

Figure 11-30. AP and lateral radiographs of a disarticulated specimen of lumbar vertebrae. Without turning back, identify the various parts.

. . . then study the ribs . . .

All the abdominal films you see will have been made with the Bucky diaphragm, and you will observe that you can see the ribs below the diaphragm much better than you do in chest films.

Calcifications in the costal cartilages, which normally are radiolucent and invisible, may cause some confusion when they are seen superimposed on intra-abdominal calcifications within the gallbladder, kidney, or adrenal gland. Rib calcifications can usually be distinguished by tracing the expected course of the rib anteriorly.

. . . and the pelvis and upper femora . . .

The shape of the shadows of the bones of the *pelvis* differs when the ray passes through PA and when it passes AP, as you can anticipate if you think of the flared and tilted wings of the ilium. These are "flattened out against the film," appearing round and wide on a supine plain film but narrow and more vertical on barium enema films made with the patient prone. This is because the ray which passes through the patient PA is much more nearly tangential to the surface of the iliac wings, so that they are more approximately filmed on edge.

The ray is usually centered on the umbilicus in making a plain film of the abdomen, so that roughly half the air-in-gut shadows will be below this point. You will therefore expect to see (superimposed on the bones of the pelvis and sacrum) the air in the cecum, sigmoid, and rectum, as well as in the small-bowel loops when they do contain air. A loop of air-containing bowel overlying the iliac wing on a supine plain film is often very difficult to differentiate from a round area of bone destruction, and the procedure is to look over several films of the area: small-bowel air changes in shape and location from film to film, but an area of bone destruction will remain in exactly the same relation to

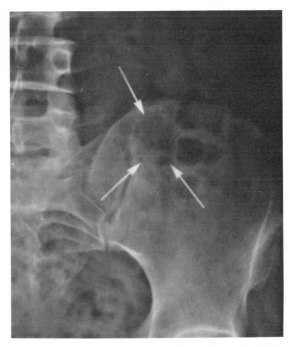

Figure 11-31. The radiolucent area of bone destruction indicated by the *arrows* did not change from film to film in relation to the margin of the sacroiliac joint. The darker air shadows lateral to it did.

the margins of the bone in which it is present (Figure 11-31).

Note that you see through the cartilaginous part of the anterior portion of the sacroiliac joint and through the symphysis pubis. Identify the spines and tuberosities of the ischia, and note that the hip joint is "seen" because it is bounded on both sides by the cortical bone of the acetabulum and femoral head, seen in tangent (Figure 11-32). Later, when you have read the section on bone, you will look at the bones on a plain film of the abdomen with a more precise eye for abnormalities, but for now leave them and go on to a study of the series of soft-tissue zones.

171

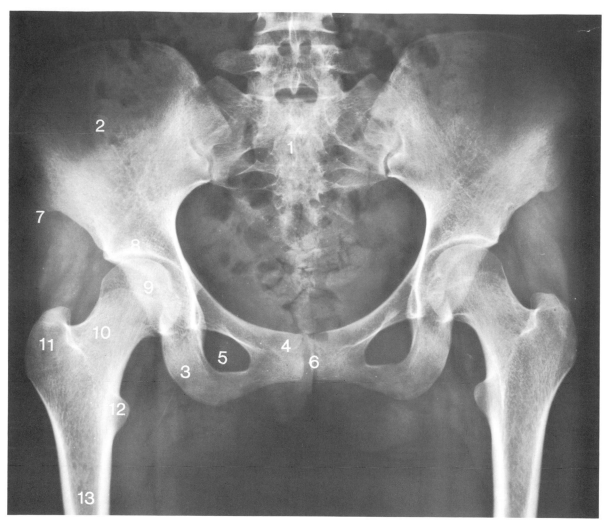

Figure 11-32. Anteroposterior radiograph of the pelvis and upper femora.

(1) Sacrum
(2) Ilium
(3) Ischium
(4) Pubis
(5) Obturator foramen
(6) Symphysis pubis
(7) Anterior superior iliac spine
(8) Acetabulum
(9) Femoral head
(10) Femoral neck
(11) Greater trochanter
(12) Lesser trochanter
(13) Femoral shaft

. . . then search the upper quadrants, flanks, and midabdomen for organ masses and calcifications . . .

Abnormality in size or shape of an organ is frequently evident from the plain film alone, but there are some differences in the degree of accuracy with which size may be judged by x-ray. The radiologic shadow of the liver is very misleading as an index to its size, for example, and it must be grossly enlarged before one can assume hepatomegaly from the plain film. Partly because of its shape and partly because of variation in the tilted position of the liver within the abdomen, pronouncements with regard to liver enlargement based on the plain film are risky. You will find that as an assay of liver size, old-fashioned palpation is a more reliable method.

The *liver,* so much larger than the spleen, normally tends to depress the organs in this quadrant. Its margin may be seen either as the inferior limit of a gray mass or as a boundary outlined by air in the transverse colon and hepatic flexure. The hepatic flexure is usually lower than the splenic flexure, but may occasionally overlap a part of the liver shadow. Radioisotope scanning, CT, and ultrasound techniques are becoming increasingly practicable for routine use in studying the liver, and metastatic lesions may be localized readily within the liver parenchyma. A characteristic pattern for cirrhosis is also recognizable at scintigraphy.

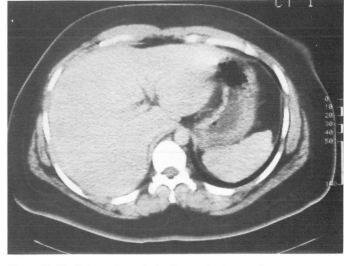

Figure 11-33. CT scan through the liver and spleen to show normal-sized organs. (Remember that there is an introduction to normal abdominal CT at the end of this chapter.)

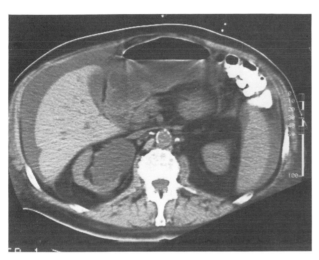

Figure 11-34. CT scan at a lower level through the kidneys shows how the right lobe of the liver decreases in size inferiorly. Did you note the fluid around the liver and spleen? This patient had malignant ascites.

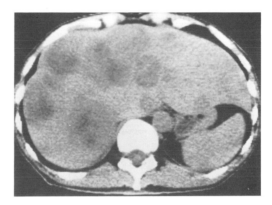

Figure 11-35. CT scan of a grossly enlarged liver, with numerous metastases from carcinoma of the prostate seen as irregular areas of decreased density

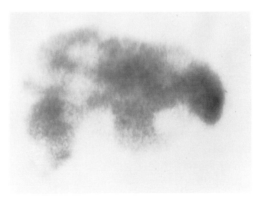

Figure 11-36. Scintigram (sulfur colloid scan) showing metastatic foci in the liver.

173

The *spleen,* on the contrary, may cast a shadow on the plain film which is unquestionably increased in size, although it has not been felt on bimanual examination. You should learn to place a good deal of reliance on a radiologic impression of splenomegaly. A very large spleen is not difficult to recognize and may reach well below the iliac crest and across the midline. A plain film suggesting splenomegaly may be confirmed today with CT, sonography, and other imaging methods, some of which may also identify pathologic conditions such as splenic trauma, neoplasm, abscess, or cyst.

The *splenic flexure* is quite variable in position. It may be indented by the tip of the spleen, overlap it partially, or extend over it as high as the diaphragm. It should not be hard for you to identify in such cases, for it will have the characteristic smooth haustral indentations of colon as opposed to the crinkled margin of the stomach shadow.

The *stomach* itself is almost never difficult to identify. In the supine film, the air in the stomach will rise into the more anteriorly placed body of the stomach, outlining the heavy rugal folds of gastric mucosa. In the prone position, whatever air is present will rise into the posteriorly placed fundus, so that on a prone plain film made with a sagittal ray the air bubble of the stomach appears as a round dark shadow with a wrinkled margin nearer the diaphragm. These differences, in fact, will also help you to decide whether a film has been made supine or prone. The same principles apply to barium studies of the stomach, as you will see later.

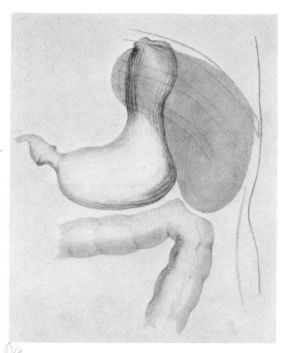

Figure 11-37. The normal stomach indented by an enlarged spleen, which depresses the splenic flexure. It is shown as it would look if you could see all three structures.

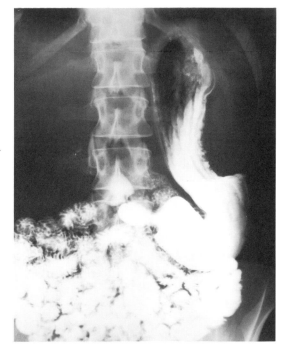

Figure 11-38. The normal stomach filled with barium and indented by an enlarged spleen.

174

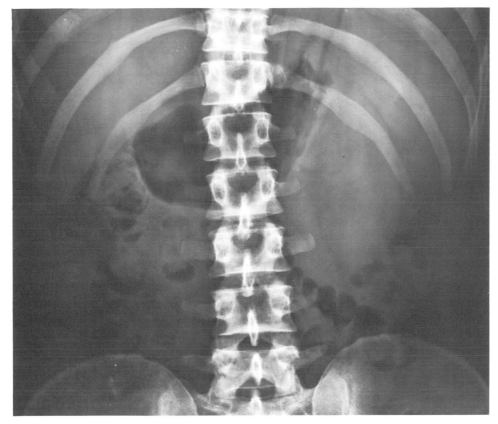

Figure 11-39. A ruptured spleen, thickened through its base, displacing the normal stomach to the right and extending down into the left flank. Note the coarse edematous rugal folds of the stomach, which probably shared in the trauma. Was this film made supine or prone?

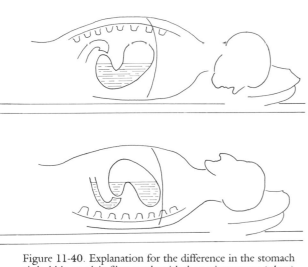

Figure 11-40. Explanation for the difference in the stomach air bubble on plain films made with the patient prone (*above*) and supine (*below*). On this page spread Figures 11-38 and 11-41 were made prone with the fundus filled with air. Figure 11-39 was made supine.

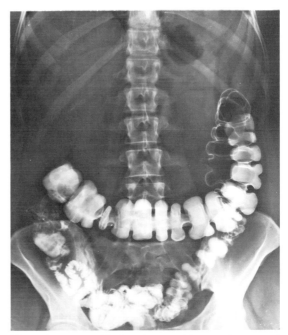

Figure 11-41. Identify the splenic and hepatic flexures and the tips of the liver and spleen. Neither liver nor spleen was felt manually to be enlarged.

175

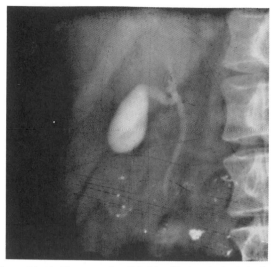

Figure 11-42. The normal gallbladder filled with physiologically concentrated opaque material (oral cholecystogram, or OCG). A fatty meal has just been given and the gallbladder is contracting, so that the cystic duct, common bile duct, and, by reflux, a part of the common hepatic duct are seen containing contrast material. Scattered flecks of dense white are leftover opaque material in the bowel.

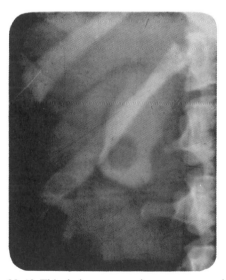

Figure 11-43. This cholecystogram shows a concentration of opaque material and a radiolucent stone composed of low-density material. It was invisible on the plain film.

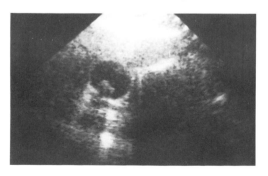

The shadow of the *gallbladder* may occasionally be seen on the plain film as a rounded shadow superimposed on the liver margin and the right kidney. It has for many years been successfully *rendered* visible by administering, by mouth, radiopaque compounds which are excreted by the liver. These materials do not concentrate sufficiently within the liver cells to visualize them, but the normal gallbladder, by extracting water and concentrating bile, also concentrates the excreted opaque substance so that contrast visualization of the gallbladder is possible. This is called *oral cholecystography* (OCG).

Only about 15 percent of gallbladder stones are shown to be calcified on plain films. *The rest are radiolucent and thus invisible on a plain film,* an important fact for you to remember. During cholecystography, in gallbladders which are still capable of concentrating the opaque substance excreted by the liver, such common radiolucent stones will appear as "filling defects," radiolucent relative to the opacified bile. Unfortunately, poor concentration in chronic cholecystitis has in the past rendered the visualization of such stones difficult or impossible.

More recently, the investigation of the gallbladder and biliary tree by ultrasonography and CT has become so successful that cholecystography is used much less, although in many cases it remains a valuable technique for recognizing diminished function. Sonography of the gallbladder and biliary tree is discussed in Chapter 14. For now, remember that it identifies stones but tells us nothing about gallbladder function.

Figure 11-44 (*left*). Sonogram showing the fluid-filled gallbladder, on the dependent posterior wall of which rest two stones. The sound beam enters through the anterior abdominal wall of this supine patient (*top of scan*). No sound waves (echoes) are reflected from the bile, so it appears black. Echoes are reflected by the stones, hence their white appearance. Note the distinct sonographic "shadows" extending posteriorly from them as areas which reflect little sound, because most of the beam has been stopped and reflected by the two stones.

Farther posterior on either side of the spine are situated the *kidneys,* the left a little higher than the right in most patients and retroperitoneal. The upper poles of both are tilted toward the midline and against the psoas muscles. You should trace their outlines as completely as possible. You will have some difficulty outlining the kidneys on a good many plain films because they are nearly always partly obscured by varying amounts of gas and stool in the bowel. If you see no kidney shadow at all on a film of good quality, without too much overlying gas, it may mean that the kidney is absent, very small, or has little or no perirenal fat, for example.

The kidneys, close to the film in the supine patient and outlined by fat, are much better described by the plain-film evidence than they can ever be on physical examination, and you will discover that a difference in size of the two kidneys, for example, or a bulge in the kidney outline, is repeatedly brought to your attention by the radiologist. A difference in length may have significance as an indication of disparity in function. Normally the kidney length should be 3.7 times the height of L2. A parenchymal renal cyst or tumor will enlarge the kidney by ballooning out the pole in which it is present, pushing the perirenal fat before it. Ptosis is common and easily recognized when you find the kidney farther down the psoas shadow than is normal. Any rotation of the kidney about its long axis will alter the shadow it casts.

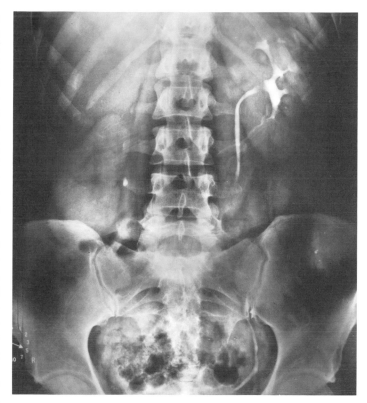

Figure 11-45. Intravenous urogram in a patient who presented with right flank pain, hematuria, and a history of passing stones. The right kidney parenchyma is denser than that on the left because the fluid-and-contrast-flow through this kidney is delayed by the obstructing dense calculus in the upper ureter. The right kidney is also ptotic. Note the discontinuous visualization of contrast in the left ureter. This is normal, since the ureter is swept by waves of peristalsis.

Figure 11-46 (*right*). CT through the midkidneys (in a different patient). Intravenous contrast has been given. Note the enhanced density of the renal parenchyma, and concentrated opaque in the renal pelves leaving the anteromedially directed hila of the kidneys. They are, of course, lying in the retroperitoneal compartment surrounded by lucent perirenal fat. Note the psoas muscle masses against the vertebral body and the aorta just anterior to it.

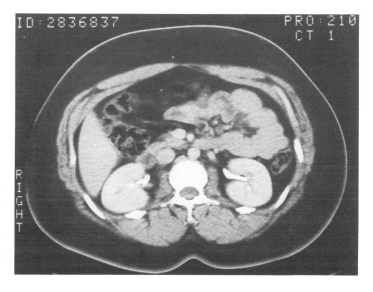

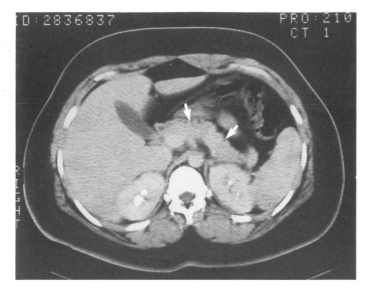

Figure 11-47 (*left*). CT scan through the pancreas (*arrows*). Note that the kidneys are sectioned through their upper-pole calyces above the indentation of parenchyma at the hilum of the kidney. (Compare with those in Figure 11-46 on the previous page.) The slender crura enclose the aorta. The gallbladder is seen as a relatively lucent area within the liver.

The kidneys are studied specifically by the use of renally excreted radiopaque contrast materials (the intravenous urogram) or by injecting similar contrast substances through catheters placed in the ureters during cystoscopy (the retrograde pyelogram). Radiographic study of the kidneys has been revolutionized by sonography, computed tomography, and other special techniques which will be discussed in more detail in Chapter 14. Your concern here is with morphology: learning to interpret changes in size, shape, and position of organs that you can identify on the plain film.

The *pancreas,* its head encircled by the loop of the duodenum, lies below and behind the antrum and body of the stomach and against the bodies of the upper lumbar vertebrae as they project forward into the abdomen. It is of course retroperitoneal and even less visible on the plain film than the kidneys, unless it contains calcifications and stones scattered through it to outline and mark its position (as in Figure 11-24). It may be indirectly bounded by other organs which normally lie close to it, and a large mass in the head of the pancreas, for example, may expand the duodenal loop and displace forward the pyloric antrum of the stomach. The pancreas may be "imaged" with sonography, CT, endoscopic retrograde cholangiopancreatography (ERCP), angiography, or MR, as you will learn later.

Your special survey of the upper *midabdomen,* then, includes some structures which you have "looked for" already, since only an arbitrary division can separate those structures which lie in the upper right and left quadrants from those which, like the pancreas, lie partly also in the midabdomen. Think of the midabdominal structures three-dimensionally, beginning with those most anteriorly placed. The *body of the stomach,* with its J-shaped streak of air in the supine patient, lies anteriorly against the abdominal wall and just above the curve of the air-containing *transverse colon.* The pyloric antrum and duodenal bulb (or cap) turn and point posteriorly so that they are best seen in the lateral view. The bulb and descending limb of the *duodenal loop,* which is partly retroperitoneal, turn downward, passing around the head of the pancreas, to the left and upward again toward the ligament of Treitz to join the jejunum. The duodenum is generally fluid filled and invisibly merged on the plain film with the shadows of other solid or fluid-containing structures near it, although you will see the duodenal loop regularly on barium studies and from it construe the position of the always invisible pancreas. Chapter 13 covers barium studies.

. . . and finally examine the flanks and lower abdomen.

Examine the *flanks* next, on both sides of the abdomen. The flank stripes may be obscured by the intense black of this area, which is often "burned out" at exposures calculated to penetrate the bones of the pelvis and spine. Even so, the flank stripes may often be seen well by placing the film against a bright light, kept handy by radiologists for the illumination of dark areas on films. The flank stripes will usually be symmetrical bilaterally in thin patients who have been positioned carefully. The dark haustrated colon should be seen lying close against the flank stripe. Free peritoneal fluid or blood may make the flank bulge out and will separate the colon appreciably from the flank stripe. In the presence of inflammation nearby, the flank stripe on that side will be seen to be smudged because of edema of the fat, rendering it indistinguishable from other water density soft tissues, such as muscle.

Study the *lower midabdomen* next; follow the known course of the ureters along the psoas shadows down to the bladder, looking for any shadow which could represent a calculus. The ureters are invisible on the plain films, but their shadows outlined with contrast material on urograms will help you to learn the variations in their position. Many plain films show small, round, calcium-dense shadows just inside the brim of the bony pelvis. These are calcified thrombi in the pelvic veins, or phleboliths, and generally lie closer to the margin of the bowl of the pelvis than any part of the ureter. Their position, then, will help you to distinguish them from calculi, and you will also be aided by the fact that calculi may be any shape at all and often have jagged points in their shadow profiles, whereas phleboliths are invariably smooth and round and sometimes show a central radiolucency, like a bead ready for stringing (Figure 11-25).

Figure 11-49 (*right*). Contrast material filling the bladder here will help you to recognize the shadow cast by the urine-filled bladder on plain films. Note the location of the ureters as they enter the bladder.

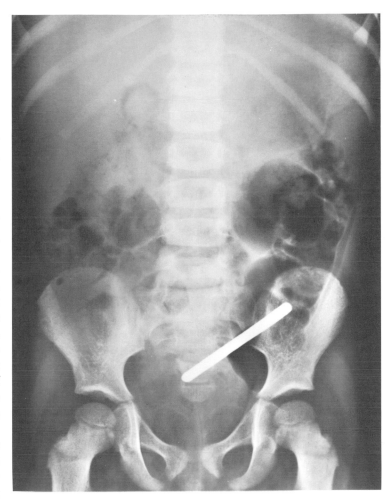

Figure 11-48. Plain film of a child admitted with fever, constipation, periumbilical pain, and an elevated white count. The clinical working diagnosis was appendicitis. At surgery the appendix was found to be retrocecal and perforated. There was inflammation and edema of the tissues of the right gutter and right flank. Note the well-seen left and the absent right flank stripe. (The white bar is an artifact.)

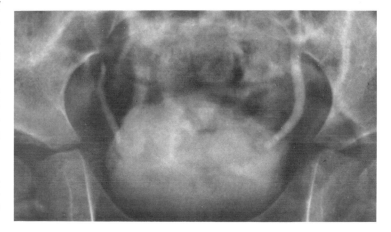

179

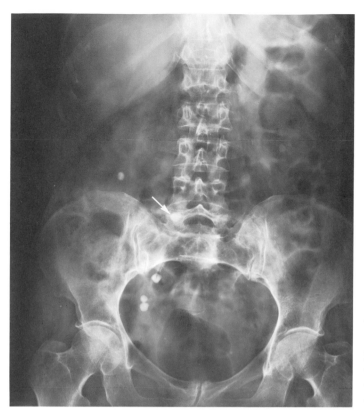

Figure 11-50. This plain film shows several calculi in the lower right ureter (*arrow* to the highest one) and a calcified mesenteric node farther lateral above the top of the iliac wing. Note the air-filled rectum superimposed on the bladder.

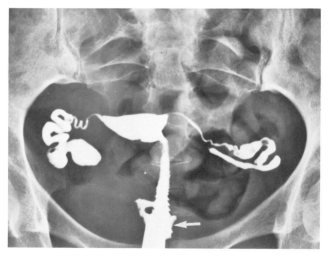

Figure 11-51. A hysterosalpingogram. The uterus and fallopian tubes have been filled with a contrast substance as a part of a sterility study. Normally there would be a spill of opaque material from the fallopian tubes into the peritoneal cavity, but none is seen here. Conclusion: outer ends of tubes closed. The *arrow* points to the injection cannula.

The lower midabdomen is a common location for calcified mesenteric nodes, and they will not usually be mistaken for ureteral stones because they tend to look like clusters of small concretions and are somewhat denser than most stones. They vary widely in position from film to film as a rule, because of the mobility of the small-bowel mesentery. They often overlap the bony structures of the vertebral column and sacrum.

The many loops of small bowel are contained for the most part in the lower midabdomen and pelvis. In the normal ambulatory adult, as we have said, they contain fluid and little or no air; but as you will be seeing plain films mostly on patients sick enough to be hospitalized, you will become accustomed to seeing some air-outlined loops of small bowel overlying the lower lumbar vertebrae and pelvis.

The soft tissues within the bowl of the pelvis, finally, include the urinary bladder and lower ureters, the sigmoid colon and rectum, the uterus and adnexae in the female, and the prostate and seminal vesicles in the male. The bladder, when it contains a moderate amount of urine, is commonly visible on the plain film as a somewhat flattened oval shadow within the pelvis. When it is greatly distended, it may rise up to the umbilicus as a uniformly gray, rounded shadow, not infrequently mistaken for a pathologic mass. The rectum will generally be visible superimposed on the shadow of the bladder and outlined with contained air or feces. The uterus, adnexae, seminal vesicles, and prostate are not visible except by special procedures of various sorts. All may be visualized and studied with injected opaque material, however. Today sonography, CT, and magnetic resonance are used to study pelvic structures and masses.

180

Computed Tomography of the Abdomen

As you discovered in Chapter 2, a computed tomogram provides you with a schema of *density* values for a particular slice of your patient, which you will learn to study with the regional cross-section anatomy in mind. An awareness of the relative attenuation of different tissues and organs, and their interfaces with fat planes in particular, helps you as you look at CT scans. As you do so, you will be better able to understand anatomic relationships and proportions by knowing that those on CT scans are *living* dimensions rather than the necessarily distorted ones in the desiccated cadaver. There are also physiological implications in some of the observations you will make in serial CT scans. For example, in scans made across the upper abdomen the inferior vena cava can be seen to distend to twice its normal size during the Valsalva maneuver (in which the patient bears down against a closed glottis, as in pronouncing a forced "G" or "K").

CT scans can be performed in the supine or prone position or with the patient lying on his side (decubitus). Usually, however, the patient is supine, as he is most comfortable and most relaxed in that position and can more readily keep still. Always remember: you are looking *up* at any CT scan from the patient's feet.

It is important for you to realize that computed tomography most of the time should be considered an adjunctive study for special problems rather than a screening procedure. Other less expensive procedures like plain films or ultrasound ought always to be used first if possible, so that the CT study, when indicated, can be employed more precisely and more economically for examination of the particular structure in question. Because of the ionizing radiation involved, the female pelvis during the childbearing era must by and large be examined by ultrasound rather than CT.

The Use of Contrast Material for Enhancement

Contrast media are almost routinely used during CT scanning for two basic reasons:

(1) The GI tract can be tagged and thus distinguished from neighboring normal structures (and abnormal masses) by having the patient swallow dilute opaque material.

(2) Intravenous administration of water-soluble contrast material will produce a temporary increase in the density of arteries, of all capillary-perfused parenchyma, and, finally, of peripheral veins during CT scanning. This is called *enhancement* and is extremely useful. Dilated low-density branching channels within the homogeneous parenchyma of the liver, for example, on an initial scan without contrast could be either fluid-filled bile ducts or blood vessels. We enhance the vascular bed with contrast medium, therefore, and if the observed channels are unchanged on a subsequent scan they are bile ducts, not vessels.

Similarly, renal-excreted contrast substances may be used, CT scanning being carried out both before and after the opaque is given so that the kidney and ureters are seen as "dense" white areas of recognizable form and in the expected locations. On the other hand, *displacement* of these structures, although they are themselves not abnormal, will provide additional information with regard to soft-tissue masses being investigated.

As you have learned thus far, computed tomography has important applications in the *chest*, where mediastinal masses can be more readily distinguished from normal structures than by conventional tomograms, and where small metastatic nodules, especially near the chest wall, can be recognized when they are not seen on routine chest films and are not detectable by any other means.

Computed tomography carried out in the abdomen is usually made transaxially at intervals of 1 or 2 centimeters, although each CT scanning study must be custom-tailored to the particular patient's problem.

Identify the liver in Figure 11-52A. Note that as you look up from the patient's feet, the liver is on your left and anterior. Ignore everything else and follow the change in shape and size of the liver down through all six sections (made at 1-centimeter intervals in this patient). Note how the dense vertebra changes shape depending on whether the cut is through the transverse processes in D and E or above or below them. The vertebral canal is visible, as is the cord within it.

Locate the aorta just anterior to the body of the vertebra and slightly to the left of the midline, with dense white areas in its periphery which are calcified plaques in its wall in the first three scans. In E and F farther down, noncalcified atheromatous plaques on the intima of the aorta can be seen as radiolucent filling defects displacing some of the circulating contrast substance. Because this series of scans was carried out after intravenous infusion of contrast material, perfused structures and vessels are slightly whiter (enhanced). Note the branching white vessels in A in the homogeneous parenchyma of the liver, which have faded away in successive sections. The intravenous contrast material used is excreted by the kidneys, so you see the renal parenchyma and calyces as whiter than other organs. Those branching linear structures near the hilum of the kidney are vessels.

The stomach in A contains fluid and probably lunch. No oral contrast material was given this patient. Note that the (perfused) wall of the stomach is denser than its fluid content, and as you look from scan to scan you cross-section first the body and then the pyloric antrum of the stomach; even the pyloric muscle, and proximal to it a peristaltic wave, are seen (in F).

The big, black, low-density areas on either side of the vertebra and posterior to the liver and spleen in A contain nothing but retroperitoneal fat. Follow those areas downward from section to section and study the kidneys, noting the initial appearance of their upper poles in B and the doughnut-shaped parenchyma around the upper calyces in C before the hilum has been reached. The two kidneys are at nearly the same level in this patient; normally the left kidney is higher. The two hila are sectioned in E, where the kidney is seen as a crescent of parenchyma curving around the anteriorly directed hila. There is a tiny cyst in the posterior parenchyma of the right kidney in F.

Now find the inferior vena cava in F, just anterior to the vertebra a little to the right of the midline. If you follow it upward you can see it in C and D clearly receiving the left renal vein, which normally crosses in front of the aorta from left to right at this level. We are just above the pancreas. Note that anterior to the left renal vein in D you can see the splenic vein joined by a gastric vein draining into the portal vein.

In sections A and B the inferior vena cava moves nearer the hilum of the liver. The dragon-shaped mass of the pancreas is seen first in section E, its tail extending toward the hilum of the spleen. Because the tail turns upward, the pancreas looks shorter in section F. See if you can figure out the identity of the two white (vascular) structures just medial and posterior to the head of the pancreas in E and F. (There are matching labeled diagrams on the next page spread to help you to check your findings.)

The two white structures in E and F are the superior mesenteric artery and vein. The artery is the smaller of the two.

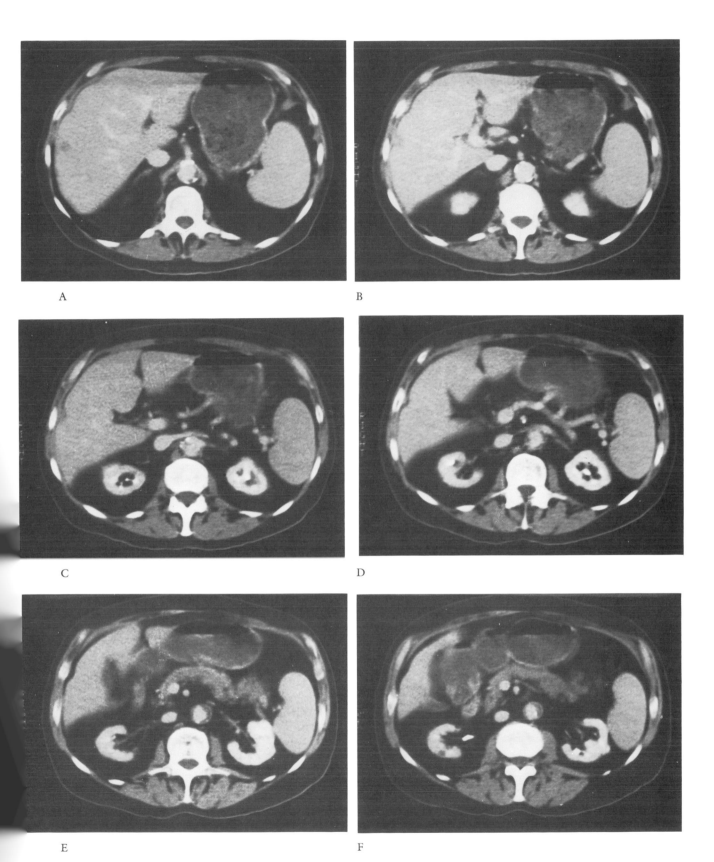

A

B

C

D

E

F

Figure 11-52. Normal computed tomograms of the upper abdomen.

Diagrams to Match CT Scans in Figure 11-52 (reprinted on opposite page)

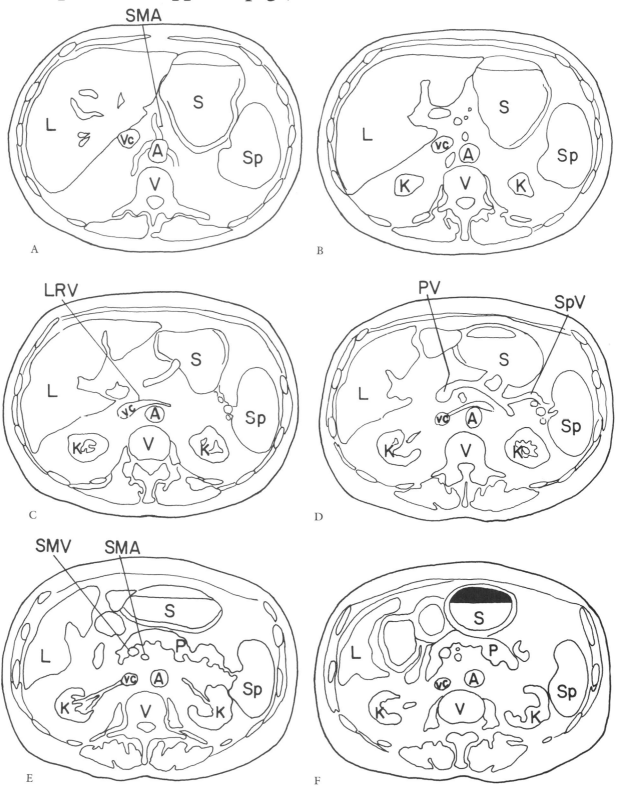

Figure 11-52 Reprinted

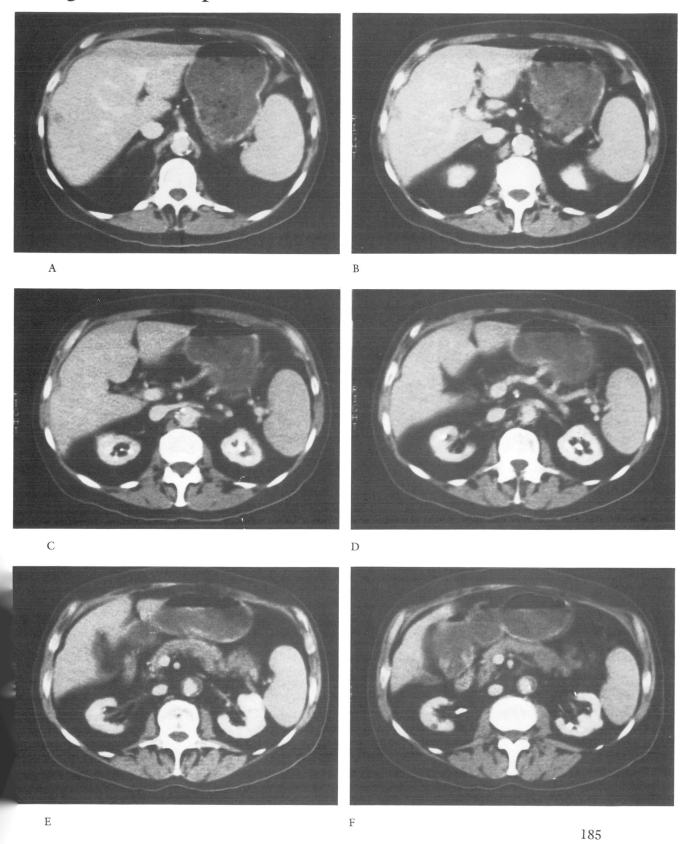

A

B

C

D

E

F

185

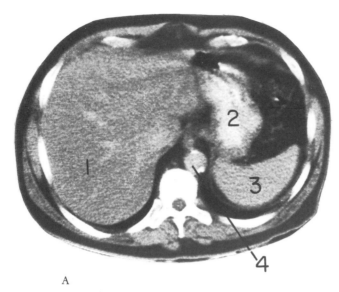

A

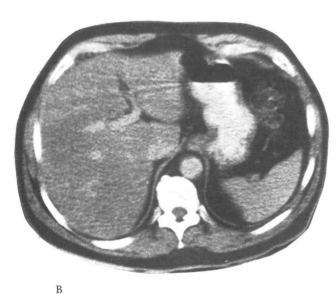

B

Now here is another series of normal abdominal CT scans for you to practice your skill on, studying all six sections and identifying serially the liver, spleen, kidneys and their calyces, aorta, inferior vena cava, left renal vein, and pancreas. Compare each structure with the same one in the patient in Figure 11-52.

By observing the density of the kidney calyces and stomach contents, decide whether intravenous or oral contrast medium was given this patient. Can you distinguish the head of the pancreas from the descending second portion of the duodenum in D? The superior mesenteric artery leaves the aorta anteriorly just above the point where the left renal vein crosses to the right. Can you find them both? Review the order in which the celiac, superior mesenteric, renal, and inferior mesenteric branches leave the aorta.

In this patient you can recognize the adrenal glands embedded in fat in sections C and D. The left adrenal looks like a flying bird and lies to the left of the aorta and posterior to the tail of the pancreas in this patient. The right is always seen just posterior to the inferior vena cava, as in C and D.

Figure 11-53. A series of computed tomograms on another patient. Use them as an exercise to test your progress. You can check the numbers listed below if you are in doubt about the identity of any structure imaged.

(1) Liver
(2) Stomach with water-soluble oral contrast medium
(3) Spleen
(4) Aorta
(5) Kidneys
(6) Duodenum
(7) Head of pancreas
(8) Left adrenal
(9) Right adrenal
(10) Superior mesenteric artery
(11) Left renal vein
(12) Inferior vena cava
(13) Diaphragmatic crura

186

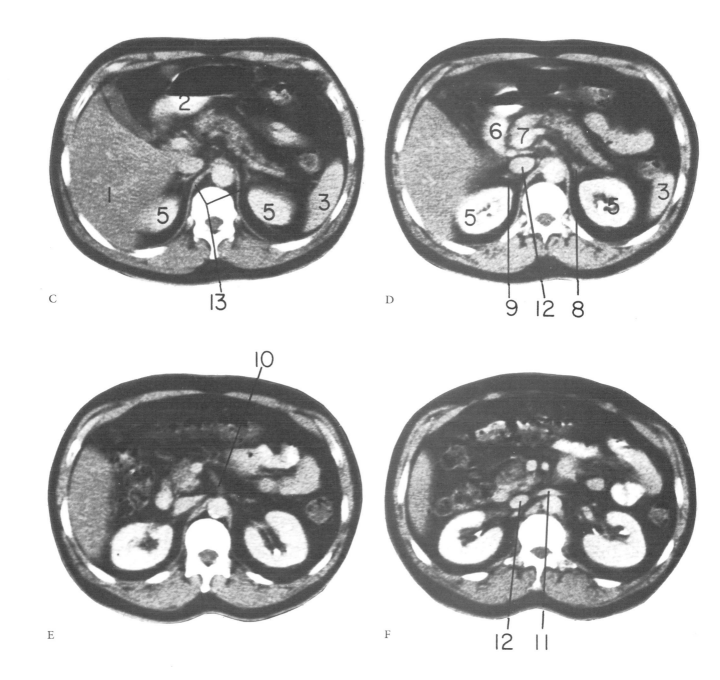

Ultrasonography

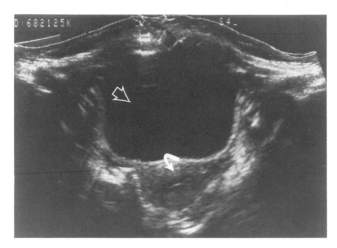

Figure 11-54. Normal transverse sonogram of the female pelvis.

Now that you have addressed yourself to the study of the plain film and to the intellectual discipline of understanding serial CT scans of the abdomen, you have certainly acquired an even more expert stereotactic feeling for considering body structures always in three dimensions. Even if you were blind, had therefore never seen an *apple* or known that such a shape existed, you would be able intellectually to reconstruct its three-dimensional form precisely from assembled slices which you had been able to touch-examine with your fingers. Now we must introduce you also to the information available through *ultrasonography*.

It is a curious fact that high-energy sound waves beyond the range of the human ear were produced experimentally some 15 years before Roentgen discovered the x-ray. No attempt was made to develop ultrasonography for medical use until after the stimulus of its use during World War II in the underwater detection of submarines. Since the 1950s, however, sonography has earned an important place in medical diagnosis and physicians find they employ it on some of their patients practically every day.

The fact that sound waves are reflected by many solid substances but transmitted readily by fluids meant that a beam of sound could be projected through water toward a submarine, and its reflection from the surface of the hull timed so that the presence of the submarine and its distance away were known.

Translated to medical use, this means that a beam of sound waves projected into the body from the surface of the skin will be transmitted forward by *sonolucent* (fluid) substances, a part of the beam being reflected back when it encounters an interface with a substance or structure of different *acoustic character*. The time needed for the signal to return *locates* the depth of the interface from which it was reflected. The rest of the initial beam continues on into and through the encountered organ or mass, reflecting more and more of the beam from other interfaces at measurable distances, until finally the last of the beam is absorbed.

Whenever the beam encounters a fluid-filled (cystic) structure inside the body, the sound is transmitted through with negligible absorption until it reaches the interface of the far wall of the cystic structure, from which it is reflected. *Sound is transmitted well through any fluid, but poorly or not at all through bone, air, and barium.*

The beam of sound is produced in pulses or periodic bursts, very brief in duration, and the same transducer then "listens" for the returning echoes until the next burst of outgoing sound.

Returning echoes are electronically converted into a video image on a monitor, echoes appearing as white dots on a black background in the technique used in this book. (In some departments the reverse technique is used: returning echoes are black on a light background.) The result is a *picture of a wedge-shaped slice of the*

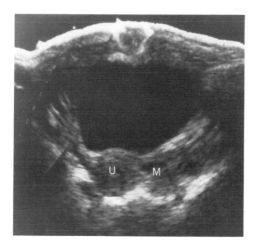

Figure 11-55. Transverse pelvic sonogram in a female patient with abdominal pain and vaginal bleeding. *U* is the uterus; *M,* a mass.

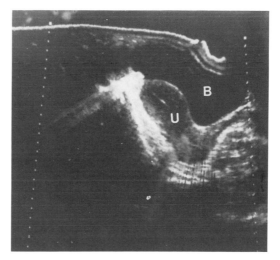

Figure 11-56. Normal longitudinal sonogram in the sagittal plane. The abdominal wall is at the top of the sonogram. *B* is the urinary bladder; *U,* the uterus. The vagina is seen extending to the right.

patient. Because of the variety of degrees of obliquity of image plane used, it is not easy to reconcile such pictures with one's intellectual awareness of cross-sectional anatomy in standard planes. In fact, the sonographer must identify the anatomic segment and image plane on each scan for the benefit of the viewer.

Unlike the important tissue injury of ionizing radiation, which has to be taken into consideration in electing to carry out any radiographic study (including CT), pulsed diagnostic ultrasound seems to have no injurious effect whatever in the range used for medical technology. This makes ultrasound a particularly valuable tool, especially in imaging pelvic structures in obstetrical and gynecological practice—and it is there that we will illustrate first the practical principles of ultrasonography. A patient being prepared for pelvic ultrasonography is instructed not to void for some time beforehand, a full urinary bladder providing a sonolucent mass (window) in the lower abdomen, which displaces undesirable air-containing loops of bowel up out of the pelvis so that a good beam of sound transmitted through the bladder will encounter the pelvic organs posterior to it.

Figure 11-54 is a *transverse* pelvic sonogram, obtained just above the pubic symphysis. The beam of sound has entered through the anterior abdominal wall (*top of figure*). You are looking up at the slice from the patient's feet. The large, uniformly black structure (*open arrow*) is the urine-filled sonolucent bladder. Posterior to it is an oval mass (*curved arrow*) representing the normal uterus. Remember: *echogenic* (or sonogenic) structures appear white and *echolucent* (or sonolucent) structures (fluid collections) appear black. Fatty tissues generally are very echogenic, and you can see their white echoes surrounding the bladder and uterus. Note the many dots representing echoes within the muscular wall of the uterus and the slitlike uterine cavity with its darker ring of endometrium.

Compare Figure 11-54 with Figure 11-55, which shows a mass lateral to the uterus. This proved to be an ectopic pregnancy in the left fallopian tube. Figure 11-56 shows the uterus in the midline *longitudinal* (sagittal) sonogram. The patient's head is to your left in every longitudinal scan. Again observe the echogenic posterior wall of the bladder and the echogenic uterine cavity.

189

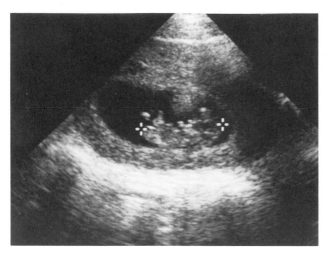

Figure 11-57. Sonogram of an intrauterine ten-week fetus. Cursors mark the crown-rump dimension.

Notice that the uterus in Figure 11-56 is empty. Compare it with the magnified uterine sonogram in Figure 11-57, which contains a ten-week-old fetus. The two cross-shaped artifacts are ultrasound markers called cursors, which are positioned by the radiologist to measure distances. After the cursors are positioned, the ultrasound machine calculates the distance between them. In this instance the crown-rump dimension measures 39.5 millimeters, normal for this aged fetus. The echogenic fetus is surrounded by sonolucent (black) amniotic fluid, contained between the muscular walls of the uterus.

In Figure 11-58 a second-trimester fetus is seen adjacent to a mass, the placenta. Note the fetal face, torso, and folded legs. Figure 11-59 is a (magnified) ultrasound view of the head of a twenty-week fetus. The detail available from fetal ultrasound makes it possible to recognize fetal abnormalities at various stages of pregnancy.

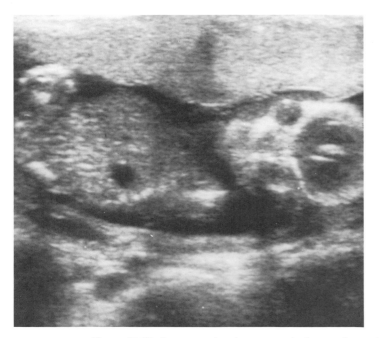

Figure 11-58. Sonogram showing a second-trimester fetus lying just below the anterior wall placenta.

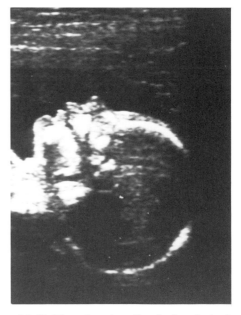

Figure 11-59. The enlarged profile of a fetus is clearly seen on sonography.

Ultrasound has many other useful applications in the abdomen, although certain parts of the body are not amenable to sonographic study because of their barriers to ultrasound transmission (air and bone). For example, the adult brain cannot be imaged by ultrasound because of the skull. The neonatal brain, however, can be imaged through a patent fontanelle, and diagnosis of hydrocephalus, trauma, and other central nervous system conditions may be made.

In the neck, ultrasound is frequently used to diagnose carotid artery atherosclerosis in patients with suspected cerebrovascular disease. Thyroid cysts can be differentiated from thyroid tumors with ultrasound, and even parathyroid masses may be discernible.

It is not possible to image pulmonary nodules and other lung masses with ultrasound because of the failure of air to transmit sound waves well. The mediastinum, however, is regularly imaged. You have seen an example of echocardiography in the heart chapter, in a patient with pericardial effusion.

The major use of diagnostic ultrasound examinations is in the abdomen and pelvis where, as in Figure 11-60, a *longitudinal* scan, the left kidney is seen lying posterior to an enlarged spleen. Note the central echoes produced by peripelvic fat in the kidney. The small black lucencies are urine in the calyces. The kidney parenchyma is surrounded by echogenic (white) perirenal fat. Note the homogeneous echo character of the spleen. The minute lucencies are splenic blood vessels.

Figure 11-61 is an enlarged *transverse* sonogram of the right kidney (*between black arrows*). The liver is seen anteriorly (*L*), and the gallbladder, a sonolucent fluid-filled oval mass, is just medial to it (*bent white arrow*). The dark echolucent quadrangle indenting the kidney from its medial surface (*open arrow*) is the renal pelvis. Renal ultrasound is used to diagnose hydronephrosis, renal cysts, and neoplasms.

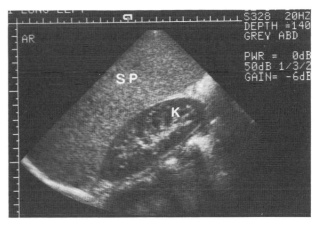

Figure 11-60. Normal longitudinal sonogram of the left kidney. *SP* is the spleen, *K* the kidney.

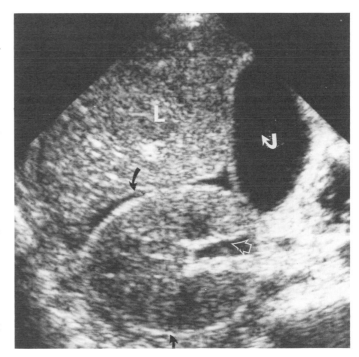

Figure 11-61. Normal transverse sonogram of the right kidney.

191

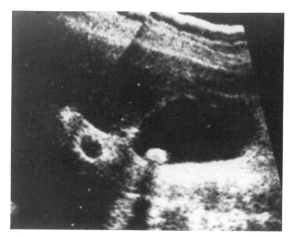

Figure 11-62A. Sonogram of the gallbladder containing a solitary calculus. Note the shadow beyond the stone, an area from which no echoes are returned.

In Chapter 2 you saw a sonogram of the gallbladder containing a solitary calculus. The stone produced a shadow behind it, because none of the beam penetrated the stone. That sonogram is reprinted here as Figure 11-62A. In Figure 11-62B you see another diseased gallbladder, half-filled with mildly echogenic sludge settled against its dependent wall. (Note that no echo-poor shadow is produced here behind it, as was the case with the stone.) Acute cholecystitis and bile duct obstruction may also be recognized with the help of sonography. In fact, ultrasound is frequently the initial procedure in patients who present with new jaundice.

Figure 11-63 is a longitudinal scan of the liver. The patient's head is to your left, and the echogenic arc (*arrow*) represents the diaphragm closely applied against the surface of the liver. The lung above the diaphragm is not well seen, but a pleural effusion would be. Ultrasound is often used to identify small pleural effusions and to localize them for diagnostic thoracentesis. Anteriorly (at the top of the scan) you see a relatively sonolucent round neoplasm in the liver parenchyma, with cursors to measure its size. The other echolucent areas are, as you would expect, hepatic blood vessels and bile ducts. Sonography of the liver easily identifies metastases as well as solitary primary tumors, liver cysts, and other conditions.

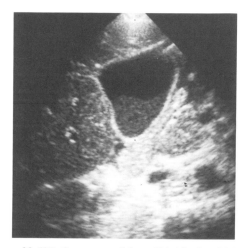

Figure 11-62B. Sonogram of the gallbladder in which relatively sonolucent sludge is seen collected against the posterior wall. It does not exhibit "shadowing"; many echoes are returned from tissues posterior to it.

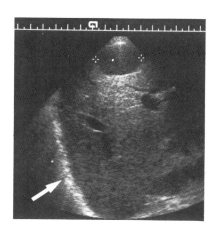

Figure 11-63 (*right*). Sonogram of the liver and diaphragm (see text).

You will see in Chapter 14 that sonography can be helpful in the diagnosis of a wide variety of other abdominal conditions. For example, in Figure 11-64, the fluid-filled aorta can be seen widening out to become an abdominal aortic aneurysm. In the remainder of the body, ultrasound can be employed to study such diverse entities as testicular tumors, popliteal artery aneurysm, and tears of the rotator cuff of the shoulder.

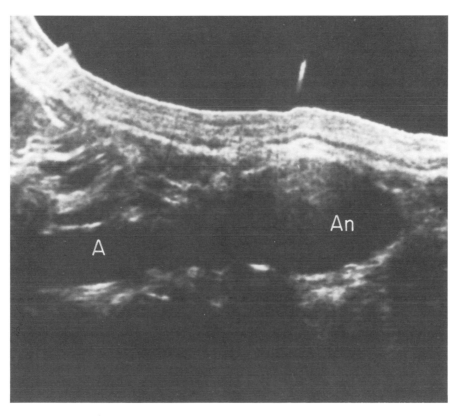

Figure 11-64. Longitudinal sonogram showing the aorta (*A*) widening to form an aneurysm (*An*).

CHAPTER 12 The Abdominal Plain Film: Distended Stomach, Small Bowel, Colon; Free Fluid and Free Air

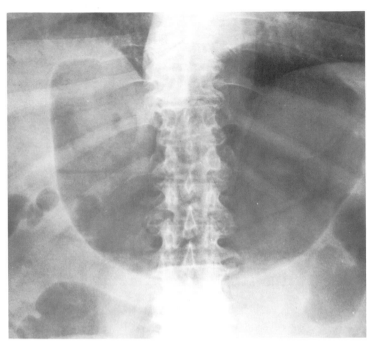

Figure 12-1. The stomach distended with air in agonal diabetic coma.

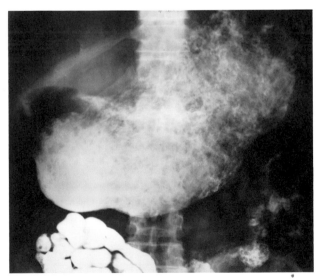

Figure 12-2. The stomach distended with food and barium mixture in a patient with gastric outlet obstruction, the result of scarring of his long-standing duodenal ulcer disease. The film was made four hours after the barium was swallowed, some of which is getting through into the small bowel. Such a patient should have been sent to x-ray only after suction and lavage.

Today perhaps the greatest usefulness of the abdominal plain film is in recognizing mechanical bowel obstruction and paralytic ileus, the subjects of this chapter.

The Distended Stomach

After you have studied the bones and the soft-tissue zones and profiles and decided whether there seems to be evidence for organ enlargement or displacement, you should *look at the whole film at once, directing your entire attention to the gas distribution and content.* Normally the air in the stomach will range from the small, round, wrinkled fundal bubble seen on the prone film to a few oblique streaks of air in the body of the stomach, which you will see in supine plain films. Visualization of the entire organ filled with swallowed air is not the rule. In Figure 12-1 you see the stomach of a patient in diabetic coma with agonal dilatation.

In pyloric obstruction the stomach may be grossly dilated, of course, and often contains a large amount of food and retained secretions. On the plain film such a stomach will appear as an ill-defined density extending across the upper abdomen, and if the radiologist tries to study it at fluoroscopy, swallowed barium appears to sink into a bog (Figure 12-2). Attempted barium study of such a stomach is futile until the stomach has been emptied, for only a clean mucosa can be examined with barium. The stomach is often seen distended with air in paralytic ileus, in diabetic coma, in air swallowing, and after nasogastric tube placement.

The Distended Colon

Abdominal plain films of hospitalized patients often show a certain amount of air in the small bowel, particularly the ileum, even though there is no clinical evidence to suggest the presence of either adynamic (paralytic) ileus or mechanical obstruction. You will find that the amount of air

194

in the intestine is increased in plain films made after any kind of painful interventional procedure (paralytic ileus). This is unfortunate, because such air usually overlies the kidneys, and the intersecting lines produced by the folded walls of air-filled bowel confuse the details of the shadows of the kidney and its draining structures.

Truly distended loops of *small bowel* may approach and even exceed the caliber of the normal colon. When they are filled with air, their distinctive mucosal markings will usually identify them; but when they are filled with fluid, they will cast vague, confluent, or sausage-shaped gray shadows across the midabdomen. Bubbles of air are often superimposed upon these shadows in the supine film.

The *colon,* particularly its distal half, usually contains some air. You may see air outlining solid fecal material within the lumen. The cecum and ascending colon often contain semisolid feces (Figure 12-3), producing a characteristic speckled shadow.

With moderate obstructive distension of the colon, the haustral indentations become shallower but are still visible. *More of the colon than is usual will be seen continuously outlined with air* (Figure 12-4). Thus, when a tumor obstructs at the level of the sigmoid, air may be seen outlining and distending all the colon proximal to that point (Figures 12-3 and 12-4). With a tumor obstructing at the midtransverse colon, the proximal half of the transverse colon, hepatic flexure, ascending colon, and cecum will be distended with air even though the left half of the colon is empty, cleared, invisible. The cecum may eventually balloon to enormous proportions in obstruction of the distal colon. All haustral indentations will be lost, and the cecum will appear as a huge air-filled structure occupying the right side of the abdomen. Still-incomplete obstruction to the forward flow of gas and feces may be temporarily overcome by retrograde instillation of fluid (cleansing enemas), as you see in the patient in Figures 12-3 and 12-4. The initial plain film on such patients will show accumulation of feces and gas above the tumor, which has narrowed the lumen. After the cleansing enemas, continuously air-filled distended colon is seen.

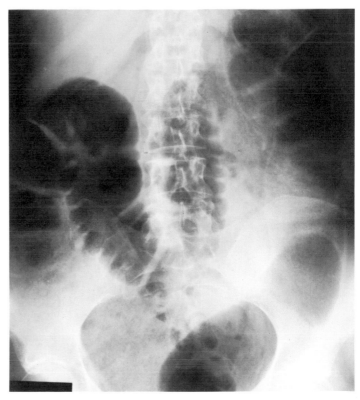

Figure 12-3 (*above*). Large-bowel obstruction in carcinoma of the sigmoid. Note the retained feces.

Figure 12-4 (*below*). The same patient after cleansing enemas, the clean colon distended with air. The ileocecal valve is competent (no air in small bowel).

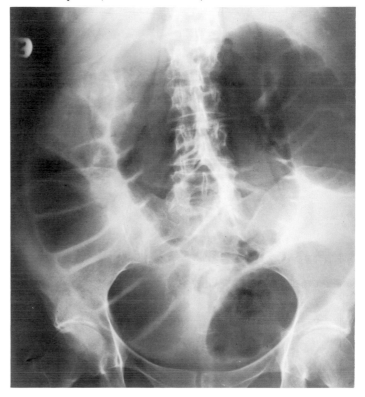

195

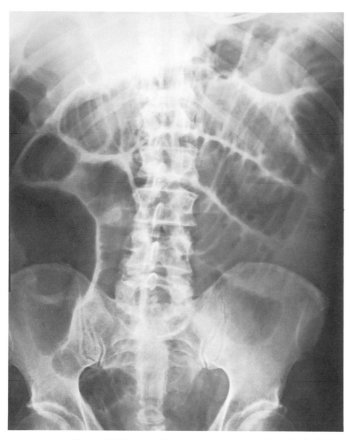

Figure 12-5. Large-bowel obstruction at the splenic flexure with decompression backward through an incompetent ileocecal valve. Note that the descending colon, sigmoid, and rectum are empty.

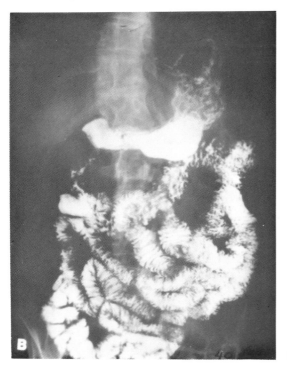

An important point in the diagnosis of all types of mechanical obstruction is that *the compensatory increase in peristalsis which develops is carried beyond the point of obstruction and results in the clearing of air from the bowel distal to that point* (that is, from that portion of the gut which *can* be cleared). Thus, in obstruction at the splenic flexure you would expect eventually to find the descending colon and sigmoid, completely empty and therefore invisible (Figure 12-5). In this way it is not impossible to make a strong presumptive diagnosis of large-bowel obstruction from a single plain film, with the next step a barium enema and demonstration of the lesion from its distal side.

In low large-bowel obstruction, air gradually fills most of the colon and, if the patient is fortunate, his ileocecal valve will become *incompetent,* allowing him to decompress his colon backward into his own small bowel (Figure 12-5).

The Distended Small Bowel

Figure 12-6 shows you the caliber of the small bowel filled with barium in a normal person and can be compared with Figure 12-7, in which obstructed and distended small bowel is seen visualized with barium and air. The *arrow* indicates the point of obstruction beyond which no barium has passed. Barium given by mouth in a patient with *colonic* obstruction could cause a dangerous barium impaction. Colonic obstruction should be ruled out by barium enema or colonoscopy in any patient whose symptoms and plain film suggest it. This is not a problem with small-bowel obstruction because the small-bowel content remains liquid proximal to the site of obstruction. The study of an obstructing colonic lesion by barium enema from its *distal* side is an entirely different matter, since the barium is readily evacuated. Sometimes in colonic obstruction a water-soluble contrast substance is used instead of barium if colonoscopy is planned.

Figure 12-6. Normal small bowel. Barium given by mouth.

Figure 12-7 shows you the caliber of moderately distended loops of jejunum with their characteristic cross striations representing the valvulae conniventes. You will say that they resemble the haustral indentations of the colon—and they do, superficially at least. They differ in their periodicity, however, being more numerous than haustral indentations and more narrowly spaced even when the small bowel is distended. They also cross the lumen from one side to the other, as opposed to haustral indentations, which indent but do not usually cross the colon and often are not precisely opposite the indentation on the other side. In addition, you will be helped in differentiating between obstructed small bowel and obstructed large bowel when you observe that small-bowel loops tend to line up in rows, three and four parallel loops of bowel appearing close beside each other (Figures 12-7 and 12-8). The colon, when it distends, almost never gives this "arranged" appearance.

In mechanical small-bowel obstruction precisely the same principle applies that was described for the large bowel: clearing of all bowel beyond the point of obstruction so that it is empty of gas, collapsed, and invisible (Figure 12-8). If you make a practice of looking for the *colon* as soon as you recognize distended small bowel, one of these days you will find yourself looking at an unknown plain film on which you can find no haustrated air shadows and hence no part of the colon. You will realize that you *must* be looking at the radiographic findings in mechanical small-bowel obstruction, the *entire* colon having been swept clear of gas and feces.

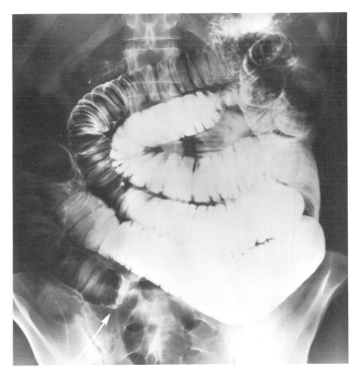

Figure 12-7. Distended small bowel above an obstructing lesion (*arrow*). Note the cleared (invisible) colon.

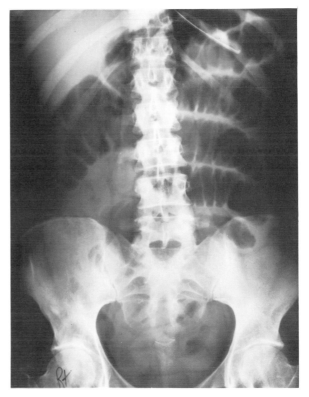

Figure 12-8. Small-bowel obstruction in a patient with inflammatory bowel disease and stricture of the terminal ileum. Note the clearing of the colon here.

197

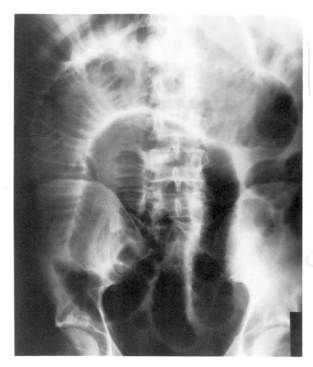

Figure 12-9. Small-bowel obstruction, many loops of small bowel distended with air, and almost complete clearing of colon. At laparotomy an adhesive band was lysed and the patient recovered.

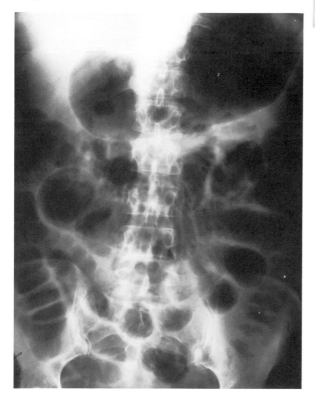

Figure 12-10. Paralytic ileus in a patient after an automobile accident. (See text.) The picture did not change on serial films made at 1 and 2 hours.

In paralytic ileus, on the other hand, both large and small bowel will be seen distended with air, since peristalsis is generally decreased. This is a far less distinctive radiologic picture than that for mechanical obstruction, and makes for indecision and a sense of confusion in trying to interpret plain films in patients with abdominal symptoms. Still, once you have learned to recognize the picture of *mechanical* obstruction when it is definitive, you will feel somewhat more comfortable about studying the equivocal findings so often seen in plain films.

Time is the important factor we forget to consider in looking at a single film. It is all too easy, when one is worried about a patient and in quest of diagnostic help, to forget that a single examination is a point on a curve and nothing more. *How long* has the obstruction in midtransverse colon been present? Has it been a complete obstruction *long enough* to allow the bowel beyond that point to become cleared of air? If not, then the presence of air in both large and small bowel may be hard to distinguish radiographically from paralytic ileus. *Serial films in patients with abdominal problems are often very informative,* indicating the developing change more clearly than any other investigative procedure.

In Figure 12-9 loops of distended small bowel are easy to identify, but no air is seen in the colon. This patient had *mechanical small-bowel obstruction* from an adhesive band in the right lower quadrant.

The patient in Figure 12-10 had *paralytic ileus.* You can identify air in the stomach, small bowel, and large bowel. Note, however, that it does not truly distend the bowel; there is a varying amount of air in the colon and small bowel, which are *discontinuously air containing.* Parts of the colon have deep haustral indentations with little resemblance to the blown-up, distended appearance seen in Figure 12-3. Contrast the *continuously distended* and elongated colon you would expect in any obstructed flexible tubular structure.

198

Differentiating Large-Bowel and Small-Bowel Obstruction from Paralytic Ileus

I. *Too much air in either colon or small bowel, but none in the other*
   —is either:
   A. Small-bowel obstruction old enough to have allowed the colon to clear
      or
   B. Large-bowel obstruction with a competent (tight) ileocecal valve.

II. *Too much air in both parts of the bowel*
   —is one of the following:
   A. Paralytic ileus
   B. Large-bowel obstruction with an incompetent ileocecal valve, allowing the patient to decompress his distended colon backward into his small bowel
   C. Small-bowel obstruction which is—
      (1) Early (colon has not had time to clear)
         or
      (2) Intermittent (knuckle of small bowel caught from time to time in hernia or behind adhesion)

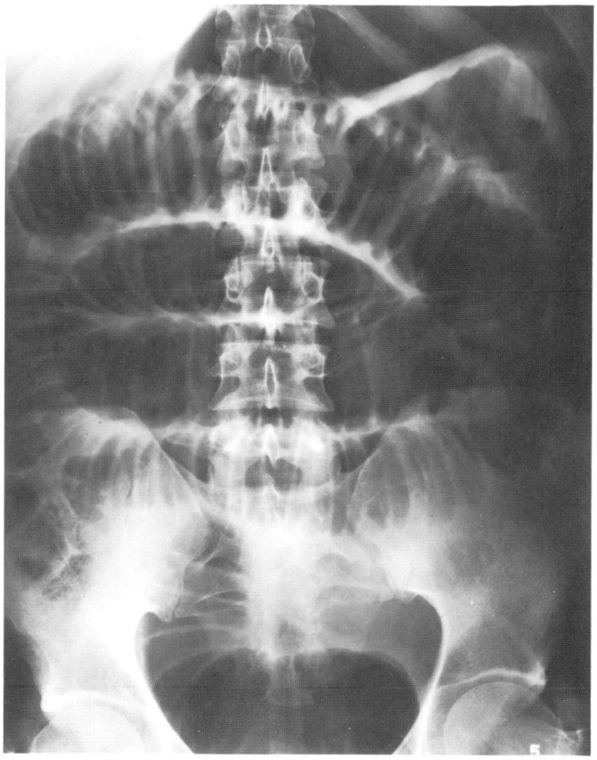

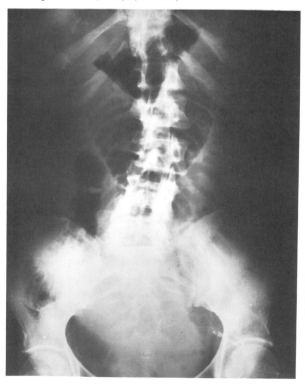

Large or Small Bowel? Mechanical Obstruction or Paralytic Ileus? Analyze Figures 12-11 and 12-12 before you read on.

When a patient is admitted with abdominal pain and his initial plain film shows both large and small bowel to be distended, the findings are equivocal, as we have said, in that they may represent either paralytic ileus or an early or intermittent mechanical obstruction. The activity of the bowel sounds, repeatedly observed over a period of time, may or may not clarify the issue. *Serial films* may show changes in the radiologic findings which provide helpful clues, however.

The small intestine always contains fluid, and when obstructed or paralyzed it accumulates additional fluid and air. On the erect plain film (Figure 12-13) the air-fluid interfaces inside distended loops of gut will appear as fluid levels, varying in length according to their size and the relative quantities of air and fluid within them. Loops entirely filled with fluid will cast ill-defined gray shadows; loops with little fluid and a great deal of air will appear on the supine film like those in Figure 12-11. Loops three-quarters full of fluid and containing a relatively small amount of air may be very deceptive, since in the erect or decubitus films they will show short fluid levels (Figure 12-14) and in the supine plain film rather unimpressive bubbles of air superimposed on the indefinite gray of the fluid (Figure 12-12).

Note that Figure 12-14 is the decubitus film on the woman in Figure 12-12. You can appreciate the fact that such a patient may not have a very startling initial plain film, and yet be sicker and in a more advanced stage of obstruction than the patient in Figure 12-11. Always remember that a plain film with obstructed, fluid-filled loops with relatively little air may indicate that your patient is dehydrated and in marked electrolyte imbalance. The patient in Figures 12-12 and 12-14 had late small-bowel obstruction from an adhesion near the ileocecal valve and marked electrolyte imbalance. She died on the table during what would have been, earlier, a very simple surgical procedure.

Figure 12-11 (*above*). (See text.)

Figure 12-12 (*below*). (See text.)

200

Except in rare cases the use of erect films of the abdomen has not proven to be of significant value in differentiating mechanical bowel obstruction from paralytic ileus. It is true that the height of the fluid levels will give you an idea of the caliber of a distended loop. The relative height of the levels, however, has proven unreliable in making the distinction between mechanical obstruction and paralytic ileus. Even normal persons with no abdominal symptoms at all may have fluid levels on erect films, since swallowed air and intestinal juices are always present.

A vital diagnosis which must not be overlooked in any patient with acute abdominal complaints is perforation of the bowel with free peritoneal air. This may be a complication of bowel obstruction. *The diagnosis of a small amount of free air cannot be made from the supine plain film* because the bubble of free air will float anteriorly under the abdominal wall and may look just like a loop of gut (if it is seen at all). On the erect film it is easy to identify free air interposed between the liver and the dome of the diaphragm, but patients who are this sick ought not to be asked to stand. On the *left-side-down decubitus film (made AP with a horizontal beam)* it is easy to identify free air between the right lobe of the liver and the lateral portion of the diaphragm. Further discussion of free air is to follow, but remember that *the diagnosis of intestinal obstruction as well as free air is a radiologic one.*

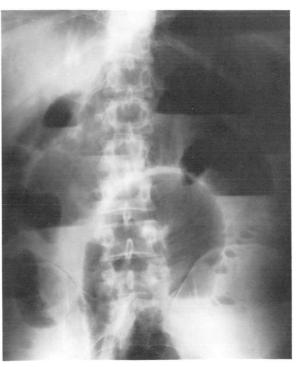

Figure 12-13. Air-fluid levels in obstructed small-bowel loops rarely help in differentiating obstruction from paralytic ileus. Levels are present in both conditions (and sometimes even in normal patients) on erect films.

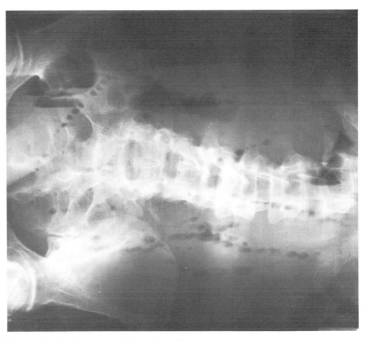

Figure 12-14. Left lateral decubitus film on the patient in Figure 12-12. Note the small bubbles of air caught against the valvulae conniventes of the obstructed small bowel, which is almost completely fluid filled.

Answers: Figure 12-11 is the plain film of a patient with small bowel obstruction showing air-filled, dilated jejunal loops and a cleared colon. Figure 12-12, by contrast, is also a plain film of a patient with small bowel obstruction, although here the air filling is minimal and all lower jejunal loops are fluid filled.

201

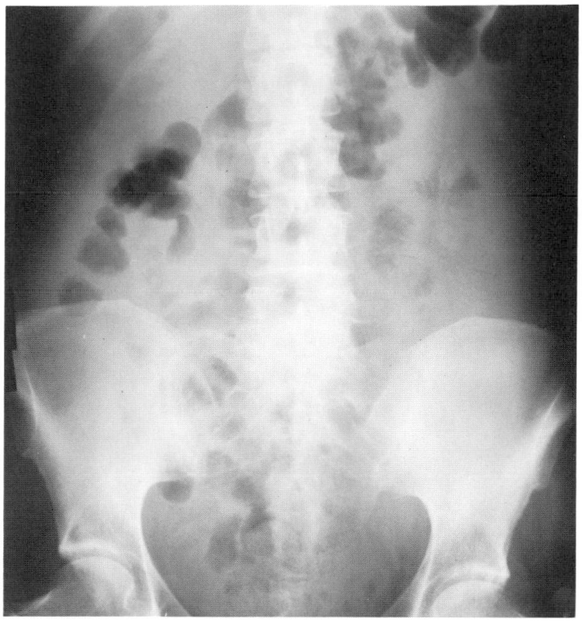

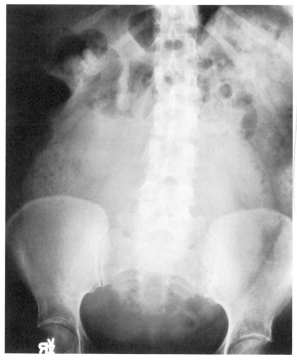

Figure 12-15. Ascites. Generalized opacity from free fluid. Since the patient is supine, loops of air containing small and large bowel float centrally under the anterior abdominal wall.

Figure 12-16. Is this ascites?

Free Peritoneal Fluid

Now direct your attention to the *general density* of the plain film. To state the oversimplified extremes first, as usual: large amounts of *free air* in the peritoneal space will increase the radiolucency of the abdomen, just as you would expect, and the film will look darker. Large amounts of *free fluid* will add to the radiodensity of the abdomen and the film will appear grayer than usual. These statements are true for the conventional exposure techniques used for radiography of the abdomen. Remember too that if intestinal loops are filled with fluid, the effect is that of adding more thickness to the patient, and for the same exposure factors such a film will also be gray and indistinct.

When there is a small amount of fluid free in the peritoneal space, it will gravitate to the most dependent part of the peritoneal cavity, which in the supine patient is the bowl of the pelvis, as you see in the diagrams in Figures 12-17 and 12-18. Such relatively *small amounts of free fluid* probably often go unobserved, because we are more or less accustomed to seeing the pelvis filled with the density of a distended bladder. Even small amounts of peritoneal fluid can be detected at ultrasound, of course.

Larger quantities of peritoneal fluid will spill over into the abdominal cavity, flowing up the flanks on either side (Figure 12-19). Fluid collected in the flank displaces the colon medially away from the flank stripe (Figure 12-21), and with even greater accumulations air-filled loops of bowel float up under the anterior abdominal wall. They are seen on the supine plain film as a cluster of radiolucent shadows in the central abdomen surrounded by the uniform gray of the peritoneal fluid (Figure 12-15).

In sum, a large amount of free fluid (ascites) is easy to recognize on plain films, but CT and sonography can show smaller amounts of fluid to be present. Note the peritoneal fluid in the CT scan in Figure 12-20 bathing the liver in a patient with malignant ascites.

Figure 12-16 could not be ascites, since air-containing gut is displaced up and laterally toward the flanks by a round mass which proved to be a large uterine myoma.

202

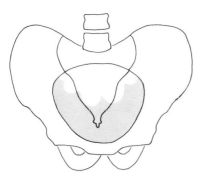

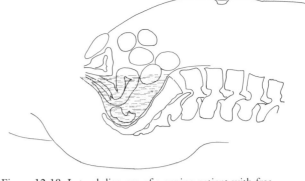

Figure 12-17. The half-moon of free fluid in the pelvis often engulfs the urinary bladder. The scalloped upper border results from loops of ileum dipping into fluid.

Figure 12-18. Lateral diagram of a supine patient with free peritoneal fluid accumulating in the most dependent part of the abdominal cavity.

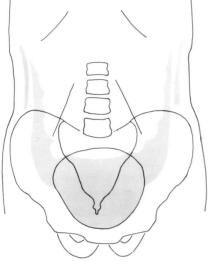

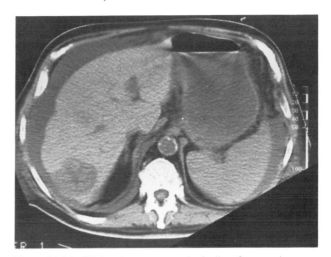

Figure 12-19. Increasing amounts of fluid flow into the flanks, displacing the colon medially as in Figure 12-21 below.

Figure 12-20. CT showing metastases in the liver from carcinoma of the colon. Note the ascitic fluid around the liver and spleen. The peritoneum was seeded with mestastases.

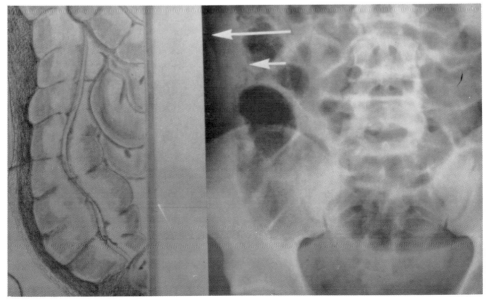

Figure 12-21. Liver rupture in this patient following trauma (automobile accident) resulted in slow bleeding, unsuspected at first. Note in diagram and supine plain film the interposition of fluid (blood in this case) between the flank stripe (*longer arrow*) and the medially displaced air in the colon (*shorter arrow*).

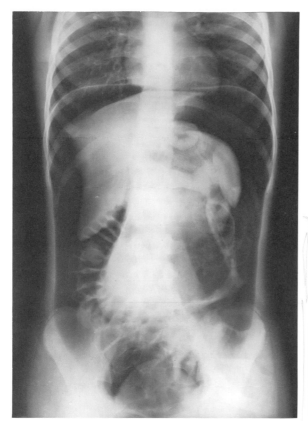

Figure 12-22. Free peritoneal air in large amounts after traumatic rupture of a viscus.

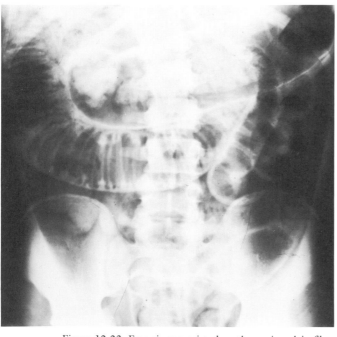

Figure 12-23. Free air appreciated on the supine plain film. Both the mucosal and serosal surfaces are seen outlined by air.

Free Peritoneal Air

A large amount of free peritoneal air strikingly outlines the organ masses of the liver and spleen, including their lateral and superior (diaphragmatic) surfaces (Figure 12-22).

Small amounts of free air may be quite as important to detect as larger amounts, for they occur most frequently with subtle or early perforation of a hollow viscus and could be missed on a routine plain film. A patient with these symptoms, if well enough to stand, will show crescents of radiolucent air interposed between his diaphragm and liver, and such a finding is occasionally first detected on an admission chest film.

The patient with a perforated viscus is often too ill to stand, however, and in any event ought not to be disturbed any more than is absolutely vital to a diagnosis. For this reason the search for free air is much more often carried out by placing the patient on his left side and radiographing him anteroposteriorly with a horizontal beam. This is called the *left lateral decubitus film* and will show even a small amount of free air lateral to the liver (Figure 12-26). *It is impossible to see small amounts of free air on a supine plain film.*

The horizontal beam can also be used in a patient too ill even to be turned on his side, as in Figure 12-24. The patient lies supine and is radiographed from side to side, a cassette being placed vertically against his flank. In this way air free against the underside of the anterior abdominal wall will be seen, even in small amounts. Figure 12-25 shows you such a horizontal-beam lateral film in a patient with a large amount of free air.

With much free air in the peritoneal space, *both the mucosal side and the serosal surface of the gut wall may be seen.* This is easy to imagine if you think of a large amount of free air into which protrude loops of air-filled bowel. *Both* sides of the wall of a loop of gut may also be seen on a regular supine plain film of the same patient (Figure 12-23). This phenomenon is not seen on a normal film.

Remember that on any of the films made with the horizontal beam (erect, left lateral decubitus, or cross-table lateral), the free air is apparent

204

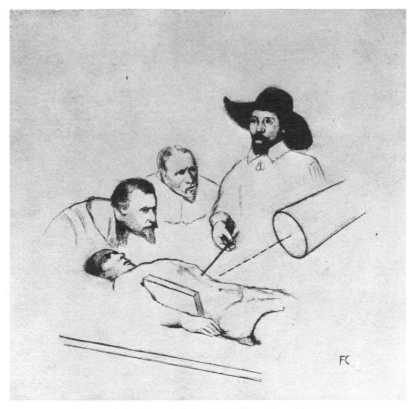

Figure 12-24. Lateral abdominal radiography with the patient supine (cross-table lateral). Dr. Tulp indicates the use of this projection to two eager residents.

because it lies against some structure not normally air-outlined (undersurface of diaphragm, lateral side of liver, anterior abdominal wall). Never forget that even a moderate amount of free air against the anterior abdominal wall cannot be recognized on the ordinary supine plain film made with a vertical beam, because the bubble of air will look just like another loop of gut. *Never request only a supine plain film to "rule out free air."*

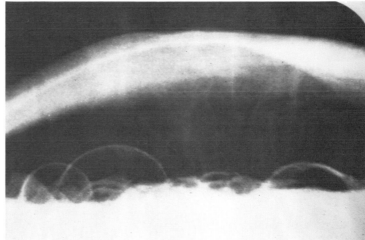

Figure 12-25. Horizontal-beam lateral radiograph made with the patient supine, as in Figure 12-24. The abundant quantity of free air under the abdominal wall outlines the serosal surface of the air-filled loops of the bowel.

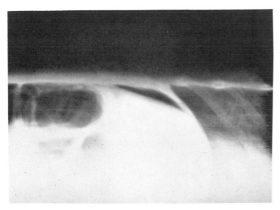

Figure 12-26. Left lateral decubitus film shows free air lateral to the liver in a patient suspected of perforated viscus, in this case a duodenal ulcer.

CHAPTER 13

Contrast Study of the
Gastrointestinal Tract

Figure 13-1. The stomach in a standing patient. Note the barium-air fluid level, peristaltic wave, pylorus (*black arrow*) and duodenojejunal junction (*white arrow*).

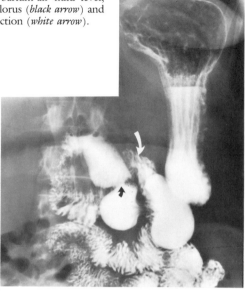

Principles of Barium Work

Diagnostic radiology is entirely based on contrasting the density of adjoining structures. Barium study of the GI tract involves the interpretation of shadows not only of whole barium sulfate fluid casts of hollow structures but also of the far more complex shadows of thin films of opaque substance caught against the mucosal irregularities of the inner surface of the gut. Such *mucosal relief studies,* as they are often called, are carried out with minimal amounts of opaque material, manipulated and spread over the surface of the clean mucosa during fluoroscopic study, *spot films* being obtained at frequent intervals by mechanically substituting a small cassette for the fluoroscopic screen.

In certain cases, and when considered desirable, the radiologist inflates the stomach or colon with air, a procedure termed a *double contrast study,* which may provide additional information, especially about superficial lesions. The technical expertise required by these procedures

and the judgment and experience needed for interpreting correctly the observed shadows constitutes one of the most sophisticated skills of the radiologist.

Nevertheless, the conclusions he draws are basically no less logical than everything else you have been learning to appreciate about the field, and in order to comprehend the reliability of the evidence offered by roentgen data obtained from barium studies, you should understand some of the fundamental implications of the various kinds of roentgen observations based on such procedures.

To that end, examine the hypothetical drawings in Figure 13-2. The gastrointestinal tract is essentially a tube, and the roentgen principles for examining it vary only in degree, even in the stomach, cecum, and rectum, where its tubular structure has been modified by nature. The simple tube in *A,* filled with an opaque substance and radiographed, would produce a shadow like the one you see in *a,* smooth bordered and uniformly dense. A polyp protruding into its lumen upon a stalk, like that in *B,* would produce a barium cast-shadow like the one in *b*. A solid tumor growing in its wall like that in *C,* and protruding into the lumen as a sessile growth, would produce a shadow like *c*.

Both of these alterations in the original normal tubular shadow are what are referred to as *filling defects*. A part of the expected luminal shadow has been subtracted, because barium has been displaced by radiolucent soft tissue.

The growth you see in *D* has entirely encircled the tubular structure being examined, so that a constriction of the lumen is produced. This is often called an *annular defect*. Whenever you see a barium shadow like the one in *d,* you ought to *reconstruct mentally* the rigid annular lesion which has produced it, supplying tumor or other soft tissue wherever the barium has been displaced. The abrupt and often angular change in the shadow where the normal luminal wall meets the margin of a tumor is frequently and aptly

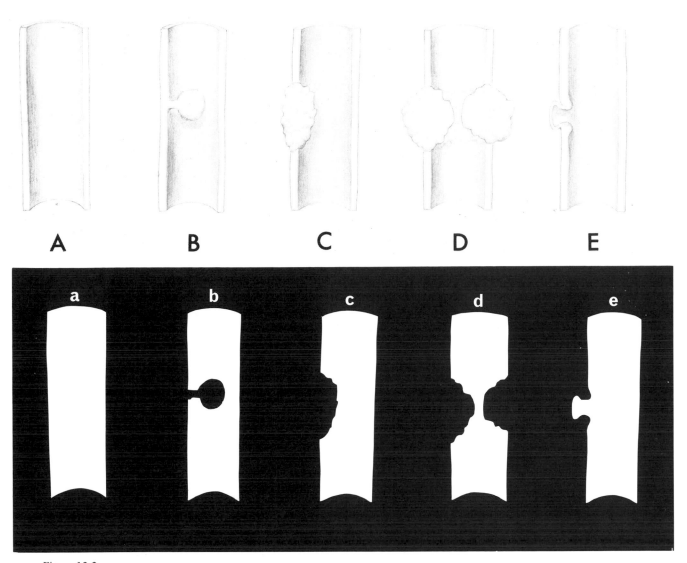

A   B   C   D   E

a   b   c   d   e

Figure 13-2

referred to as a *shelf* or *shoulder,* and its consistent appearance on film after film in the same location is to be interpreted as reliable evidence of rigidity of some sort in the otherwise distensible wall of the gut. *E* and *e* represent the appearance of a benign ulcer crater in the wall of the gut, which extends the luminal shadow and is surrounded by a *collar* of regenerating mucosa, seen in tangent about the neck of the crater.

You will find that a filling defect and its shelf-like margin are often so precisely the same from film to film in a series made during the barium study that they may be superimposed on each other over a bright light. If on two or more such films one can bring into perfect register the margin of a filling defect suspected of representing a malignant tumor, then the probabilities that it *is* a tumor are greatly enhanced. If, of course, two such films do not superimpose, it may mean either that the area in question is not rigid, and therefore changes slightly, or that the two films were made in different projections.

207

Normal Variation versus a Constant Filling Defect

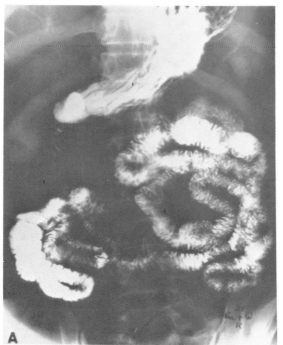

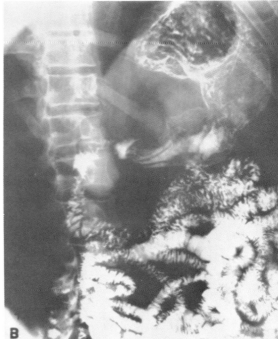

The variation of barium shadows within the gastrointestinal tract is well illustrated by these films made during an *upper GI series* with small-bowel follow-through (Figure 13-3). A, made prone half an hour after 10 ounces of barium suspension had been swallowed, shows the stomach nearly empty and the jejunum and upper ileum filled. B, made 15 minutes later in an oblique position, shows most of the small bowel filled, and C, made an hour after the administration of barium, shows the right colon filling. Transit time from stomach to right colon varies but is about 1.5 hours in a fasting normal patient. (Later on, the presence of barium in the hepatic flexure and transverse colon would interfere with refilming of the stomach and duodenum.) Cholecystography had been done that morning and the patient had continued to fast.

You may be inclined to reject the possibility of demonstrating any structure consistently in so changeable a barium pattern, but look carefully at Figure 13-4, two spot films of the stomach

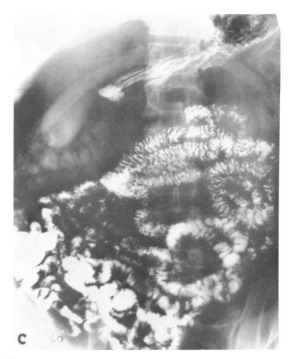

Figure 13-3. Normal upper gastrointestinal series, large films only. Smaller films made in several projections and spot films made during fluoroscopy would complete the series.

208

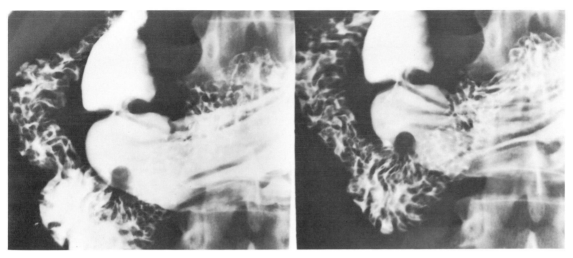

Figure 13-4. Can you spot the consistently present filling defect? (See text.)

and duodenum of a patient who had guaiac-positive stools. She had no hemorrhoids, negative findings on sigmoidoscopic and barium enema study, was not anemic, and enjoyed excellent health. (Answer later.)

If up to now barium studies have tended to confuse you, if you have wondered how any firm conclusions at all can ever be derived from them, this is the time to tell you that the assurance of his interpretations is possible to the radiologist largely because he has been able to demonstrate a finding *repeatedly*. No finding present on a single film only is worth very much, and the resident in training in radiology soon finds that positive diagnostic observations made from barium studies must be *consistently demonstrable* if they are to be believed. So variable and shifting are the shadows presented by opaque sub-

stances within the constantly changing gastrointestinal tract that only those consistently present should be taken seriously. A transient finding seen on only one film may represent an area of spasm, a peristaltic wave, or food. This is no less true for other spheres of roentgen investigation, to be sure—nor for that matter for other branches of medicine. Any single positive test, always negative thereafter, is unlikely to weigh much in the balance of evidence, and the principle is no different for the more complex investigative procedures.

(The small round filling defect near the pyloric canal on both spot films of the patient in Figure 13-4 was consistently present both at fluoroscopy and on films. At endoscopy it was found to be a benign polyp.)

The Components of the Upper GI Series

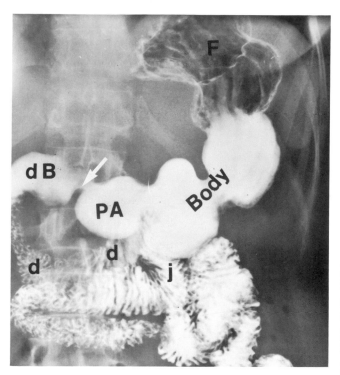

Figure 13-5. Prone film of barium-filled stomach with fundus (*F*), body, pyloric antrum (*PA*), pyloric canal (*arrow*), duodenal bulb (*dB*), C-loop of duodenum (*d*'s), and jejunum (*j*) identified.

The student who looks at radiographs of the barium-filled stomach for the first time often has some difficulty identifying the various parts of the stomach, in particular the pyloric canal, and this difficulty generally stems from the fact that each of the conventional views of the stomach is made in a different projection with the patient differently positioned.

The fluoroscopist usually begins with the patient standing, and examines the esophagus and stomach with a small amount of barium to study the mucosal relief pattern. Then he tilts the power-driven fluoroscopy table into the horizontal position and arranges the patient prone and turned slightly up on his right side. The patient drinks more barium (through a straw) and is turned into the lateral and then into the supine position. Spot films are made at intervals whenever the radiologist sees anything on the

screen he wishes to record. Next, large films are made by an x-ray technologist in a series of specified projections. These generally include one made straight prone, one prone but turned slightly to the right (the right anterior oblique), one made in a straight lateral projection with the patient on his right side, and one made supine with the patient rolled to the left slightly so as to fill the antrum of the stomach with air. The radiologist may elect to study the stomach by *air-barium double contrast* for certain suspected conditions. He does this by giving the patient effervescent materials with the barium.

Study the series of normal stomachs in various positions on this and the following pages. Note the varying shape of the stomach and of the duodenal bulb, as well as the deep indentations in both curvatures (peristaltic waves, which progress when seen at fluoroscopy). You can figure out the position of the patient and the projection of the film by noting (1) the appearance of the spine, and (2) the presence of barium or air in the fundus of the stomach. If the spine is seen to be *symmetrical* (pedicles on either side of the spinous process), then the film was made either AP or PA with the beam in the sagittal plane (frontal view). If the *bodies of the vertebrae* are seen completely separated from the complex posterior structures, you are looking at a *lateral view* and can see the anterior and posterior walls of the stomach. If the spine is seen with the complex posterior structures overlapping the posterior third of the body of the vertebra, you are looking at an oblique film. You can easily decide whether it is a prone oblique or a supine oblique film, because in any prone film the fundus will contain air, whereas in any supine film barium flows back into the more posterior fundus. Decide for each of the following films whether the patient was filmed prone, lateral, or supine, and whether the film is frontal, lateral, or oblique. The pylorus is located for you in each study by an *arrow*. You will find the answers at the bottom of page 213.

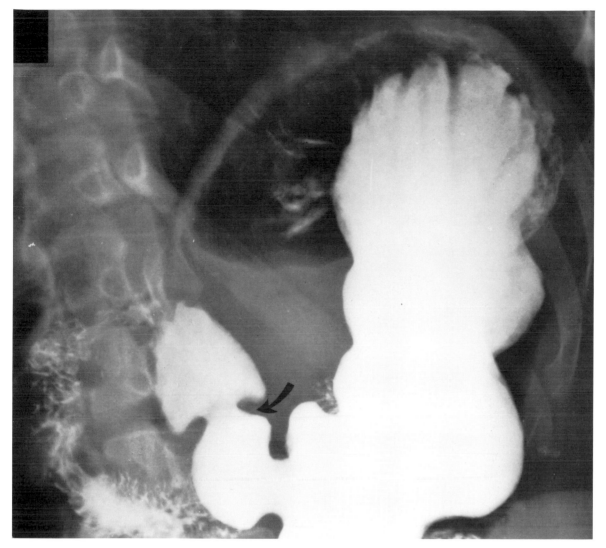

Figure 13-6

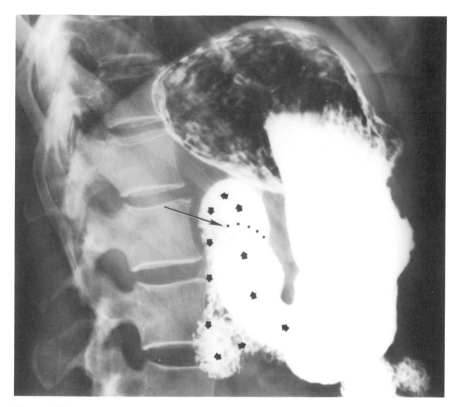

Figure 13-7

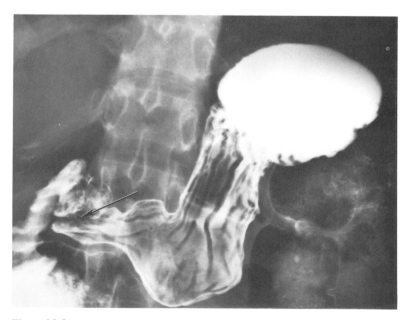

Figure 13-8

212

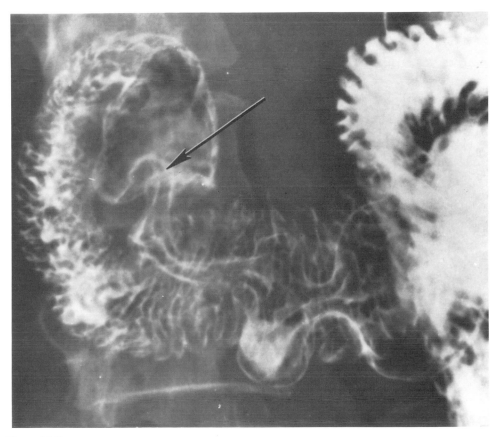

Figure 13-9

Answers

Figure 13-5 is a frontal prone film. Note air in the fundus.

Figure 13-6 is a right prone oblique film with air in the fundus (the highest part of the stomach in the prone patient). The pyloric canal (*arrow*) and the normal, nondeformed duodenal bulb are seen.

Figure 13-7 is a right lateral film. The spine is clearly seen in the lateral projection, the patient lying on his right side, air filling the high fundal bubble. Note that ulcer craters on the posterior gastric wall might be well seen in this view. The *long arrow* indicates the site of the pyloric canal; the *short arrows* indicate the direction of fluid flow.

Figure 13-8 is a supine film. Most of the barium has flowed back into the now-dependent fundus, and air is seen inflating the barium-coated body and pyloric antrum. The *arrow* indicates the pyloric canal.

Figure 13-9 is a detail view of a supine oblique. The patient is rolled up to the left, and air is flowing through to inflate the duodenal bulb. Again, the *arrow* indicates the pyloric canal.

213

Rigidity of the Wall

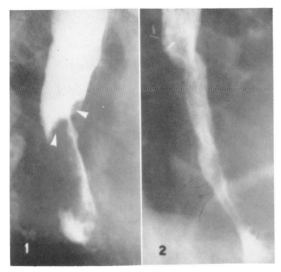

Figure 13-10. A patient with dysphagia. 1: Carcinoma of the esophagus narrowed the lumen to a tunnel a few millimeters wide and 10 centimeters in length, a rigid segment which never changed either at fluoroscopy or on the other films. *Arrows* indicate the tumor shelf. 2: Appearance after radiation therapy.

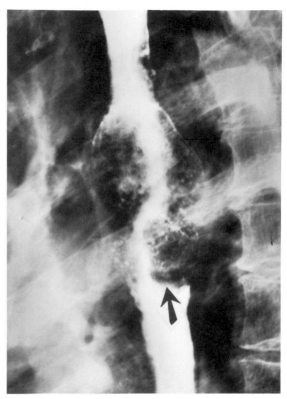

Figure 13-11. Another patient with carcinoma in the mid-esophagus. Note the irregular rigid lumen. *Arrow* indicates shelf of tumor.

In studying the gastrointestinal tract, the radiologist looks for a mucosal relief pattern which seems to him to be within normal limits of variation. He searches specifically for *ulcer crater niches* and *filling defects*. He then fills the succeeding parts of the gut with barium, testing their *distensibility* and looking for areas of *rigidity,* which may indicate even without any apparent ulceration that the wall is invaded by new growth or scarred by inflammation.

The recognition of an area of rigidity in the gut wall is more difficult in many ways than the recognition of a crater, because the wall of the gut varies so much from part to part normally and because early infiltration with sheets of tumor cells does not render the wall entirely rigid but rather limits its elasticity, much in the way that a sheet of rubber changes with age. If you can imagine a remarkably distensible organ like the stomach, into the wall of which has been set a piece of rubber which has lost some of its elasticity, you will have a fair idea of the behavior which can be expected from such a segment under the fluoroscope. Barium pushed against it will fail to produce quite the prompt bulging expected. Barium pushed upward into normal gut shows a marginal pattern of wrinkles or folds as the flexible wall is mechanically displaced; the rigid or infiltrated segment will fold sluggishly and less deeply. Peristalsis too will be altered, and as one watches the normal passage of ringlike constrictions along the organ, one sees that they are resisted by the suspicious segment, which indents less readily with the passage of the wave. Flexibility of the wall is limited by the infiltration of tumor cells, by edema, or by postinflammatory changes, as the case may be. Decisions with regard to the flexibility of gut wall, then, are based on the manner in which the stomach or intestine is seen to distend with barium, to respond to manipulation, and to contract physiologically.

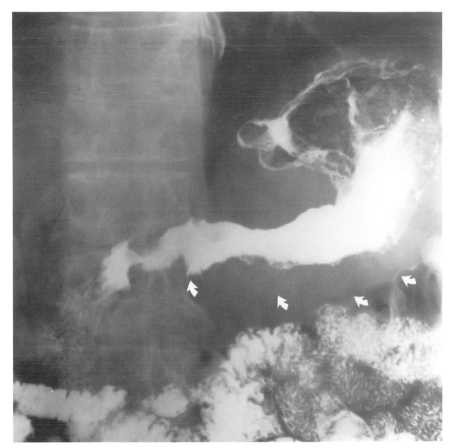

Figure 13-12. Barium study of a patient with advanced scirrhous carcinoma of the stomach (linitis plastica). *Arrows* indicate the thick tumor-invaded wall.

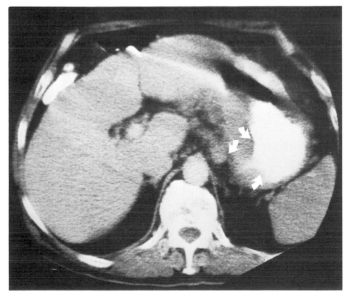

Figure 13-13. Same patient at CT. *Arrows* indicate the thick tumor-invaded wall of the stomach which is displacing barium.

215

Filling Defects and Intraluminal Masses

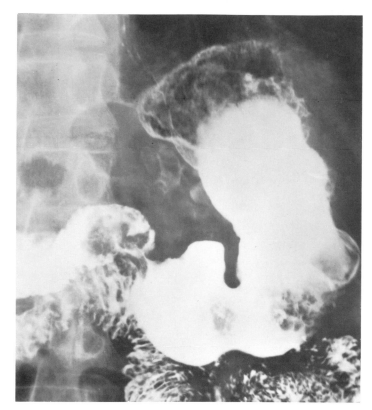

A

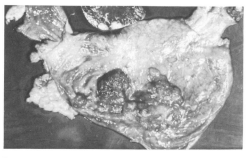

B

Figure 13-14. A (*left*): Filling defects along the greater curvature in a patient with "anemia." There is also a defect inside the duodenal bulb. The patient refused endoscopy. B (*above*): The open stomach at postmortem. Polypoid lesions along the greater curvature proved to be adenocarcinoma. There was also a larger carcinomatous polyp found prolapsed into the duodenal bulb.

Intraluminal masses, which you see illustrated on these pages, may take many forms. Polyps range in size from a millimeter to several centimeters (Figure 13-14). Polypoid tumors may fill the lumen of the gut (Figure 13-15). Barium passing between the tumor and the normally distensible wall of the gut will outline the tumor, showing the normal mucosal markings stretched over the tumor. These can often be seen as a double moulage, the one distinguishable from the other, like those in Figure 13-17, where the normal mucosa of the posterior or anterior wall is seen streaming across the coated lesser curvature tumor.

Intraluminal masses can sometimes be seen to be free floating in the barium, unattached to any wall. Occasionally, matted intraluminal masses are formed of foreign substances like hair or vegetable fibers, becoming too large to be passed and eventually causing symptoms. These are called bezoars (Figure 13-16) and are similar to the hair balls animals vomit. They can usually be differentiated from intraluminal soft-tissue masses because barium mixes with the matted

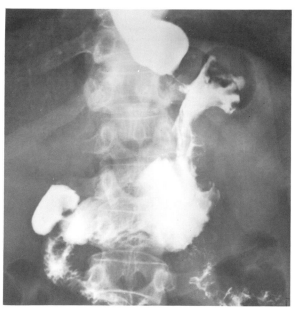

Figure 13-15. Constant, rigid filling defect in the upper part of the stomach. Note the infiltration of the cardia; the esophagus does not empty. At postmortem: adenocarcinoma, primary in the stomach.

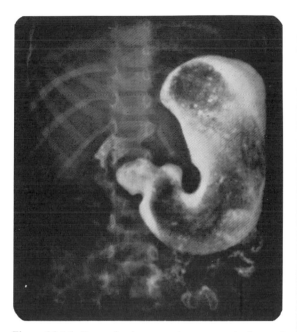

Figure 13-16. Bezoar in the stomach, composed of matted hair, in a little girl known to chew the ends of her pigtails.

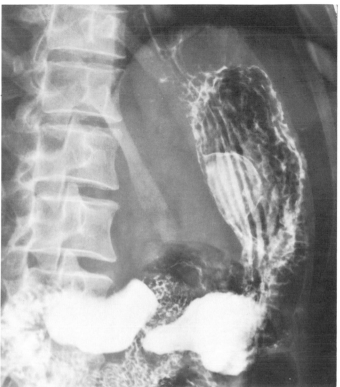

Figure 13-17. Benign tumor projecting into the lumen of the stomach from its sessile base high on the lesser curvature. The normal rugal folds either behind it or in front of it are seen outlined with barium.

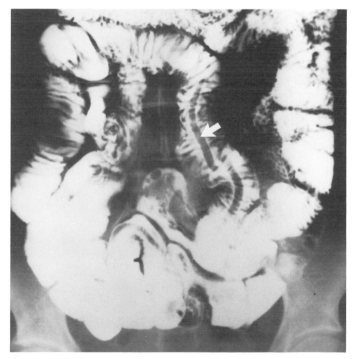

Figure 13-18. Ascaris infestation of small bowel. The worms are seen as long intraluminal filling defects (*arrow*) in the small bowel.

bezoar, giving an appearance quite different from tumor coated on the outside with barium.

Figure 13-18 shows another sort of intraluminal mass. You can see now why it is so vital to have the patient fast overnight before a gastrointestinal examination with barium: the mucosa must be perfectly clean and the lumen clear of food and feces.

From the teaching you have had about *endoscopy* you may wonder if it is really necessary for you to learn much about barium studies. As a matter of fact, endoscopy and radiographic examination of the gastrointestinal tract are *complementary*. Certain patients may benefit from a combination of these studies; others may need only one or the other. For example, the young patient suspected of having duodenal ulcer disease is usually diagnosed accurately with an upper GI series, which is quicker and more comfortable for him than endoscopy. On the other hand, in suspected acute gastritis causing hemorrhage, the patient is better studied by endoscopy because the subtle mucosal changes cannot be seen with barium. A barium enema would be the appropriate study for a patient with suspected low large-bowel mechanical obstruction, whereas the superficial lesions of early ulcerative colitis may be easier to detect by sigmoidoscopy. Remember too that the small bowel cannot be visualized endoscopically and *must* be studied with oral barium and a small-bowel follow-through.

Gastric Ulcer

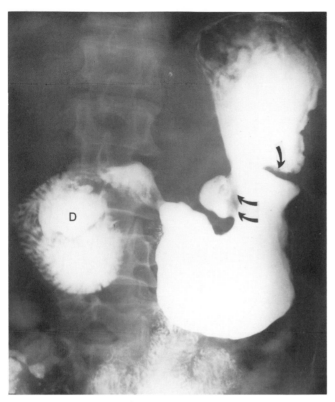

Figure 13-19. Large benign ulcer crater projecting from the midlesser curvature. Note the radiolucent collar of granulation tissue (Hampton's line, *twin arrows*) across the base of the ulcer. Upper *single arrow* indicates a partial constriction of the lumen by an area of spasm along the greater curvature in response to the large active ulcer. *D* is a diverticulum, arising from the medial wall of the descending limb of the duodenal loop.

In the last of the five hypothetical tubular structures in Figure 13-2 an ulceration has occurred in the wall of the tube, forming a small additional hollow space into which the opaque substance can flow. The term generally applied in radiologic parlance to this type of shadow is *niche,* and you will find that term used commonly in reference to the projecting shadow of a barium-filled ulcer crater in the esophagus, stomach, or duodenum. Only when seen in profile, of course, will it be a projection from the normal margin of the gut wall.

When a barium-filled crater is seen en face, it appears as a spot of white more dense than the surrounding shadow because it is frequently encircled by a rolled-up margin of granulation tissue. Ulcer craters which are filled with blood clot

or food particles at the time of examination with barium will not be visualized at all. As they heal, they fill in from the sides, becoming sharp and thorn-shaped in profile and finally disappearing altogether.

Because the tubular gastrointestinal tract is flexible, fills and empties in response to waves of peristalsis, and has opposing walls coated with barium, there are myriad small angular barium shadows in most of the films you examine. To find among them one which can with confidence be labeled a niche requires that it have certain characteristics. In the first place, a niche is deeper than most of the valleys between the folds of mucosa. Therefore its shadow will be *denser,* because it contains a slightly greater thickness of barium. Because it is an ulcer it will have no mucosal pattern, and because it is generally surrounded by inflammatory reaction it will be less flexible than the rest of the gut wall. The shadow of the niche accordingly will be *constant in shape and size.* It will be *consistently demonstrable* in the same place from film to film, and all these characteristics enable the radiologist to find and identify it in the course of his study.

There are numerous other details which help him in interpreting his findings. For example, when he observes that the nearby mucosal folds in the stomach *converge toward a demonstrable ulcer crater,* he may report that the ulcer is almost unquestionably benign, because in differentiating the two types of ulcer in the stomach, the *convergence of folds* has proven to be the most reliable indication of benignity.

You will hear much about the differentiation of benign and malignant ulcers in the stomach, and you will also find that a benign ulcer of long standing may be so embedded in scar tissue, so rigid, and so reluctant to heal on medical management that it is believed to be malignant by the referring physician, radiologist, and surgeon, and only the pathologist with his microscopic evidence can establish the fact that it is benign. Of course most patients with ulceration of this type should have endoscopic biopsy during the workup. The majority of benign gastric ulcers, however, *are* convincingly benign at upper GI series and do not require either endoscopy or biopsy.

Keep in mind that:

(1) Most gastric ulcers are benign (90 percent).
(2) Size and location of a gastric ulcer crater are *not* an index of malignancy. Convergence of folds, the shape of the crater, its projection beyond the stomach lumen, and its propensity to heal *are* reliable characteristics of benign ulcer craters.
(3) *Every* "benign" *gastric* ulcer must be followed by x-ray until it has disappeared because failure to heal may be a sign of *carcinoma in situ*. This does not apply at all to duodenal ulcers, which are uniformly benign and do not require either endoscopy or reexamination.
(4) There is no need to gastroscope the large number of gastric ulcers which are *convincingly benign* by x-ray. Only the problematic or clearly malignant ones or those that fail to heal require endoscopy and biopsy. Many physicians order endoscopy for patients who do not really require that procedure for diagnosis and management.
(5) Most acute upper GI bleeders stop bleeding spontaneously in 6 hours. Gastroscopy is certainly indicated if they do not, or if the probability that they are bleeding from varices or alcoholic gastritis is indicated by the history.

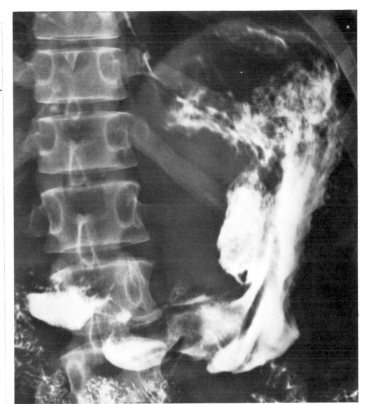

A

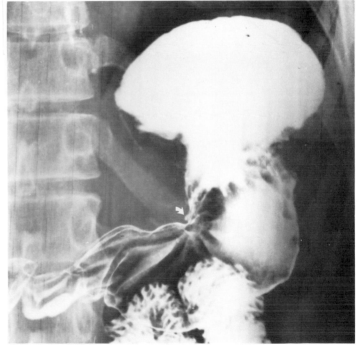

Figure 13-20. Natural history of healing in a large benign gastric ulcer. In B, a film made six weeks later than A, the healing thorn-shaped crater might easily be missed. The convergence of folds toward the small remaining crater reinforces its probable benign character.

B

219

The Clearly Malignant Ulcer

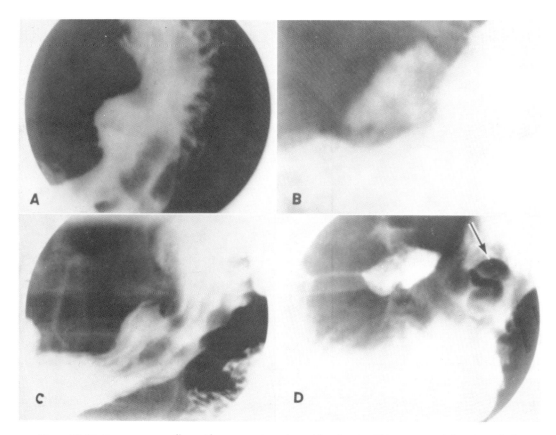

Figure 13-21. Four proven malignant lesser curvature ulcers. The ulcer is *within a mass*, and there is marked distortion and infiltration of the surrounding mucosa (D, *arrow*). All four would probably be labeled malignant by the radiologist, but should certainly have endoscopic biopsy.

Any radiologist would recognize the ulcer craters above as malignant. They do not project beyond the lumen but are ulcerations within a mass. Convergence of folds up to the margin of the crater is not present, and folds are irregularly interrupted by the surrounding tumor mass. Of course *these* patients should be endoscoped and biopsied so that the surgeon can plan his procedure and management.

Duodenal Ulcer

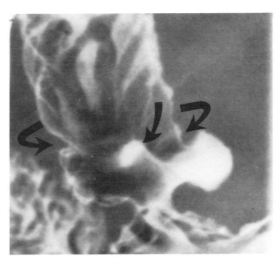

Figure 13-22. Classic location of a duodenal ulcer (*center arrow*) on the posterior wall, midcap. Note the indentation on the greater and lesser curvature sides of the cap (*bent arrows*), the beginning of scarring that will produce a typical cloverleaf deformity as the proximal and distal portions of the cap distend in response to constriction about the ulcer (prestenotic and poststenotic dilatation).

What is true about the identification of stomach ulcers is true about duodenal ulcer craters, in that they are consistently demonstrable collections of barium. In the duodenum, however, the problem is somewhat different, since instead of a wide sac the structure to be examined is a narrow tube with a bulb or ampulla at its commencement just distal to the pyloric canal. Although the crater itself is demonstrated in much the same way as it is in the stomach, still more important and informative in the long run are the changes due to scar tissue formation in this characteristically recurrent condition.

The most common location by far for the crater is in the center of the posterior wall of the bulb. Duodenal ulcer disease has a recurrent course and after several episodes of ulceration and healing, permanent strands of scar tissue develop, which constrict the lumen of the duodenal bulb and limit its free distensibility. These limiting bands of scar tissue produce distinctive changes in the shape of the shadow of the barium-filled bulb, so that its cavity seems to be divided into several cavities bulging outward from the central point at which the ulcer crater has been present or may still be seen. This appearance has been called the *cloverleaf deformity* of the duodenal bulb or cap (Figure 13-22).

This is only one of the scarring patterns in long-standing duodenal ulcer disease and is by no means present in all of the advanced cases you will see. Another common pattern of scarring is the gradual development of a stenosed apex of the cap, eventually producing a high degree of obstruction. Still other patterns of scarring may flatten one side of the bulb asymmetrically.

Several chapters could be written on the subject of duodenal ulcer disease, and you will gradually become familiar with the problems of diagnosing this entity. One very important point to remember is that in its early episodes a duodenal ulcer crater is quite easy to demonstrate with barium. After scar formation has become fairly well advanced, however, the crater itself becomes more and more difficult to visualize with each successive attack, and at length the radiologist will find it almost impossible to demonstrate the crater in spite of unquestioned reactivation suggested by the patient's symptoms. Of course, the permanent deformity does not change. For this reason *reexamination with barium is definitely not indicated with each new attack* in a patient with a well-established diagnosis of *duodenal ulcer disease,* made either from the presence of a crater or from typical scarring.

Once the diagnosis has been made, the clinician does well to be guided by the patient's symptoms alone. Only with a significant change in the patient's long-standing symptoms or with increasing evidence of obstruction need reexamination be carried out. Remember that the diagnosis can be made from either a crater or typical scarring, and that the patient needs to have the usually recurrent nature of the disease explained to him so that he will not seek reexamination with barium during each episode, thereby exposing himself needlessly to additional ionizing radiation.

Examples of Duodenal Ulcer Disease

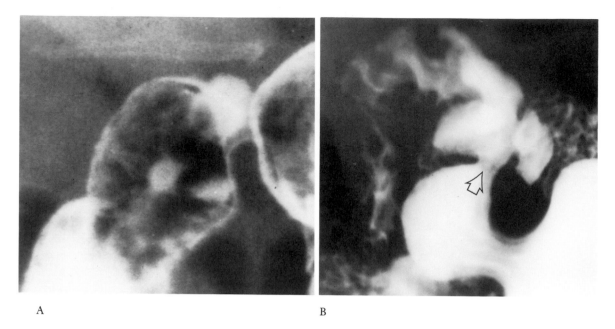

A   B

Figure 13-23. A: Duodenal ulcer crater in the classic location on the posterior wall in a patient radiographed supine with air filling the cap and, as yet, no deformity. B: Deformed cloverleaf cap. *Arrow* indicates the pylorus.

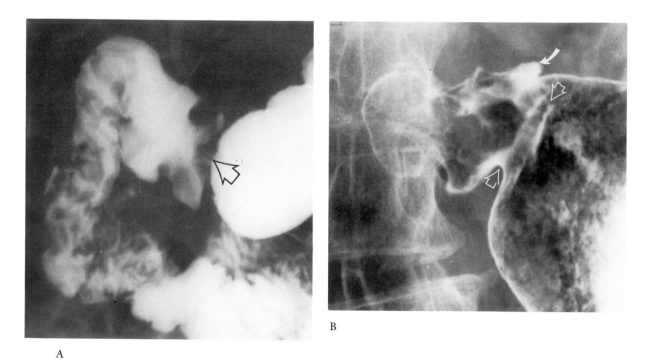

B

A

Figure 13-24. A: Cloverleaf deformity of the cap in duodenal ulcer disease, probably active, but a crater is not demonstrated. *Arrow* indicates the pylorus. B: Duodenal ulcer disease in a patient whose crater is located eccentrically just beyond the pylorus on the lesser curvature side of the cap (*curved arrow*). The wide, patulous pyloric canal is indicated by *open arrows*. Scarring has flattened the cap and resulted in the eccentric canal.

Figure 13-25. Large ulcer crater (*white arrow*) at the apex of the cap. Scarring produced by craters in this location is likely to lead to eventual obstruction. *Black arrow* indicates the pyloric canal.

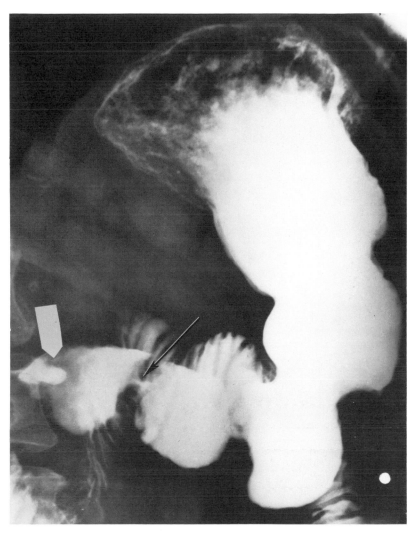

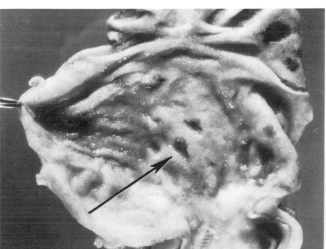

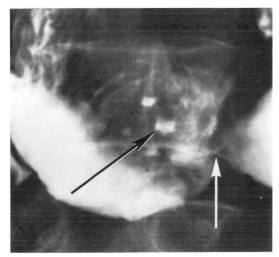

Figures 13-26 (*left*) and 13-27 (*right*). Surgical specimen and radiograph of a patient with multiple ulcer craters on the posterior wall of the duodenal bulb. *Black arrow* indicates the large central crater, around which the others are arranged in a circle. *White arrow* indicates the pyloric canal.

223

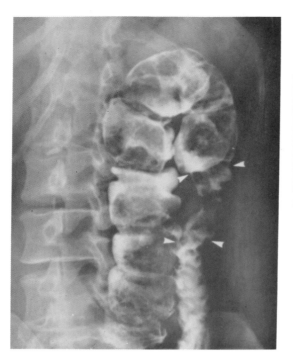

Figure 13-28. An annular area of narrowing just distal to the splenic flexure was constant on all films obtained during a barium enema. Note the evidence of low-grade obstruction in the relative dilatation of the transverse colon and splenic flexure, which contain scybala (fecal boluses) outlined by barium. The descending colon below the lesion shows the pattern expected after evacuation. Carcinoma was found at surgery.

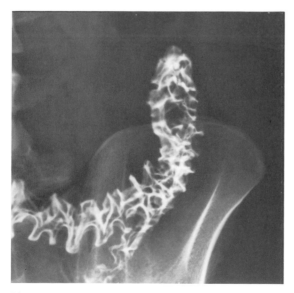

Figure 13-29. Normal empty splenic flexure after evacuation of barium enema.

224

The Barium Enema

The cecum and rectum, like the stomach, are expanded sections of the gut. They are difficult to examine and present special problems for the radiologist. The colon can only be examined properly after it has been thoroughly cleansed. This usually requires catharsis, although patients in whom catharsis is contraindicated may be studied after two days on a low-residue diet followed by two days on a liquid diet and cleansing enemas. The cecum should not be considered as seen in its entirety until there is retrograde filling of either the appendix or the terminal ileum. This is a vital point in patients with unexplained anemia, in whom carcinoma of the cecum must be ruled out.

Carcinoma of the rectum should be diagnosed by the clinician on physical examination and proctosigmoidoscopy. Because of the great distensibility of the rectal ampulla, the radiologist knows that it is easy for him to miss completely a sizable carcinoma in this location, obscured by the barium surrounding and concealing it.

During the conventional single-column barium enema patients are examined as the barium is being instilled by gravity into the rectum, sigmoid, descending colon, transverse and ascending colon and cecum. In the supine position the flexures are studied in various degrees of obliquity. When the colon is filled, multiple overhead films are obtained. Then the patient is allowed to evacuate the barium, after which a prone film is made to show the emptied large bowel and its mucosal relief pattern.

The radiologist, searching for intraluminal tumor masses in the colon, may allow the patient to evacuate most of the barium and then insufflate the colon with air so that a *postevacuation air-fill study* can be filmed. Or he may elect to use the *double contrast method* from the start of the examination, instilling a small amount of barium and then air as needed. A double contrast study is especially useful in identifying small polyps and mucosal lesions. In planning the workup of your patient you may wish to discuss with the radiologist the advisability of the barium enema or colonoscopy or both, and in what order.

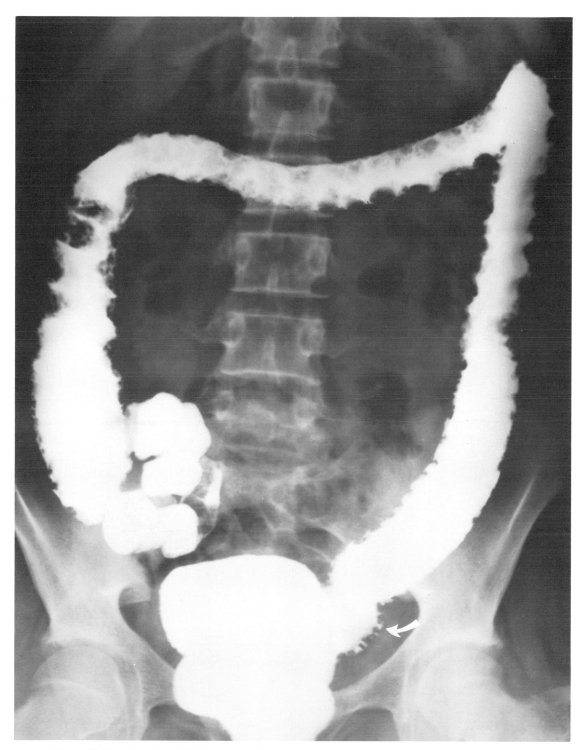

Figure 13-30. Ulcerative colitis in a young boy. Here ulceration is seen from cecum to rectum. *Arrow* indicates the classic "collar button" shape of ulcer. Note also that there is shortening of the colon (straightened flexures), loss of normal haustral markings, nodular indentations (pseudopolyps), reflux into the terminal ileum, and that the cecum is much smaller than normal because of scarring.

Filling Defects and Intraluminal Masses in the Colon

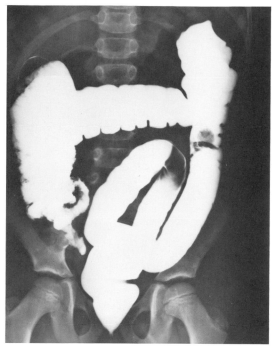

A

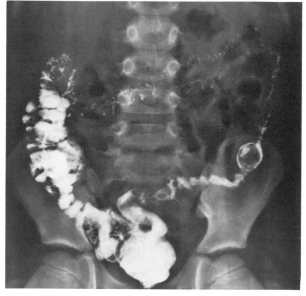

B

Figure 13-31. Polyp in the descending colon in a boy with bloody stools and crampy left abdominal pain. Note that the polyp is seen demonstrated in three different ways, always in the same location. In A it is seen as a radiolucent filling defect in the opaque barium column. In B, after evacuation, the polyp is seen because it prevents collapse of the barium-coated walls of the colon, as is seen above and below it. In C the polyp, coated with opaque material, is seen outlined by air.

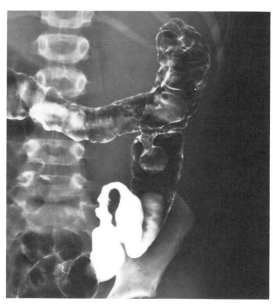

C

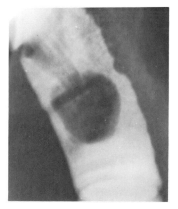

Figure 13-32. Polyps within the colon may be demonstrated as radiolucent filling defects displacing the contrast substance. Note stalk, which is well seen in this patient.

226

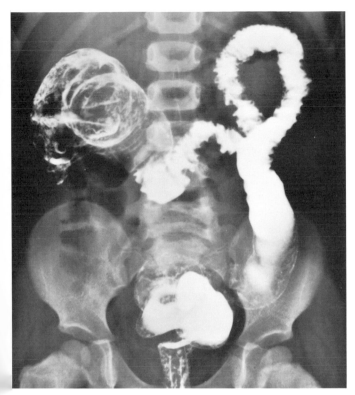

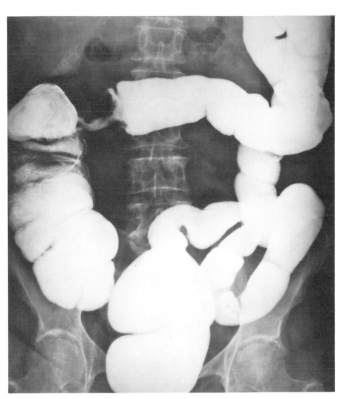

Figure 13-33. Intussusception. The intraluminal mass at the hepatic flexure is composed of the patient's own cecum and terminal ileum telescoped inside the colon by forceful peristalsis. Early in the illness intussusception may often be reduced by barium enema without manipulation. When it is reduced, the normal anatomical relationships will be seen.

Figure 13-34. The constant annular lesion near the hepatic flexure proved to be a carcinoma, as expected.

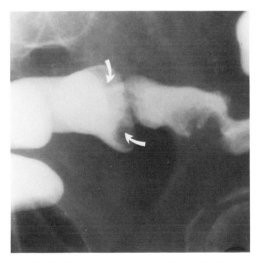

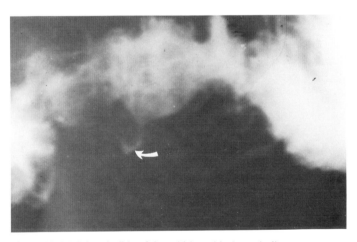

Figure 13-35. Carcinoma of the midsigmoid. The normal sigmoid suddenly showed an annular constriction which was rigid and identical in all films. *Arrows* indicate the tumor shelf.

Figure 13-36. Diverticulitis of the midsigmoid. *Arrow* indicates barium extravasation into the middle of an intramural abscess on the inferior wall of the sigmoid. Contrast the uninterrupted mucosal markings with the absence of mucosal pattern in the carcinoma in Figure 13-35.

227

The Sigmoid Colon

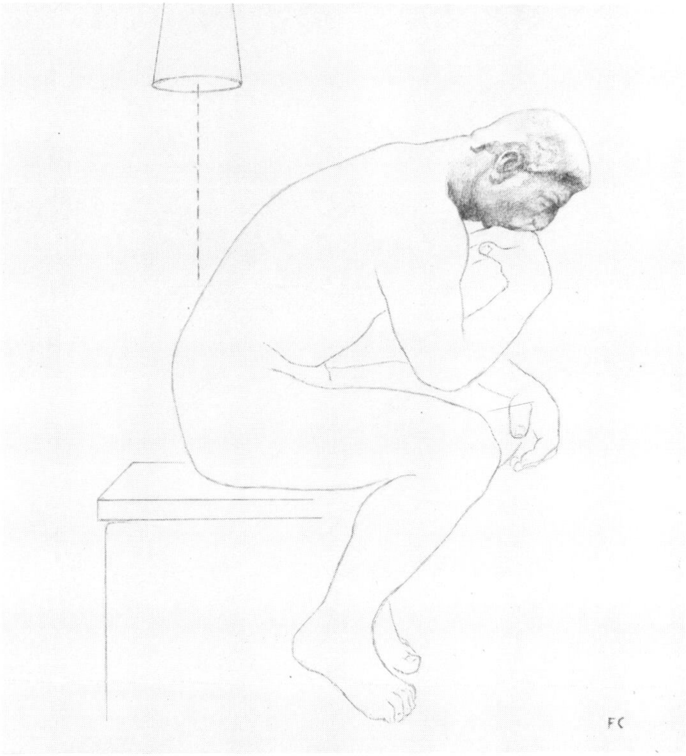

The rectosigmoid colon, because of its great redundancy and overlap in the pelvis, is very difficult to "unroll" and therefore to visualize in every part. A number of ingenious maneuvers have been designed to help locate malignant lesions in the sigmoid. Patients have been examined head down at a sharp incline on a table, so that the loops of bowel are pulled up out of the pelvis by their own heavy barium content and the sigmoid is straightened. Patients are routinely examined in oblique projections and laterally, and many radiologists use a view in which the central ray is directed obliquely caudad in the sagittal plane in a prone patient. The patient may also be examined sitting up, the ray directed downward through the back, as in Figure 13-37. New projections are constantly being evolved for the better visualization of opaque-filled structures. The cooperation of the patient makes a great deal of difference in the success of these procedures. For this reason it seems to us that it ought to be a rule with physicians to explain to the patient briefly beforehand approximately what is going to be done.

Figure 13-37. A special position in which the patient may be examined in order to unroll the sigmoid colon and reveal abnormalities concealed by its usual redundancy.

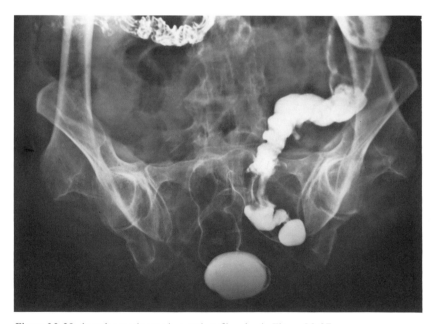

Figure 13-38. Annular carcinoma in a patient filmed as in Figure 13-37. The lesion was not seen on routine barium enema.

Contraindications to Barium Studies

Some contrast studies are virtually harmless; others have well-recognized contraindications. So many studies incur little risk and minimal discomfort and have become so routinely a part of the diagnostic plan, however, that perhaps too few physicians could list half a dozen conditions in which a gastrointestinal series or a barium enema, for example, should *not* be carried out, or in which it would be better to postpone the procedure and the preparation for it. Barium sulfate in water suspension is itself inert, and none of it is absorbed during its passage through the gastrointestinal tract; but almost any such study involves the taking of numerous films and perhaps repeated fluoroscopic inspections over a period of several hours. The process is fatiguing for the patient, particularly for one who is acutely ill. The anxiety of the patient is always a vital part of the hazard of the procedure. Such anxiety is allayed to an appreciable extent by intelligent preparation: a referring physician, if he will take the time, can always explain in advance a little about the procedure.

The patient suspected of having a recent myocardial infarction should *not* be sent to the radiology department prematurely for an extended and fatiguing procedure, and the patient with symptoms suggesting any kind of large-bowel obstruction should *not* be given barium by mouth, as it becomes dehydrated in the colon. Furthermore, the preparation of the patient for a colon study requires thorough cleansing of the bowel, usually by catharsis and cleansing enemas, and such measures would sometimes be contraindicated clinically in the debilitated, elderly, dehydrated patient, or the patient in severe electrolyte imbalance.

In sum, then, the complex barium contrast study should not be requisitioned without consideration of the entire clinical problem, nor should it be undertaken when the patient is not in reasonably safe condition to undergo it. You would do well to observe one example of each of the major investigative procedures for yourself, so that you will understand not only what it may require of your patient in terms of energy, stamina, and patience, but also the degree to which his cooperation may be required for the success of the procedure. A patient who is paralyzed will not be able to stand for certain parts of a gastrointestinal examination which are usually carried out in that position. A patient who speaks no English will be particularly difficult to examine; he must hold his breath on command during the exposure of films, and if he does not understand and continues to breathe, the films obtained will often be valueless. Obviously, this kind of difficulty may be prevented by your discussing the procedure with the radiologist before it is carried out. *If intelligent consideration for the patient is the primary concern of both radiologist and referring physician, undesirable developments resulting from any sort of procedure will be kept to a minimum.* (Needless to say, this applies no more to radiology than to any other branch of medicine.)

CHAPTER 14 Imaging the Abdominal Organs

In this chapter we shall study techniques for imaging the individual organs of the peritoneal cavity and retroperitoneum. The chapter is subdivided by organ system, and the most common disease conditions requiring diagnostic imaging are discussed. The indications for performing various imaging examinations will be reviewed and many examples shown.

Today such a wide variety of techniques is available for imaging the abdomen that it is often difficult for the young physician to decide which is most appropriate for a given clinical problem. It is our hope that this chapter will provide some initial direction. Of course, our comments apply to current recommendations; with the passage of time imaging technologies will change. Certain examinations may increase or decrease in popularity, and new ones will become available. For example, in the future magnetic-resonance scanning may replace computed tomography for the diagnosis of many abdominal conditions.

If on completion of this chapter you feel somewhat lacking in confidence in planning certain imaging algorithms, remember that consultation with the radiologist is always possible and will prove useful to you in the selection of imaging examinations for your patients.

The Liver

The liver can be imaged with a variety of techniques including plain films, ultrasound, radioisotope scan, computed tomography, magnetic-resonance scan, and angiography. You have already seen the liver shadow on plain films. The determination of hepatomegaly on plain films, however, is generally unreliable and can be made with certainty only when the liver is massively enlarged. Plain films may show liver calcifications and air within the biliary tree or abscesses; they will not show soft-tissue abnormalities such as fluid-filled cysts and liver tumors.

Ultrasound can easily diagnose dilated bile ducts in patients with obstructive jaundice, as well as cysts, abscesses, and tumors, which appear as focal areas of decreased or increased echogenicity. But the detail is less than with CT, the accuracy of diagnosis varies with the skill of the operator, and some anatomic portions of the liver are difficult to evaluate with ultrasound.

A radioisotope liver scan is performed after an intravenous injection of a radioisotope-labeled sulfur colloid (usually technetium). The colloid particles are phagocytized by the reticuloendothelial (Kuppfer's) cells of the liver and spleen, and then imaged with a gamma camera. A normal liver scan is shown in Figure 14-1. Cysts, abscesses, and tumors which displace the normal reticuloendothelial system will appear as "cold spots" (focal areas of diminished or absent radioactivity) on isotope liver scans. Unfortunately, small lesions, especially those 1 centimeter in diameter or less, may be overlooked.

At present, CT with intravenous contrast material is the procedure of choice for examining the liver parenchyma. It can identify a wide range of hepatic pathology with excellent detail. In the future magnetic-resonance scanning will no doubt assume an important role in the diagnosis of hepatic disease. Today hepatic angiography is reserved primarily for those patients who need detailed evaluation of their hepatic vasculature, including the portal venous system.

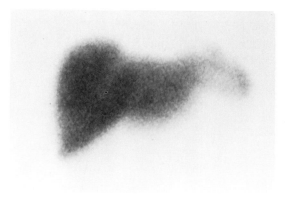

Figure 14-1. Normal radioisotope liver scan.

230

Liver Metastases

You may wish to examine the liver for possible metastases in a patient with a recently diagnosed primary cancer which is known to spread to the liver. (The most common arise from the lung, breast, colon, rectum, stomach, and pancreas.) Approximately 30 percent of patients with liver metastases have normal liver chemistries at the time of initial staging; therefore, imaging the liver should not be neglected if the laboratory values are normal. In addition, you may image the liver in a patient with known metastatic disease in whom you wish to reevaluate the liver after therapy.

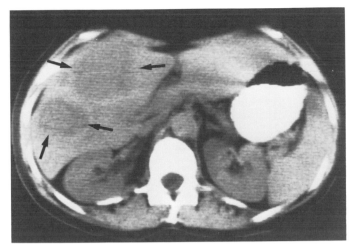

A

CT with intravenous contrast material is presently the most accurate, readily available technique for identifying liver metastases. Both large and small lesions can be recognized and their location pinpointed. The entire liver can be evaluated in a single examination. The remainder of the abdomen is also shown, and not only may extrahepatic metastatic sites be seen, but the primary tumor may be shown as well.

Metastatic tumors are generally of lower CT density than the surrounding contrast-enhanced hepatic parenchyma (Figure 14-2A). They are less well circumscribed than liver cysts and a measure of their CT attenuation would show it to be much higher than that of cysts (you will remember that the density of cysts is similar to that of water). Also, CT can usually determine by location and size whether a single metastatic tumor is amenable to surgical resection.

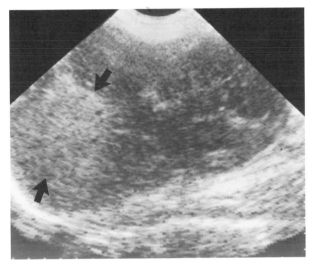

B

Ultrasound can show large metastases in portions of the liver which are easily examined by this technique. Generally they are echogenic as compared with normal liver parenchyma (Figure 14-2B) and are not echolucent like liver cysts. As with the radioisotope liver scan, small metastases, especially those less than 1–2 centimeters in diameter, will be overlooked by ultrasound. Ultrasound and nuclear medicine scanning (Figure 14-2C) are used primarily for follow-up of known metastases which are large enough to be seen on these two examinations.

Figure 14-2. Liver metastases as they appear on three different imaging modalities (same patient with metastatic colon cancer). A: Low-density areas at CT (*arrows*). B: Echogenic mass at ultrasound (*arrows*). C: Focal areas of decreased isotope uptake on liver scan.

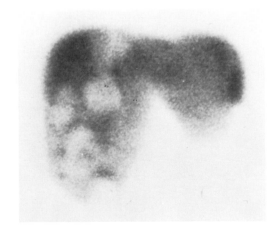

C

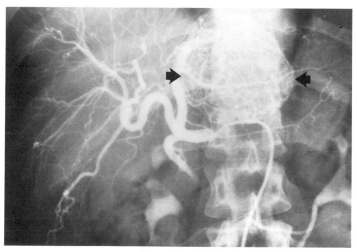

A

B

Figure 14-3. Benign hepatic adenoma in a 36-year-old woman. A: CT scan shows a hypervascular left lobe of liver mass (*arrow*). B: Hepatic arteriogram confirms a hypervascular mass (*arrows*) with tumor vasculature.

Primary Tumors of the Liver

Primary tumors of the liver often present with right upper quadrant pain; a mass or hepatomegaly may be detected on physical examination. Liver chemistries may be normal or abnormal. Benign tumors such as hepatic adenoma and focal nodular hyperplasia are more common in young and middle-aged women who have been taking birth control pills or hormonal replacement therapy. Hepatocellular carcinoma, or hepatoma, is more common in cirrhotic patients.

At ultrasound, primary tumors will appear as echogenic masses, distinguishing them from cysts. On radioisotope liver scans, most appear as cold spots, the exception being a benign tumor such as focal nodular hyperplasia which contains functioning Kuppfer's cells that concentrate isotope. CT with intravenous contrast material is the procedure of choice for imaging liver tumors. Most will appear as solid masses having less CT density than the surrounding liver parenchyma. Hypervascular tumors, however, may show increased CT density. Liver tumors tend to have ill-defined margins and sometimes necrotic centers and calcification. CT accurately localizes tumors within the liver, usually making it possible to determine whether resection is possible or not. Preoperatively, hepatic angiography is also performed to delineate the major hepatic arteries and veins. If certain major vascular structures such as the portal vein or inferior vena cava are encased, resection may not be possible.

Figure 14-3 shows the CT examination and the hepatic arteriogram of a 36-year-old woman with a benign hepatic adenoma of the left lobe of the liver. It is hypervascular on both examinations. Compare the bizarre arterial pattern within the tumor with the normal arteries in the right liver lobe. This pattern is typical of "tumor vasculature."

Figure 14-4 shows the liver scan, CT, and arteriogram of a 58-year-old man with a hepatoma of the left lobe. Note the large, round cold spot between the right lobe and the spleen on the radioisotope scan. At CT the mass has less density than the surrounding parenchyma. And, as predicted by the CT scan, the mass is shown to be "hypovascular" on the late phase of a celiac arteriogram.

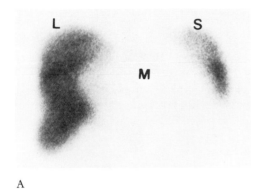

A

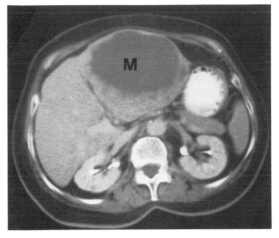

B

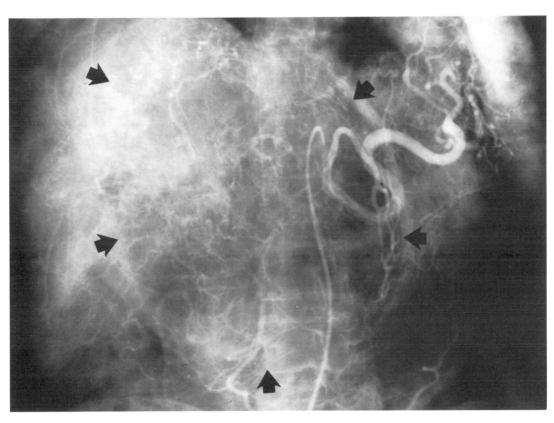

C

Figure 14-4. Hepatoma of the left lobe of the liver. A: Isotope scan shows a large area of absent uptake (*M*) between the right lobe of the liver (*L*) and the spleen (*S*). B: CT demonstrates a large, low-attenuation mass in the left lobe. C: Celiac arteriogram confirms a large hypovascular mass (*arrows*) in the left lobe of the liver.

233

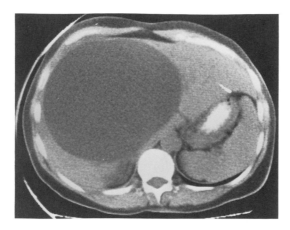

Figure 14-5. Enormous fluid-filled liver cyst. It proved to be an echinococcal cyst in a patient who had just completed a long journey around the world.

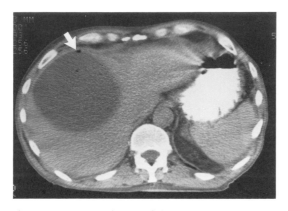

Figure 14-6. Large abscess of the right liver lobe. *Arrow* points to a dot of gas produced by the responsible gram-negative organism.

Figure 14-7. The five steps involved in percutaneous needle aspiration and catheter drainage of a hepatic abscess. A: Localization needle positioned in center of abscess. B: Percutaneous placement of a small caliber catheter within the abscess. C: Heavy-duty exchange wire inserted through catheter; localization needle removed. D: Small caliber catheter replaced with large caliber drainage catheter over exchange wire. E: Wire removed; patient ready for abscess drainage.

Hepatic Cyst and Abscess

Two nonneoplastic liver masses which may be easily diagnosed with cross-sectional imaging techniques are hepatic cysts and abscesses. Both may present with right upper quadrant pain, and a mass or hepatomegaly may be detected on physical examination. Patients with abscesses, having signs of fever and septicemia, usually appear sicker than those with cysts.

On radioisotope liver scans, cysts and abscesses appear as focal cold areas, and they may be single or multiple. Liver scans cannot differentiate cysts from abscesses, or either from liver tumors. At ultrasound a hepatic cyst appears as a sharply defined round mass which is echo free compared to the normal echogenic liver parenchyma. A liver abscess may be echo free or echogenic depending on the density and consistency of fluid within the abscess. Its outline may or may not be spherical.

The best imaging technique for diagnosing liver cysts and abscesses is CT. Both will be less dense at CT than the normal hepatic parenchyma. Cysts will look similar to their appearance in other organs, with a sharply defined margin and spherical shape (Figure 14-5). Abscesses may look similar to cysts, but they will be correctly identified if the CT scan also shows collections of gas (Figure 14-6), produced by gasforming organisms. Hepatic abscesses may also vary from a spherical shape.

When no gas is seen and an abscess is suspected in a liver lesion that appears to be a cyst at CT, then percutaneous needle aspiration is performed (Figure 14-7A). If an abscess is confirmed, it may be drained percutaneously, under CT guidance, using a series of needles, exchange wires, and catheters, until a suitably large drainage catheter has been placed (Figures 14-7B to E).

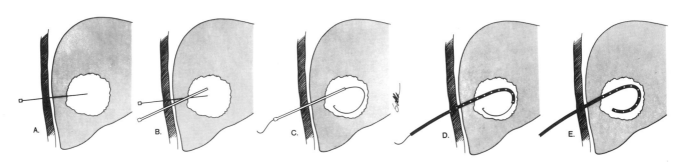

Liver Trauma

The liver may be injured by either blunt or penetrating trauma. The former is common in motor-vehicle accidents and falls; the latter in stab wounds, gunshot injuries, and hemorrhagic complications of liver biopsy. When serious liver trauma is apparent clinically, and the patient is bleeding rapidly and unstable, he should be taken directly to the operating room. If necessary to confirm the need for laparotomy in an unstable patient, a peritoneal lavage examination will quickly determine the presence of hemoperitoneum. *An unstable trauma patient should not be taken to the radiology department for a diagnostic procedure.*

Diagnostic imaging of a suspected hepatic injury is indicated when the patient can be stabilized and the diagnosis is in doubt. CT is the procedure of choice. It can detect hepatic injuries with a high degree of accuracy and also determine whether hemoperitoneum is present. A small intrahepatic hematoma which remains within an intact liver capsule and does not bleed into the peritoneal cavity can often be treated conservatively, without surgery. Follow-up CT exams can be performed to assess healing.

An *intrahepatic hematoma* (Figure 14-8) resulting from an intrahepatic laceration often has a stellate configuration. This injury is common with blunt trauma. A *subcapsular hematoma* (Figure 14-9) appears as a crescent-shaped mass immediately below the liver capsule. It is often the result of penetrating injuries. CT for suspected abdominal trauma is performed with intravenous contrast medium to better show lacerations and hematomas. The normal hepatic parenchyma will be enhanced with contrast medium, but the hematoma will not. Consequently, at CT hematomas appear less dense than the surrounding hepatic parenchyma. Occasionally emergency angiography may be indicated in the liver trauma patient when a bleeding injury is more amenable to angiographic embolization than to surgery.

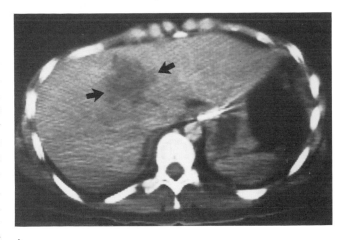

A

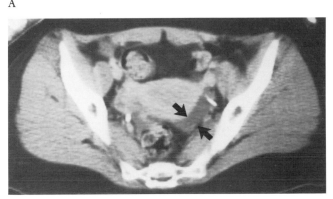

B

Figure 14-8. Hepatic laceration after blunt trauma. A: CT reveals a low-density intrahepatic hematoma (*arrows*) within a stellate liver laceration. B: A lower CT scan through the pelvis shows free blood (hemoperitoneum) in the pelvis (*arrows*).

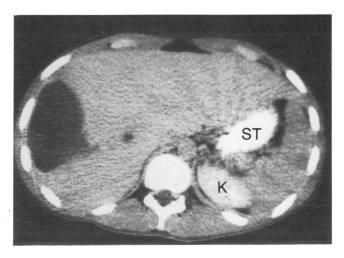

Figure 14-9 (*right*). Large subcapsular hematoma of the right liver lobe in a nine-year-old child with very little body fat. ST: Stomach opacified with oral contrast medium. K: Left kidney opacified with intravenous contrast medium. Low-density streaks overlying the spleen are rib artifacts. The patient did *not* have hemoperitoneum.

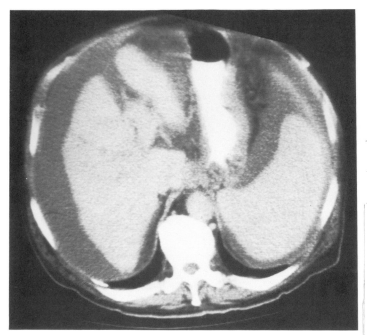

Figure 14-10. Cirrhosis of the liver with splenomegaly and ascites. Note the large amount of low-density fluid in the peritoneal cavity.

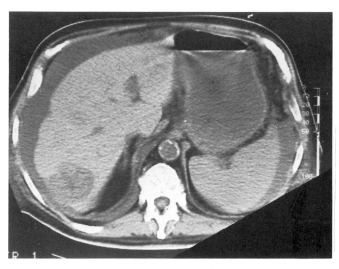

Figure 14-11. Malignant ascites from metastatic colon cancer. Low-density liver metastases are also evident.

Cirrhosis and Splenomegaly

Diffuse parenchymal diseases of the liver such as acute hepatitis may not produce any changes in the liver which can be detected by conventional imaging procedures. Posthepatitic cirrhosis, however, and cirrhosis resulting from chronic alcoholism may be detected when these processes alter liver size, contour, or density—the latter ranging from fatty infiltration to advanced fibrosis. These changes are best imaged with CT.

Normally the liver has a slightly greater CT density than the spleen. This ratio is reversed with fatty liver infiltration, which may be diffuse or focal. Later, in advanced cirrhosis, the liver will appear small in size and irregular in shape because of fibrous scarring, segmental atrophy, and the appearance of regenerating nodules. The CT scan may also show splenomegaly and ascites.

Note the large spleen, small scarred liver, and copious peritoneal fluid in the CT scan of a 56-year-old alcoholic woman shown in Figure 14-10. No intravenous contrast was used for this scan; it might have opacified large venous structures (gastroesophageal varices, caused by portal hypertension) around the stomach and esophagus.

The patient in Figure 14-11 also has ascites (in this case malignant ascites from metastatic colon cancer), but the spleen is normal in size. Did you notice the liver metastases?

Splenomegaly can usually be detected by physical examination. When the diagnosis is uncertain, spleen size may be estimated from plain abdomen films, a radioisotope spleen scan, ultrasound, or CT. In addition to confirming splenic enlargement, the last three procedures may show the etiology—whether a splenic tumor, abscess, cyst, or other process.

Splenic Trauma

The spleen is the most frequently injured organ during blunt abdominal trauma. Splenic injuries are commonly seen after motor-vehicle accidents and falls, especially when lower left rib fractures are present. CT is the procedure of choice for imaging patients with suspected abdominal injuries. In one quickly performed examination all of the organs of the abdominal cavity and retroperitoneum can be visualized, and injuries can be detected with a high degree of accuracy.

In the past, radioisotope spleen scanning and splenic angiography were performed when splenic trauma was considered. Neither of these procedures is as accurate as CT, and both show only the spleen. Ultrasound can detect splenic injuries and hemoperitoneum but with less accuracy than CT. You may, however, consider requesting a portable ultrasound when the patient is too unstable to be brought to the radiology department for a CT scan. Another alternative would be a peritoneal lavage examination, which would indicate immediate laparotomy if positive.

Figure 14-12 shows the CT scan of a young man injured in an automobile accident. Although he was stable hemodynamically, a CT scan was performed because of left upper quadrant pain. It showed a subcapsular hematoma (low-density crescent) lateral to the spleen, with several small areas of hemorrhage within adjacent splenic lacerations. In none of the CT sections was free blood detected in the peritoneal cavity, an indication that the splenic capsule was intact. Remember, a patient such as this could have a misleading negative peritoneal lavage examination.

Figure 14-13 shows CT scans of a 15-year-old boy who was thrown over the handlebars of his bicycle. An upper abdominal scan (A) shows a splenic fracture; a lower scan (B) shows gross hemoperitoneum (low-density fluid collections in both paracolic gutters lateral to the ascending and descending colon). The patient was taken directly to the operating room for splenectomy. With a lesser degree of splenic injury in a child or teenager, and absence of hemoperitoneum, conservative treatment without surgery may be indicated; serial CT scans can be used to document healing.

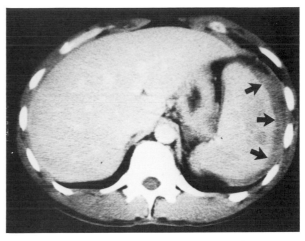

Figure 14-12. Subcapsular splenic hematoma. The *arrows* indicate the crescent-shaped blood collection.

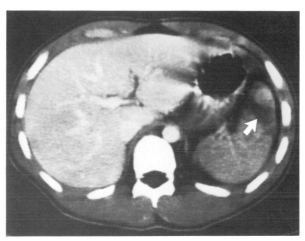

A

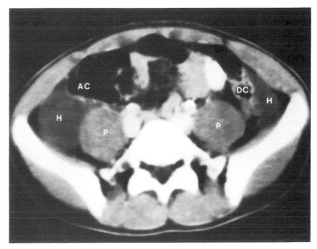

B

Figure 14-13. Spleen fracture after blunt trauma. A: *Arrow* points to the lower-density blood within the splenic fracture. B: Gross amounts of hemoperitoneum (*H*) are shown in both paracolic gutters lateral to the ascending (*AC*) and descending (*DC*) colon and psoas muscles (*P*).

Cholelithiasis and Cholecystitis

Two tests are available for diagnosing chole-lithiasis, oral cholecystography (Figure 14-14—you may also wish to review Figures 11-42 and 11-43 on page 176), and gallbladder ultrasound (Figure 14-15). Currently ultrasound is the

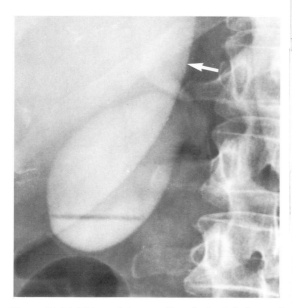

Figure 14-14. This upright spot film obtained during oral cholecystography shows a row of radiolucent stones layering (floating in a layer of similar-density bile) within the gallbladder. The *arrow* points to a right breast shadow. Supine films may miss small stones; consequently, upright films are always obtained by the radiologist at oral cholecystography.

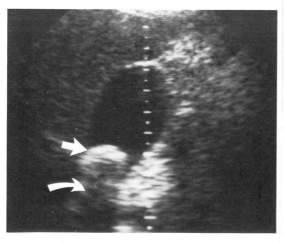

Figure 14-15. Positive gallbladder ultrasound showing echogenic stones (*straight arrow* indicates strong white echoes) in the dependent portion of the gallbladder, as well as acoustic shadowing (*curved arrow* indicates black shadow) behind the stone echoes.

more popular examination because it can be performed quickly, it does not require radiation or any patient preparation other than fasting, and the accuracy of diagnosis of gallbladder stones approaches 98 percent. Because this examination may not be successful in very obese patients and in those in whom copious amounts of bowel gas interfere with the transmission of sound waves, oral cholecystography is still performed.

Oral cholecystography must be arranged in advance, the radiologist supplying the patient with the oral contrast agent in the form of tablets. The dose is calculated according to body weight. The patient, fasting after a light supper, swallows the tablets of opaque drug the evening before the examination. Cleansing cathartics are not used because they interfere with the absorption of the contrast substance from the small bowel.

The absence of a gallbladder shadow on the films obtained does not necessarily imply depressed function. A number of factors still influence the successful resolution of the test. The patient may not, after all, have taken the tablets as he was instructed to do. If he took them, he may not actually have fasted—in which case the gallbladder would have contracted, emptying itself of the opaque material. If he indeed refrained from food, he may have had some nausea or diarrhea in reaction to the contrast material, preventing its retention in the small bowel long enough to allow for absorption. For these reasons the fallibility of the test is customarily checked in negative cases by reexamination a day later. The patient adheres to a very light diet overnight, takes a *second measured dose* (*not* a double dose, which can be dangerous), and the following morning a second set of films is obtained.

Failure to visualize the gallbladder after properly performed oral cholecystography on two successive days may mean, then, that one of several different pathologic conditions is present. It *may* mean that liver function is depressed and the drug is not being excreted. (Cholecystography is contraindicated in frankly jaundiced patients, and with a serum bilirubin over 3 milligrams per 100 milliliters it is usually considered that the test is unsatisfactory.) Or the absence of a gallbladder shadow may mean that faulty absorption in the small bowel interfered with arrival of the opaque substance in the bloodstream.

Another possibility is that any of several sorts of obstruction may be present. Obstruction may be *gastrointestinal* (pyloric or duodenal), so that small-bowel absorption is delayed or interfered with. Or it may be *biliary,* in which case bile does not reach the gallbladder to be concentrated (and visible—bile as first excreted is too dilute for resolution on the radiograph). Obstruction of the cystic duct, for example by a stone, will prevent bile from entering the gallbladder and there will be no visualization. Obstruction of the common bile duct from within (as by a stone lodged at the ampulla of Vater, or an intraductal tumor) or compression from without (as in pancreatic carcinoma) will cause jaundice and consequent failure to visualize even a normal gallbladder.

Finally, chronic cholecystitis may cause nonvisualization because functioning of the organ is affected. It is important to remember that even when the gallbladder is successfully visualized, disease of the gallbladder may be present, especially when cholelithiasis is demonstrated. In sum, then, after properly performed oral cholecystography (with a repeat dose) nonvisualization of the gallbladder must be taken seriously, but the problem may not be the gallbladder itself. Even when there is visualization, mild cholecystitis may be present.

In patients whom you suspect of having *acute cholecystitis,* two examinations will be helpful for diagnosis. Controversy remains at this time over which of the two is the better. A diagnosis of acute cholecystitis may be made with ultrasound when gallbladder stones are seen and the patient notes pain when pressure is exerted over the gallbladder by the ultrasound probe. This is the ultrasound counterpart of the surgical Murphy sign. Other ultrasound findings include demonstration of a thickened gallbladder wall and pericholecystic fluid. *Cholescintigraphy* images the gallbladder with intravenously injected hepatobiliary iminodiacetic acid (HIDA, as well as PIPIDA and DISIDA) congeners. These are excreted by the hepatocytes into the biliary system, from which they flow into the bowel. Normally

there is reflux of the isotope up the cystic duct into the gallbladder (Figure 14-16). As the cystic duct is nearly always occluded in acute cholecystitis, there is generally no visualization of the gallbladder, even on delayed images (Figure 14-17).

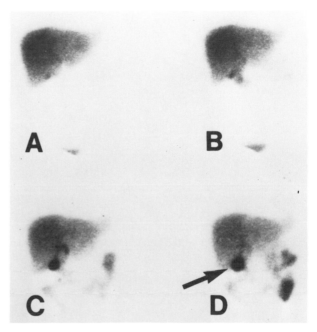

Figure 14-16. Normal HIDA scan showing isotope only in the liver initially (A), then in the biliary tree (B and C), with later concentration of isotope in the gallbladder (*arrow*) in D.

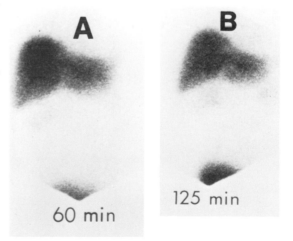

Figure 14-17. Abnormal HIDA scan showing no isotope in the gallbladder on films delayed as long as 60 minutes (A) and 125 minutes (B). This patient proved to have obstruction of the cystic duct due to acute cholecystitis.

239

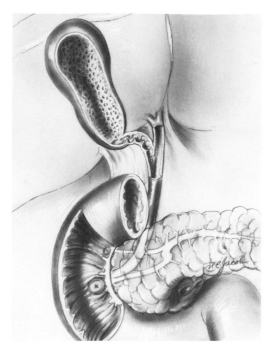

Figure 14-18. Drawing of the biliary tree and pancreas. The gallbladder has been reflected upward.

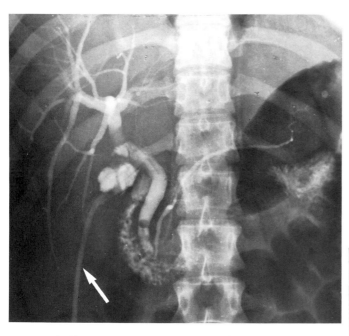

Figure 14-19. Intraoperative T-tube cholangiogram. This procedure was performed immediately after cholecystectomy and common duct exploration to evaluate the patency of the biliary tree and search for any retained common duct stones. The *arrow* points to the T-tube, which terminates in the common bile duct and through which contrast material was injected. The intrahepatic biliary tree is opacified and contrast material refluxes into the pancreatic duct, behind the dark, air-filled stomach. Also there is opacification of the duodenal lumen, where the common bile duct empties. The

Obstruction of the Biliary Tree

A drawing of the biliary tree and pancreas is provided for you in Figure 14-18. In the porta hepatis, trunks from the right and left liver lobes join to form the hepatic duct. The short hepatic duct is joined by the cystic duct draining the gallbladder to form the common bile duct. This structure drains into the bowel at the duodenal papilla (papilla of Vater), which has a common orifice for the termination of both the common bile duct and the main pancreatic duct. The accessory pancreatic duct drains into the duodenum through a separate orifice.

The common bile duct can be opacified directly by injection of contrast medium through an indwelling T-tube drainage catheter, as shown in Figure 14-19. This procedure may be performed intraoperatively or postoperatively, in patients who have had placement of T-tube drainage following common duct exploration. The anatomy of the biliary system can be fully displayed and any residual common duct stones easily identified. Note the round filling defects (stones) in the distal duct. The majority of patients whose biliary system you may wish to study will not have had surgery, however, and therefore will not offer such easy access for administration of contrast medium; you will have to employ other imaging techniques.

One of the most common reasons for imaging the biliary system is to determine whether it is dilated or not. And <u>dilatation</u> of the common bile duct and intrahepatic biliary tree is most easily detected by <u>ultrasound.</u> This would be the appropriate first imaging procedure in a patient presenting with new jaundice. If the biliary system *is not dilated* at ultrasound, then you should test for hepatocellular processes such as hepatitis to account for the patient's jaundice. If the biliary system *is dilated,* then you should consider causes for mechanical obstruction of the major bile ducts, such as a common duct stone and pancreatic carcinoma. Less common causes would include bile duct stricture and tumor. In

round radiolucencies in the distal common bile duct represent residual common duct stones, which were removed following detection by this x-ray examination.

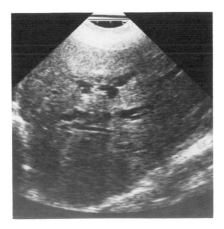

A

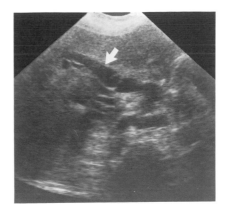

B

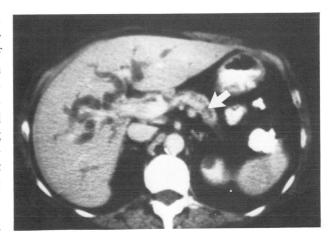

C

addition to recognizing biliary dilatation, ultrasound may show a common duct stone or pancreatic mass. Nevertheless, the fine detail of ultrasound imaging is limited, and bowel gas and body habitus may make ultrasound evaluation of the common bile duct difficult. Consequently, if the ducts are dilated but the level of obstruction is uncertain, additional imaging procedures such as CT, percutaneous transhepatic cholangiography (PTC), and endoscopic retrograde cholangiopancreatography (ERCP) may be required.

The patient illustrated in Figure 14-20 is a 52-year-old woman who presented in an emergency room with new, painless jaundice. Two images from her initial ultrasound examination showed dilatation of the intrahepatic biliary radicles (A) as well as dilatation of the common bile duct itself (B). Dilated intrahepatic ducts appear as branching, tubular structures at ultrasound, coursing parallel to the routing of the portal venous system. The common duct diameter can be measured at ultrasound, and extrahepatic biliary obstruction can be diagnosed when the common duct measures more than 4 to 5 millimeters. This patient's common bile duct measured 1.2 centimeters in diameter. CT confirmed dilatation of the intrahepatic ducts and the common bile duct (C and D) and showed a dilated pancreatic duct. The patient proved to have a small tumor of the ampulla of Vater.

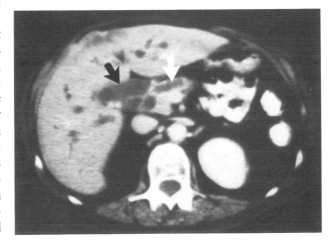

D

Figure 14-20. Patient with painless jaundice due to obstruction of the common bile duct by a small tumor at the papilla of Vater. A: Parasagittal liver ultrasound, showing dilatation of the intrahepatic biliary radicles. The echogenic curving diaphragm is located to your left. B: Transverse liver ultrasound, showing the dilated common bile duct (*arrow*). C: CT scan, showing marked dilatation of the intrahepatic biliary radicles. The pancreatic duct is also dilated (*arrow*). D: Lower CT scan, showing marked dilatation of the common bile duct (*black arrow*) and the pancreatic duct (*white arrow*).

241

Percutaneous transhepatic cholangiography is carried out by injection of a water-soluble contrast material through a fine needle introduced directly into the liver through the skin. The dilated biliary tree is shown in great detail and the site and cause of biliary obstruction is usually readily apparent.

In Figures 14-21A and B you see CT studies carried out on a female patient aged 65, who had been hospitalized for evaluation of jaundice and a history of bouts of abdominal pain over the previous 20 years. Ultrasonography (not illustrated here) indicated dilated bile ducts as well as the presence of pancreatic pseudocysts. A CT examination was requested for further evaluation. Note the dilated biliary radicles in Figure 14-21A and the dilated common bile duct in Figure 14-21B. The patient's long history of pain suggested either cholecystitis with the passage of gallstones or pancreatitis or both. (She was not an alcoholic.) Her development of obstructive jaundice was worrisome and could have been caused by stones in the common bile duct or by the development of carcinoma in the head of the pancreas.

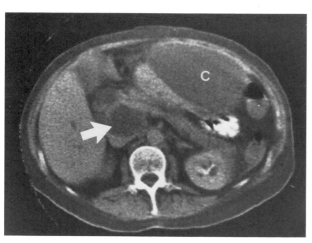

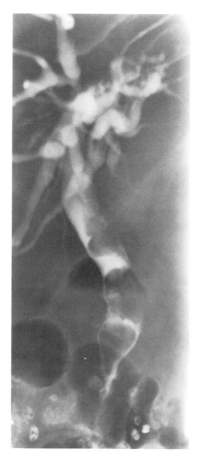

Figure 14-21. A and B are CT scans of another patient with obstructive jaundice. Note the dilated intrahepatic biliary radicles, dilated common bile duct (*arrow*), and pancreatic cyst (*C*). C: Percutaneous transhepatic cholangiogram of the same patient, showing the large stones within the common bile duct which caused biliary obstruction.

The next step in this patient was, logically, a percutaneous transhepatic cholangiogram, which you see in Figure 14-21C. Several large filling defects are visible in the dilated common bile duct. At surgery several large stones were removed successfully and the pancreatic pseudocyst arising from the tail of the pancreas was drained externally.

An embellishment of PTC is percutaneous transhepatic biliary drainage (PTD), a therapeutic procedure for patients with inoperable causes of obstruction, such as unresectable pancreatic carcinoma or sclerosing cholangitis. Via a similar percutaneous approach, under fluoroscopic control a multi–side-hole catheter is placed across the site of obstruction so that bile can flow freely into the duodenum.

Figure 14-22 diagrammatically illustrates the steps in that procedure. In A we can see a tumor encasing the common bile duct and causing mechanical biliary obstruction. A percutaneous biliary needle-catheter combination has been advanced into the biliary system in B. After removal of the needle in C, a small-caliber flexible guide wire, which had been inserted through the biliary catheter, is shown after having been advanced through the obstructing stenosis. In D the biliary catheter has been withdrawn from the guide wire and replaced with a larger-caliber, multi–side-hole drainage catheter. The catheter has been advanced over the guide wire until its tip is within the duodenum. The guide wire is removed in E. The drainage catheter is then clamped outside the skin surface. Now the patient has a route for internal biliary drainage. When unresectable tumors obstruct the biliary tree, this palliative treatment can eliminate symptoms due to jaundice.

In Figure 14-23 we see the results of a percutaneous biliary drainage procedure. Water-soluble contrast material has been injected through the external portion of the drainage catheter, opacifying the intrahepatic biliary radicles and proximal common bile duct. Although the distal duct (*arrows*) is markedly narrowed around the tube by the unresectable pancreatic carcinoma, there is free flow of contrast and bile into the duodenum through the drainage catheter. This patient's jaundice was entirely relieved.

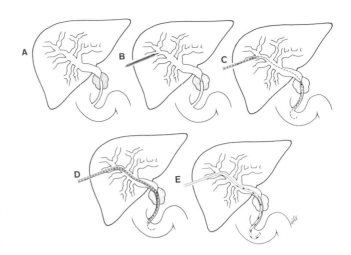

Figure 14-22. Technique for percutaneous transhepatic biliary drainage. (See text.)

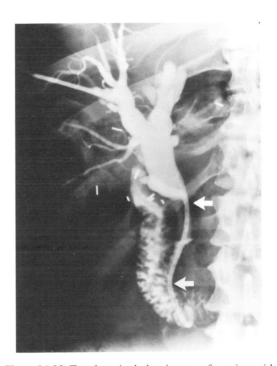

Figure 14-23. Transhepatic cholangiogram of a patient with a percutaneous biliary drainage catheter transversing a pancreatic carcinoma. (See text.)

243

The Pancreas

Prior to the advent of ultrasound, CT, and magnetic-resonance scanning, the pancreas was considered to be one of the "concealed" organs of the abdomen, imaged only indirectly. With the newer cross-sectional imaging modalities we can visualize pancreatic tissue directly, and the pancreatic duct itself can be opacified by endoscopic retrograde cholangiopancreatography (ERCP).

The pancreas is not visible on plain films, but pancreatic calcifications may be evident in some patients and are usually diagnostic of chronic pancreatitis. When large pancreatic masses are present, they may be detected indirectly at upper gastrointestinal series by anterior displacement of the barium-filled stomach and widening of the duodenal loop, which wraps around the head of the pancreas.

Arteriography does not opacify the pancreatic parenchyma as brightly as the parenchyma of other organs such as the liver, spleen, and kidneys. Rather, the angiographic diagnosis of pancreatic disease is based on the demonstration of encasement of, or tumor vessels associated with, the major blood vessels adjacent to the pancreas and the pancreatic vessels themselves.

Although better seen by CT, the pancreatic parenchyma can be visualized directly with ultrasound in most patients. Normally pancreatic tissue is more echogenic than the adjacent liver, and alterations in echogenicity may be important signs of pancreatic disease. Ultrasound may show pancreatic masses, pseudocysts, biliary obstruction, and evidence of pancreatitis.

Pancreatic anatomy can be clearly delineated with CT, which shows the pancreas arcing anteriorly over the spine, its head adjacent to the duodenum and its tail extending toward the spleen. (See Figure 11-52E, page 183.) The pancreas may look smooth or slightly lobulated. In order to differentiate pancreatic tissue from the adjacent blood vessels and duodenum, both oral and intravenous contrast materials are used.

ERCP (Figure 14-24) involves cannulation, under fluoroscopic guidance, of the common bile and pancreatic ducts via the ampulla of Vater during upper endoscopy. Generally this requires the combined efforts of the endoscopist and the radiologist. Contrast material injected into the common bile duct can show pathology at this level when the common bile duct is totally occluded from above. When the ultrasound, CT, and/or angiographic diagnosis of suspected pancreatic disease is uncertain, ERCP with contrast injection into the pancreatic duct is often conclusive.

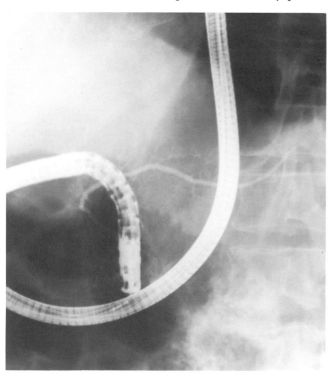

A

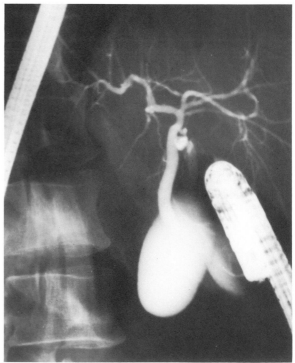

B

Figure 14-24. Endoscopic retrograde cholangiopancreatography (ERCP). The pancreatic duct (in A) and the common bile duct (in B) have been cannulated and injected with contrast medium.

Pancreatic Tumors

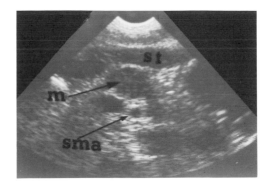

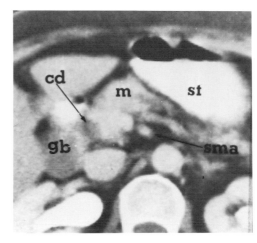

B

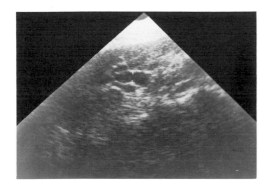

A

Carcinoma of the pancreas may be a difficult diagnosis to make. The symptoms of abdominal pain, weight loss, and early satiety are often nonspecific, and the small size of some tumors may make them impossible to image. When pancreatic cancer is clinically suspected, the diagnostic procedure of choice is computed tomography. If the patient is jaundiced, ultrasound is usually performed first to determine if biliary obstruction is present; ultrasound may even show the pancreatic mass (Figure 14-25).

At ultrasound, pancreatic cancers appear as masses or bulges, more echogenic than the remainder of the organ (Figure 14-25B). At CT, pancreatic cancers also appear as masses disturbing the normal organ contours (Figure 14-25C). Although the tissue density of pancreatic carcinoma is similar to that of the normal pancreatic parenchyma, CT can show more subtle alterations in pancreatic shape and size than ultrasound. CT may also show secondary findings better, such as pancreatic duct dilatation (as you have previously seen in Figures 14-20C and D). It may also show signs of local and distant abdominal metastases.

C

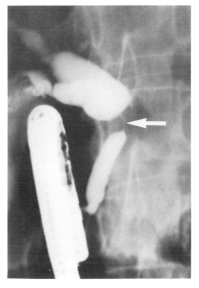

D

Figure 14-25. Obstructive jaundice caused by a small pancreatic carcinoma. A: The initial ultrasound survey showed that the common bile duct was dilated to a diameter of 9 millimeters (measured by ultrasound cursors, the two white crosses placed on the lateral margins of the duct). B: Transverse ultrasound showed a mass (*m*) between the stomach (*st*) and superior mesenteric artery (*sma*). This would be the location of the pancreatic head. C: CT scan through the same level confirmed a mass (*m*) between the stomach (*st*) and the superior mesenteric artery (*sma*). An *arrow* points to the dilated common bile duct (*cd*). The gallbladder (*gb*) is also indicated. D: Endoscopic retrograde cholangiopancreatography identified a marked stenosis (*arrow*) of the common bile duct, which was encased by pancreatic tumor. Note the marked dilatation of the common duct proximal to the stenosis.

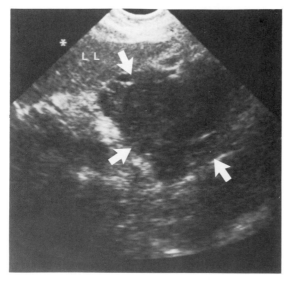

A

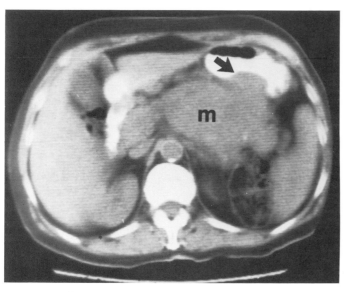

B

Figure 14-26. Islet cell cancer of the pancreas. A: Transverse ultrasound shows a large mass (*arrows*) in the body of the pancreas behind the left lobe (*LL*) of the liver. The mass is less echogenic than the liver or surrounding fat. B: CT confirms a large mass (*m*) in the body of the pancreas, which indents the contrast-filled stomach posteriorly (*arrow*). C: Selective splenic arteriogram shows that the mass is hypervascular (*arrows*); this would be more typical of an islet cell pancreatic tumor than a pancreatic carcinoma. D: Venous phase of the splenic arteriogram shows marked collateral circulation through veins (varices) of the lesser and greater curvature of the stomach (*c*'s) because of splenic vein occlusion by the tumor. The portal vein (*pv*) remains patent. This patient has *prehepatic portal hypertension* and could bleed from gastric varices.

Under CT guidance (following the advancing needle tip with serial CT scans), biopsy of pancreatic masses by percutaneous needle aspiration may be obtained in order to provide a tissue diagnosis. This technique allows confirmation of cancer when the diagnosis is in doubt. In addition, tumors deemed unresectable by CT may be biopsied so that a patient can be started on appropriate radiation and/or chemotherapy, without the further stress of a laparotomy biopsy.

When there is any doubt about the CT identification of a pancreatic mass, ERCP is usually performed as the next imaging procedure. It may confirm a CT suspected mass by showing encasement of, or occlusion of, either the pancreatic duct or the common bile duct. This will of course depend on whether the mass is located in the head, body, or tail of the pancreas. (In Figure 14-25D the ERCP examination shows that the common bile duct is encased by the mass detected in the head of the pancreas at CT.)

Angiography is used less than it once was for the diagnosis of pancreatic carcinoma, although it is often performed for preoperative staging after a pancreatic tumor has been detected by CT. If a pancreatic cancer encases a major blood vessel such as the portal vein, it is usually unresectable. As blood vessel encasement is generally better shown by angiography than by CT, many surgeons refer their patients for preoperative angiography.

At angiography the vascularity of the tumor may also be better appreciated than with CT. Pancreatic carcinoma is nearly always *hypovascular,* whereas islet cell tumors, such as insulinomas (Figure 14-26), are usually *hypervascular.* This may not be such an important differentiation to make by imaging, because most islet cell tumors usually present with symptoms and signs of their associated hormonal syndromes. You will generally know that your patient has an islet cell tumor—be it insulinoma, gastrinoma, or glucagonoma—by clinical and laboratory findings, even before you refer your patient for CT.

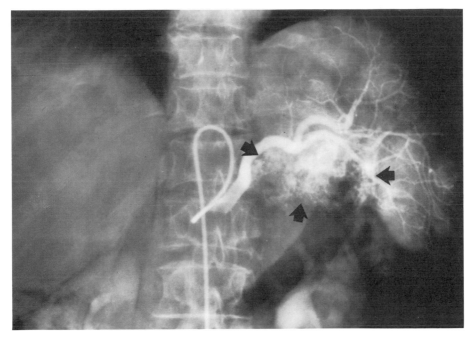

C

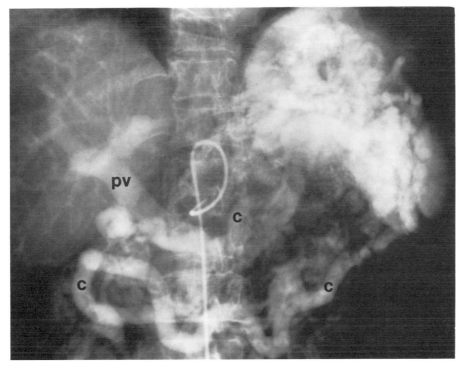

D

Pancreatitis and Pancreatic Abscess

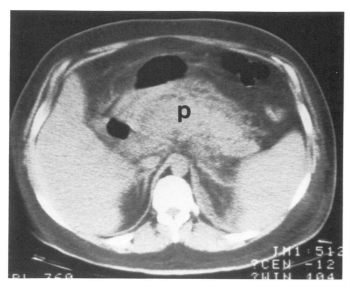

Figure 14-27. CT scan of an alcoholic patient with pancreatitis. Note the marked enlargement of the pancreatic shadow (*p*) and irregularity in the outline of the pancreas as compared with the CT scan of the normal pancreas in Figure 11-52E, page 183.

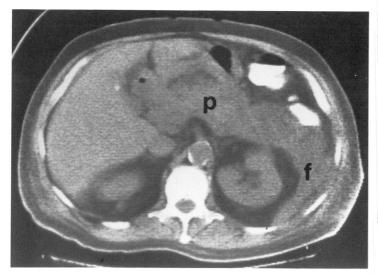

Figure 14-28. Another patient with pancreatitis. The CT scan shows an increase in pancreatic size and irregularity of the pancreatic outline (*p*). Note the large amount of fluid (*f*) in the left anterior compartment of the retroperitoneum.

Making a diagnosis of acute pancreatitis may not require any imaging at all. The diagnosis may be obvious from the clinical findings of epigastric pain and tenderness, nausea, vomiting, and elevation of serum amylase. The causes include alcoholism, obstruction of pancreatic duct drainage (by a distal common bile duct stone, for example), trauma, recent surgery, and certain therapeutic drugs. Imaging is recommended when the diagnosis is in doubt or when complications of pancreatitis, such as pseudocyst and abscess formation, are suspected.

Acute pancreatitis is nearly always associated with edema and enlargement of the pancreas. This is best demonstrated with CT (Figure 14-27), which usually also shows irregularity of the pancreatic outline. In mild cases, however, the CT examination may be entirely normal, or it may show only mild enlargement. In severe cases peripancreatic fluid (Figure 14-28) may be visible, as well as evidence for pancreatic phlegmon, consisting of a large inflammatory mass of pancreatic and peripancreatic tissues. The ultrasound findings of acute pancreatitis also include pancreatic enlargement and an overall decrease in the echogenicity of the organ. Pseudocysts are easily detected with ultrasound.

A dreaded complication of acute pancreatitis is pancreatic abscess formation, which is suspected clinically when the patient also presents with fever and septicemia. The pathognomonic finding is the presence of gas bubbles in the pancreatic bed. Although best shown by CT (Figure 14-29A), when only a small amount of gas is present, this finding may be seen on a plain abdominal film (Figure 14-29B) when copious gas is present.

In fact, a plain-film study of the abdomen, including an upright or lateral decubitus view, is the appropriate first step in the imaging workup of suspected pancreatitis. Pancreatic calcifications may be identified, providing evidence for previous pancreatitis. Free air in the peritoneal space would indicate a perforated viscus, such as a perforated peptic ulcer, which may mimic the clinical signs of pancreatitis.

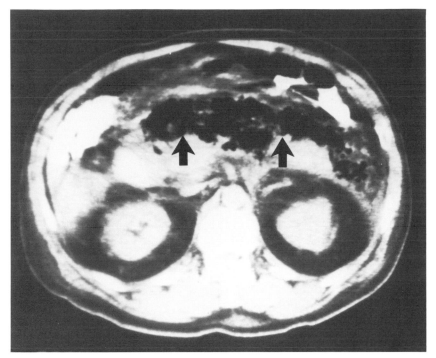

A

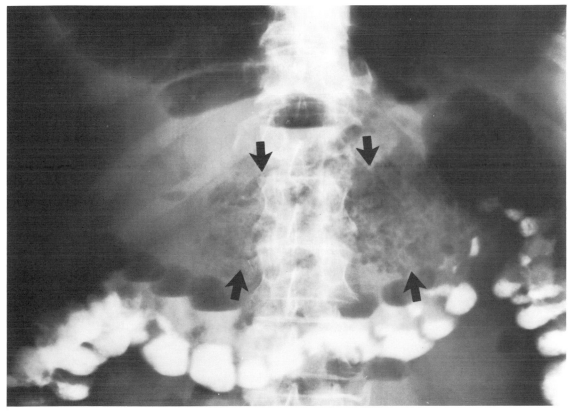

B

Figure 14-29. Pancreatic abscess. A: CT scan shows a large collection of gas in the anterior pancreatic bed (*arrows*). B: A collection of speckled air densities (*arrows*) in the pancreatic bed can also be seen on the plain abdominal film.

249

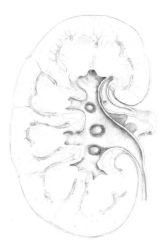

Figure 14-30. Drawing of the normal kidney anatomy in the coronal plane.

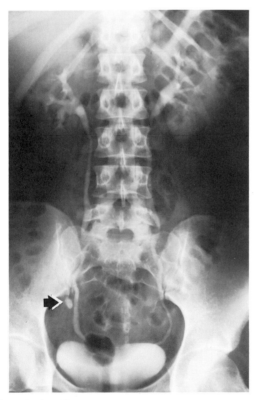

Figure 14-31. Almost normal intravenous urogram. The distal right ureter is displaced slightly medially within the bowl of the bony pelvis by what later proved to be a calcified right ovarian teratoma (*arrow*). The intrarenal collecting systems, left ureter, and bladder are normal.

The Urinary Tract

With a few exceptions, the study of kidney disease should begin with the excretory examination, the intravenous urogram. For this examination an intravenous infusion of iodinated contrast material is followed by a series of x-ray films which show the opacified kidneys, ureters, and bladder. The intravenous urogram should be considered a morphologic examination rather than a functional examination, because one cannot equate the density of contrast material seen on the x-ray films with overall kidney function. Rather, kidney function is a highly complex matter comprising many interrelated processes: glomerular filtration, tubular excretion, and water reabsorption. The density of contrast substance in the draining structures and parenchyma of the kidney must be interpreted in the light of any variation in the *fluid flow through the kidney* as well as any fluctuations in renal physiology.

The contrast materials most widely used are excreted by the kidney almost entirely in the glomerular filtrate. Less than a minute after the intravenous infusion is started, enough opaque substance is present in the glomeruli and tubules of the renal parenchyma to give an appreciable whitening to the kidney shadow on an abdominal film. This has been called the nephrogram phase of urography and is the proper time to observe the size and shape of the kidney. The rule in studying the morphology of the kidneys on plain films and nephrograms is that *the normal length of the kidney is 3.7 times the height of the second lumbar vertebra in that patient.* This measures approximately 8 to 15 centimeters in adults.

The calyces, pelves, ureters, and bladder are viewed in sequence following the nephrogram phase. These draining structures may be seen to fill, at the earliest, within minutes of the nephrogram phase; the filling increases to a peak and then gradually fades. The entire length of the ureters is not normally seen filled on any single film, since they are constantly being swept by peristaltic waves. After 20 to 30 minutes the collecting system will be seen too faintly for further study and all the visible opaque will be collected in the urinary bladder. Of course the kidneys continue to excrete the remaining opaque until the bloodstream is cleared.

The density of the opaque material seen in the collecting system will be decreased if there is ureteral obstruction. The contrast substance will be delayed in its time of appearance, and the filming sequence will have to be lengthened accordingly.

The *conventional intravenous urogram* commences with a preliminary plain film, which is always examined by the radiologist before the injection of contrast material, screening for calcification or stones which might be obscured by the contrast. (Ninety percent of kidney stones are radiopaque and dense enough to be seen on the plain film.) Then films are made at intervals, each being reviewed by the radiologist until he is satisfied that the examination has been completed for that patient. Thus every intravenous urogram is essentially a custom-tailored study. If the abnormality revealed on the first films suggests the need, additional special views may be obtained while the contrast material is still present. Even conventional tomography of the kidneys (nephrotomography, not CT) may be performed.

Pyelography (either *retrograde,* in which visualization of the urinary collecting system is achieved via a cystoscope, ureteral catheterization, and injection of contrast medium, or *antegrade,* via percutaneous puncture of the collecting system) can be performed when the intrarenal collecting systems and ureters cannot be opacified by intravenous techniques. Pyelography shows only the collecting systems (renal pelves and associated structures) and yields no information with regard to the parenchyma of the kidney itself.

Sonography is extremely useful and widely employed in the evaluation of kidney disease, and has become the method of choice in screening for obstructive nephropathy (especially in renal failure) and in differentiating kidney cyst from solid tumor. *CT* and *angiography* are also employed when indicated.

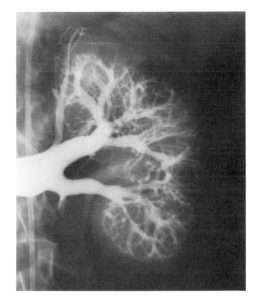

Figure 14-32. Normal left renal venogram.

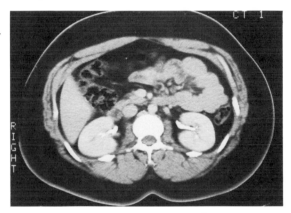

Figure 14-33. Normal CT scan through the midkidneys.

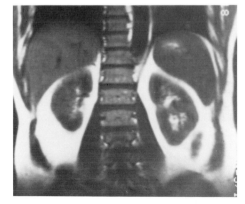

Figure 14-34. Normal coronal MR scan through the midkidneys.

251

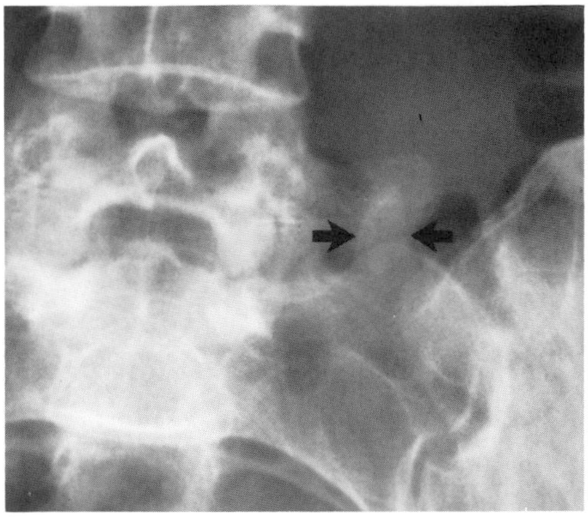

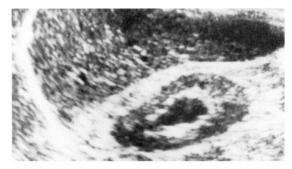

A

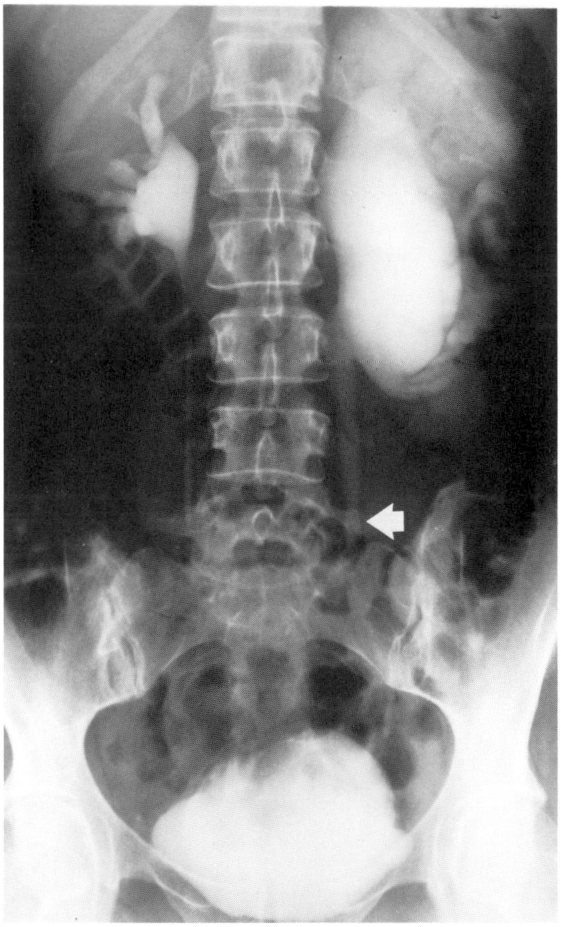

B

Figure 14-35. Partially obstructing left ureteral stone. A: Plain film shows a calcified stone (*arrows*). B: Urogram shows left hydronephrosis; *arrow* indicates the site of obstruction.

Obstructive Uropathy

Fluid flow out of the kidney may be prevented in numerous ways, but among the commonest is an obstructing *ureteral calculus*. Since 90 percent of renal calculi are radiopaque, the chance of recognizing the presence of a calculus on the initial plain film of an intravenous urogram is excellent, and the study for stone should begin there (Figure 14-35). With one ureter obstructed by stone and nonopaque-containing urine backed up above it, a delay in the appearance of contrast medium in that kidney is to be expected; sometimes several hours are needed before the nephrogram finally appears. This has been called the late white kidney of acute renal obstruction. Ultimately opacification of the ureter down to the point of the obstruction will occur as excreted opaque mixes with retained urine. The degree of dilatation of the intrarenal collecting system and ureter proximal to the site of obstruction (degree of hydronephrosis) will depend on the degree of obstruction (partial versus nearly complete) and the length of time that obstruction has been present.

The obstructed kidney can be readily diagnosed by ultrasound if significant hydronephrosis has occurred. The fluid-filled dilated calyces on the hydronephrotic side will produce an echo-free center for that kidney on sonogram (Figure 14-36), as compared to the normal side showing an echogenic center of renal sinus fat (Figure 14-37).

Figure 14-36. Parasagittal ultrasound showing the liver and right kidney of a patient with right hydronephrosis. Compare the dark, echolucent, fluid-filled center of the kidney with the normal right kidney ultrasound in Figure 14-37.

It is surprising that any function remains in a chronically obstructed kidney; in advanced hydronephrosis the kidney will be converted into a thin-walled sac with only a slender rim of renal parenchyma remaining. Figure 14-38 is a late urogram film which shows bilateral obstruction in an infant with a low congenital defect in the drainage of both ureters. Note the marked dilatation of the ureters. A lesser degree of obstruction is evident in Figure 14-39.

Obstruction to outflow of urine from the kidney is of course only one way in which the fluid flow through the kidney may be decreased. Interference with the blood supply to the kidney also decreases fluid flow through that kidney, and if this occurs on one side, the other kidney takes over the workload and excretes a much larger amount of urine than normal.

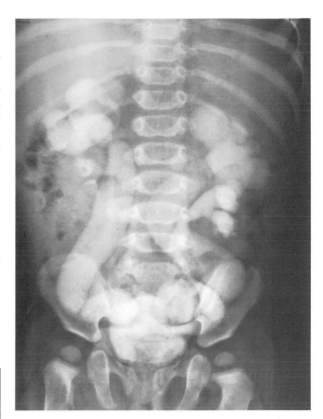

Figure 14-38. Advanced bilateral hydronephrosis in a child with congenitally defective drainage of the lower urinary tract.

In sum, then, *in studying plain films and intravenous urograms* you must carefully assay the size and shape of the two kidneys, the outline of parenchyma for each and its homogenity, the appearance of the collecting structures and their rate of filling and emptying. *Failure of the kidney to visualize* should make you ask whether there is evidence for—
(1) No blood getting into the kidney (renal artery compromised);
(2) No blood getting out (renal vein thrombosis);
(3) Blocked drainage (such as a ureteral stone); or
(4) Destruction of the nephron system.

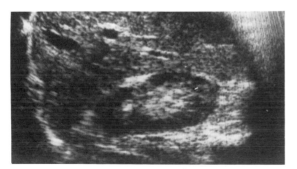

Figure 14-37. Parasagittal ultrasound of a normal right kidney. Note the echogenic (white) kidney center; the echoes are produced by normal, central, renal sinus fat.

Figure 14-39 (*right*). Early bilateral hydronephrosis caused by external compression from a pelvic mass.

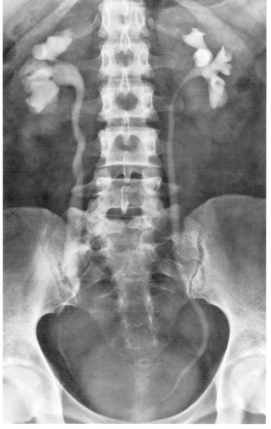

Cystic Disease of the Kidneys

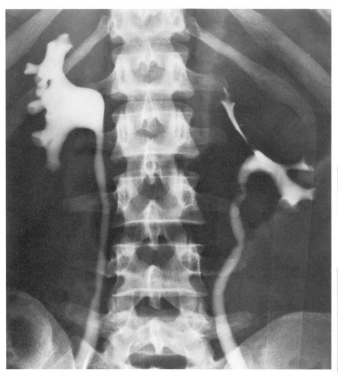

Figure 14-40. Retrograde pyelogram after injection catheters have been withdrawn. Note the stretching of upper and middle calyces in the left kidney around a "mass," which proved at ultrasonography to be a cyst.

Because the kidneys secrete fluid, they are subject to the development of retention cysts of various kinds. Although these do not fill with excreted opaque because they are walled-off collections of fluid, their presence in the kidneys distorts the parenchyma and the draining structures on urography in a characteristic fashion (Figure 14-40). Even more precise is the recognition of cystic renal masses by either sonography (Figure 14-41) or CT (Figures 14-42 and 14-43). A renal mass discovered clinically, by plain films or by urography, should be studied at once, with sonography as the less invasive procedure, CT being used only when sonography is impossible. Ultrasound can usually differentiate between a fluid-filled cyst and a solid renal tumor.

In the patient with no hematuria, determination by sonography that a renal mass is cystic (with good through transmission, a sharp far wall, and no interior echoes) is usually sufficient evidence to terminate the study. Few cysts require treatment. Cyst puncture (Figure 14-44)

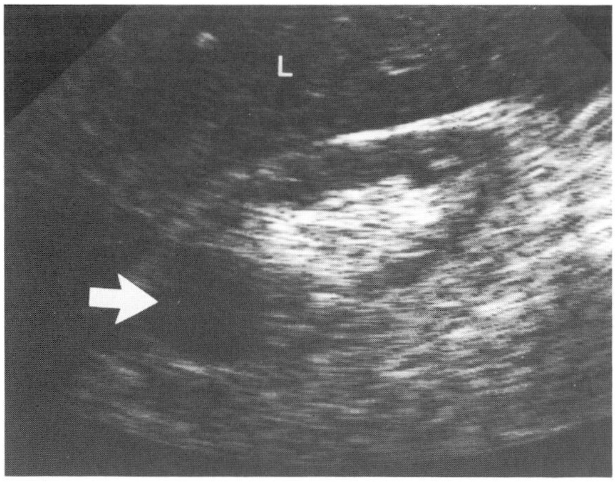

Figure 14-41. Sagittal ultrasound of the right kidney in a different patient showing an upper pole cyst (*arrow*), which appears as an echolucent (black) round mass in the upper pole of the right kidney. The liver (*L*) is located just anterior to the kidney.

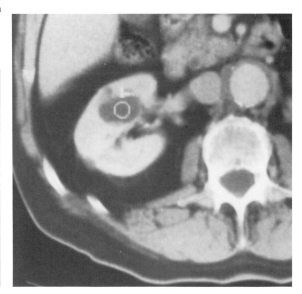

Figure 14-42. Coned-down CT scan of a right renal cyst. It appears as a round, sharply defined area of diminished CT attenuation (darker), as compared to the renal parenchyma. The white circle overlying the cyst represents a cursor positioned for computer sampling of CT density. This sample measured 3 Hounsfield units; a value which is similar to water and is typical of a benign cyst.

can be carried out for confirmation; obtaining a clear aspirate proves the diagnosis. The patient with hematuria must have additional diagnostic procedures (CT, aspiration, angiography), however, before the diagnosis of simple cyst can be accepted.

Polycystic kidneys (Figure 14-45) have so classic and pathognomonic an appearance on both sonogram and CT scan that those procedures are used for screening in families of patients with polycystic disease.

Infection

The physician ought not to routinely request intravenous urography on adult patients with urinary tract infections. Of course, the indications for urography in all patients with flank pain suggesting stone and those with hematuria are perfectly clear, but in the adult patient with only urinary tract infection the examination is often futile. Children with pus in their urine always need urography at the time of initial workup, on the other hand, as they may have a congenitally obstructing lesion or vesicoureteral reflux.

Most kidneys chronically infected from childhood do show important morphologic changes, demonstrable either on urography with tomograms or with CT. These alterations consist of an overall decrease in size of the affected kidney and/or localized thinning of the parenchyma where pitting and scarring are to be seen on the surface of the surgical specimen. When you examine a plain film, always make a habit of estimating kidney size and shape and trace its normal smooth, plump outline. Perinephric abscesses are easy to diagnose by both ultrasound and CT, and one of these procedures should be carried out as soon as the diagnosis has been suggested clinically.

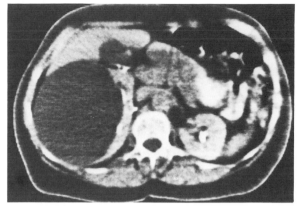

Figure 14-43. CT scan of a patient with an enormous right renal cyst. Notice the splaying of the right renal parenchyma around the cyst and just medial to it. The remainder of the right kidney parenchyma has a crescent shape.

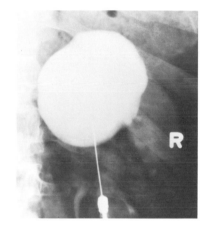

Figure 14-44. Percutaneous cyst puncture. To confirm that an ultrasound-diagnosed cyst was indeed benign in a patient with microscopic hematuria, a percutaneous needle aspiration was performed. A spot film (the patient is lying prone, and therefore the film is correctly marked with an *R*) shows the cyst cavity opacified with water-soluble contrast medium. Analysis of the aspirated cyst fluid showed no evidence of blood or malignant cells.

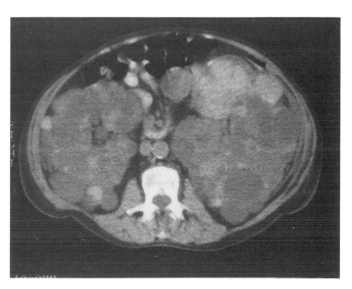

Figure 14-45. CT scan of a patient with polycystic kidneys.

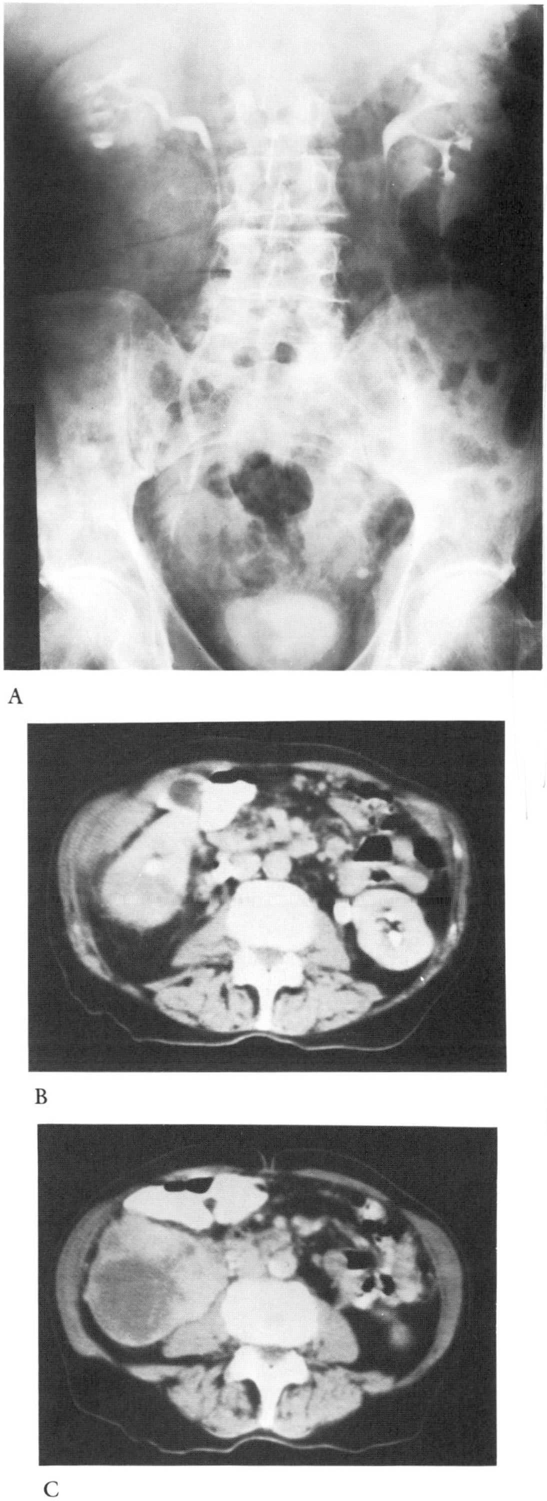

A

B

C

Figure 14-46. Renal cell carcinoma. A: Intravenous urogram, showing a lower pole right renal mass which displaces the proximal right ureter medially. B: CT scan through the midkidneys reveals a low-attenuation mass posteriorly in the right kidney. C: Slightly lower CT scan shows a large right renal tumor with a low-density necrotic center.

Renal Tumors

When a renal mass is discovered by clinical examination, plain films, or intravenous urography, and sonography indicates that the mass is not classically a cyst (poor through-transmission of sound waves as occurs with solid masses, an irregular margin, or internal echoes), the mass is considered to be a solid tumor and the patient is referred for computed tomography. CT performed with intravenous contrast material can characterize tumors with better detail than ultrasound. It can show the degree of vascularity, the presence of a necrotic center, and the presence or absence of local invasion of adjacent structures such as the renal vein and inferior vena cava. If the mass shown at urography is very large and irregular or shows invasion of the intrarenal collecting system, or if hematuria is present, the patient may be referred directly to CT, bypassing sonography.

In masses which seem cystic at sonography but have thick walls on CT, one must suspect a tumor that is partially necrotic or has central hemorrhage. Percutaneous needle aspiration can be carried out and may provide specific tissue diagnosis. If the aspirated fluid is bloody or dark and no tissue diagnosis can be made, then surgical exploration is indicated; tumors are known to arise occasionally in the wall of a benign cyst, and when they do, they may present with hemorrhage.

The patient illustrated in Figure 14-46 is a 62-year-old man with right flank pain and microscopic hematuria. His urogram (A) shows a large right lower pole renal mass which produces a bulge in the medial kidney margin, splays the collecting structures away from it, and displaces the ureter medially. Because of the hematuria, the patient was referred directly to CT and a large lower pole tumor was confirmed (B and C). It has a low CT attenuation and irregularly margined center that is seen with central tumor necrosis; this finding is common with renal cell carcinoma (hypernephroma), which this proved to be.

Renal arteriography or venography frequently is indicated to better define invasion of the renal veins and the inferior vena cava. A case illustrating the latter will be presented later, in the section on the inferior vena cava. In addition, angiography can better show the vascularity of the tumor itself. The arterial and venous phases of the selective right renal arteriogram of another patient with renal cell carcinoma are shown in Figure 14-47. They depict a markedly hypervascular tumor which does not invade the right renal vein.

As very vascular tumors are often associated with significant blood loss at surgical resection, a popular angiographic technique is preoperative embolization of the renal artery on the affected side. Through the same small-caliber catheter used for arteriography, the radiologist carefully injects small pieces of particulate material, frequently pieces of Gelfoam (surgical gelatin), while watching on a fluoroscope. Figure 14-47C shows the right renal artery after embolic occlusion. Ischemic kidney pain is extremely severe. Consequently, preoperative embolization is performed on the morning of surgical resection, just after preoperative medication and just prior to surgical resection.

Intravenous Opaques

Radiographic opaques used intravenously and excreted by the liver or kidney very occasionally produce undesirable reactions, and all physicians should be aware that intravenous administration of contrast substances may result in such episodes while the patient is being examined.

Reactions may be quite mild—with pallor, sweating, a feeling of warmth, nausea, vomiting, and anxiety—and the injection should be stopped at once. These effects probably occur in 1 to 5 percent of all such studies.

Reactions may also, very rarely, be severe: fatalities (generally due to cardiovascular collapse in anaphylactoid reactions) are reported to occur once in 40,000 to once in 140,000 cases. (It is interesting that the incidence of all types of reaction is similar to that of penicillin.) For this reason no such studies should be carried out without ready availability of an emergency cardiopulmonary support system.

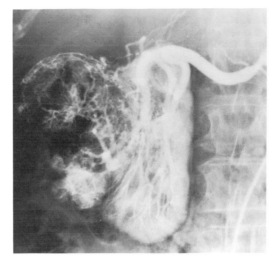

A

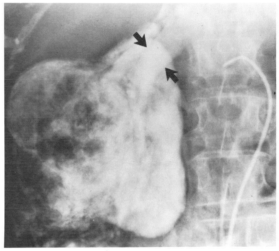

B

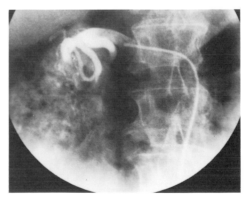

C

Figure 14-47. Arteriography of another patient with renal cell carcinoma. A: Arterial phase of a right renal arteriogram shows a large vascular tumor. B: Venous phase shows no evidence of tumor invasion of the right renal vein (*arrows*). C: Right renal arteriogram after embolic occlusion.

Renal Trauma

Renal trauma may be suspected in patients with hematuria and/or flank pain occurring after any kind of accident. The trauma may be slight (contused kidney, self-curing) or catastrophic (fractured kidney, torn major renal blood vessels). Varying degrees of trauma between these extremes may or may not require surgical repair. Consequently it is important not only to make a diagnosis of renal trauma, but to stage the degree of renal injury.

The best imaging procedure for examining patients with suspected renal injury is CT (Figure 14-48). Not only can CT recognize a smaller degree of injury than can be seen with intravenous urography, but it can also stage the injury as well, differentiating contusions and small cortical lacerations, which can be treated conservatively, from more severe injuries needing surgery. Of course one would correlate the CT findings with the clinical status of the patient, expediting renal surgery in the unstable patient and carefully monitoring those being treated conservatively. In addition, CT is faster than intravenous urography, requires less patient manipulation, and uses less radiation. In the same CT examination, and taking no extra time, the other abdominal organs, lumbosacral spine, and pelvis can be evaluated.

When CT is not available, intravenous urography may be performed and may show a variety of findings. With renal artery injury the kidney will usually not opacify. When renal lacerations have extended into the collecting system, extravasation of contrast medium may be seen around the kidney and within the laceration itself. With small cortical lacerations and perirenal hemorrhage, the renal outline will become less apparent and the psoas margin on that side may disappear. Injuries of the ureters and bladder may be clearly shown at urography.

Renovascular Hypertension

There are several ways in which the arterial supply to the kidney can be compromised. Acutely, this can be caused by an embolus to a renal artery, the patient presenting with acute flank pain. Rarely, the lumen may be reduced by extrinsic pressure. The cause more often is atherosclerotic disease producing a renal artery stenosis or occlusion. Gradually atherosclerotic plaques narrow the lumen and eventually occlude it. Another arterial disease causing renal ischemia is fibromuscular disease of the renal arteries.

With any of these conditions the restriction of arterial supply may affect a main renal artery or

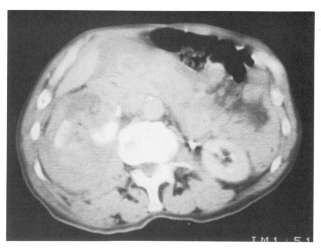

A

B

Figure 14-48. CT of a right renal laceration. A: The diagonal lucency through the right kidney represents hematoma within a laceration; the hematoma is lower in density than the opacified renal parenchyma. Surrounding the kidney is a ring of hematoma (*arrows*) within the perirenal space. B: Lower CT scan of the same patient, showing separation of the lower pole renal parenchyma into two portions, both engulfed in perirenal hematoma.

any of its branches; the entire kidney may become ischemic, or only a small part of it. The entire excretory capacity may be proportionally reduced, or only a small part of it. Renal ischemia with increased excretion of renin by the tissue distal to a renal artery stenosis or occlusion has been demonstrated to be the cause of hypertension in a small percentage of the population. As this is a treatable cause, it is an important one to diagnose. Renovascular hypertension should be considered in young patients with hypertension as well as in patients with hypertension of new onset, hypertension and an abdominal bruit, hypertension and renal failure, and hypertension with an elevated peripheral renin level.

When renovascular hypertension is suspected clinically, the patient should be referred for arteriography. Although intravenous urography may show delayed appearance of contrast medium and decreased kidney size with renal ischemia, it is such a poor screening procedure for renovascular hypertension that it is not recommended. If a renal artery stenosis or occlusion is found at arteriography, then selective catheter sampling of blood from both renal veins must be performed. In order to make a diagnosis of renovascular hypertension, the physician must show a significant elevation in the renal vein renin level in the kidney with the arterial stenosis or occlusion (Figure 14-49). It is important to do this, because many patients with essential hypertension may coincidentally have a renal artery stenosis; in this situation there would be no antihypertensive benefit to fixing the renal artery stenosis. Patients with true renovascular hypertension will generally benefit from repair of a renal artery stenosis or a bypass graft about a renal artery occlusion. In some patients with an end-stage kidney, nephrectomy may be required to cure the hypertension.

The limited role of radiologic procedures in the workup of the hypertensive patient is important for every physician to understand, since most hypertensive patients one will see in a lifetime of practice will have essential hypertension and normal intravenous urograms. Only very rarely will one see a patient with renovascular hypertension, and then one will have to eliminate other forms of hypertension before ordering renal arteriography. Coarctation of the aorta

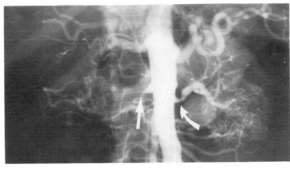

A

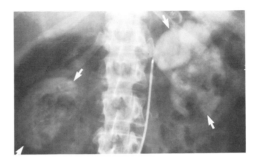

B

Figure 14-49. Aortogram of a patient with renovascular hypertension. A: Early phase, showing a total occlusion of the right renal artery (*straight arrow*) and a stenosis (*curved arrow*) in the proximal left renal artery. B: Later phase, showing a small, poorly opacified right kidney, as compared to the left. Venous sampling of the right renal vein demonstrated a significantly elevated renin level.

should be recognized from unequal limb pressures on physical exam, and endocrine-related adrenal hypertension should be suspected from the clinical presentation and laboratory values. Although adrenal masses can be identified by CT, this procedure is carried out subsequent to the laboratory evidence. Certainly the physician should not routinely order urography on patients with hypertension of some duration who respond well to antihypertensive medication.

In patients with renovascular hypertension caused by a renal artery stenosis, a popular new radiologic alternative to renovascular surgery is transluminal angioplasty. Via a percutaneous femoral artery puncture, a balloon-tip catheter is directed into the affected renal artery, advanced across the stenosis, and then inflated to dilate the stenosis. The success rate is similar to that of surgery and there often is a dramatic return to the normotensive state. This technique is especially useful in older patients who are poor surgical risks.

The Urinary Bladder

The urinary bladder is routinely opacified and filmed at intravenous urography, and you have seen several examples already. Conditions such as bladder cancer and bladder stones which produce filling defects in the bladder lumen thus can readily be detected at intravenous urography. In addition, masses adjacent to the bladder that displace it can also be identified. Figure 14-50 shows a portion of the intravenous urogram of an elderly man with benign prostatic hypertrophy; the bladder floor is elevated by the enlarged prostate gland.

Improved opacification of the bladder can be obtained by direct installation of contrast material into the bladder through a catheter inserted via the urethra. This procedure is called a *retrograde cystogram*. Figure 14-51 shows an example in a patient with a large nodular bladder cancer. Retrograde cystography may also be indicated when bladder opacification is required in a patient with renal failure whose kidneys are unable to concentrate contrast material, and in a patient whose bladder does not opacify because of bilateral ureteral obstruction.

Multiple trauma patients with bloody urethral discharge are routinely examined with a retrograde cystourethrogram to diagnose possible injuries of the urethra or bladder. This is performed carefully with a small-caliber injection catheter and fluoroscopic control. In the unstable trauma patient it may need to be done portably in the emergency ward. Figure 14-52A illustrates the retrograde cystogram of a multiple trauma patient with a bladder rupture. Note the teardrop shape of the bladder, caused by compression of the lateral bladder walls by bilateral pelvic hematomas. You can see extravasation of urine and contrast material into the pelvic soft tissue outside the bladder wall, and also into the peritoneal cavity. As is typical, the extravasation is easily identified, but the exact site of bladder rupture is uncertain. A CT examination (Figures 14-52B through E) was performed after cystoscopy for evaluation of the abdominal organs. No other injuries were found, although the extravasated contrast material and urine in the peritoneal cavity beautifully show the extent of this space on the four CT scans reproduced.

Remember that the bladder mucosa is well seen at cystoscopy and if a small bladder cancer is suspected, but not seen at intravenous urography, cystoscopy is usually performed. Further-

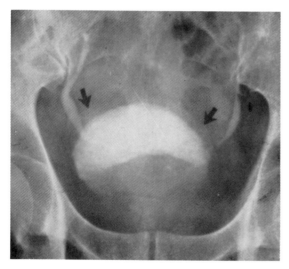

Figure 14-50. Coned-down view of the bladder in a patient with prostatic hypertrophy. The filling defect elevating the floor of the bladder represents an enlarged prostate. *Arrows* indicate the thickened bladder wall.

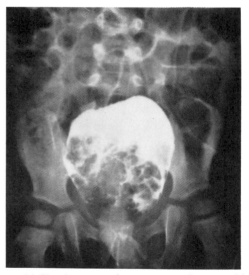

Figure 14-51. A retrograde cystogram shows multiple radiolucencies within the bladder, outlined by contrast material. These represent a nodular sarcoma of the bladder in this pediatric patient.

more, urography shows the lumen of the bladder only, not the thickness of the bladder wall. Ultrasound, CT, and magnetic-resonance imaging have been helpful in the diagnosis of bladder lesions that affect the bladder wall and surrounding tissues more than the lumen. For example, in the staging of bladder cancer, CT can show the extent of involvement of the bladder wall and the presence or absence of invasion of the surrounding pelvic structures.

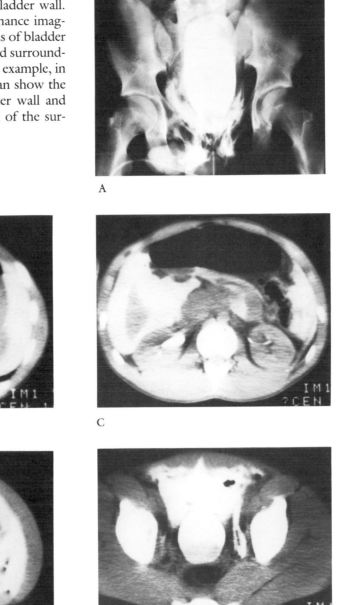

Figure 14-52. Multiple-trauma patient with a bladder rupture. A: Cystogram film shows a teardrop-shaped bladder and extravasation of contrast medium. B: CT scan of the upper abdomen after intravenous contrast medium shows opacified fluid (urine opacified with contrast medium leaking into the peritoneal space via the bladder rupture) in the peritoneal space, surrounding the liver, stomach, and spleen. C: CT scan through the midkidneys shows opacified fluid surrounding the tip of the liver and in the left paracolic gutter. D: Lower CT scan shows opacified urine in both paracolic gutters. E: CT scan through the pelvis shows contrast medium extravasation into the anterior pelvic soft tissues and peritoneal cavity.

The Adrenal Glands

Computed tomography and ultrasound have significantly advanced the imaging diagnosis of adrenal disease. Prior to these techniques, patients were subjected to lengthy and uncomfortable angiographic procedures in order to determine if adrenal masses or enlargement were present. Although ultrasound can readily detect large adrenal masses, patients with suspected adrenal disease are usually referred for a CT examination because its finer anatomic resolution can identify even small adrenal abnormalities. In fact, CT is the procedure of choice and appropriate first imaging examination to perform in your patients with suspected adrenal disease.

At CT the normal left adrenal gland is triangular in shape, whereas the right is crescent shaped. You have seen normal examples already at the end of Chapter 11. The indications for adrenal CT include paroxysmal hypertension suspicious for pheochromocytoma, clinical findings of Cushing's disease or other adrenal cortex hypersecretion syndrome, and a new flank or abdominal mass which could represent an adrenal carcinoma or neuroblastoma. Finally, the adrenal glands are routinely examined with CT in patients undergoing staging of lung and breast cancers, which frequently metastasize to the adrenal glands.

Bilateral enlargement of the adrenal glands is seen at CT with adrenal hyperplasia. Unilateral enlargement usually signifies a benign or malignant adrenal mass, such as a pheochromocytoma or cortical adenoma. Metastatic disease, however, may cause enlargement of one or both adrenal glands. Consequently it is imperative to correlate the CT examination with the clinical findings. The patients illustrated in Figures 14-53 to 14-55 all have right adrenal enlargement. In Figure 14-53 the patient had an aldosteronoma, in Figure 14-54 a pheochromocytoma, and in Figure 14-55 metastases from a bronchogenic carcinoma.

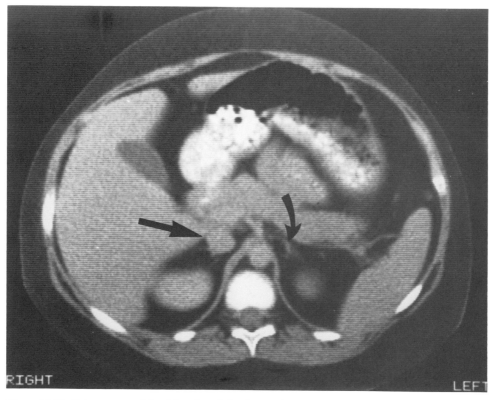

Figure 14-53. Enlargement of the right adrenal gland (*straight arrow*) due to the presence of an adrenocortical tumor, an aldosteronoma. *Curved arrow* points to the normal-size left adrenal gland.

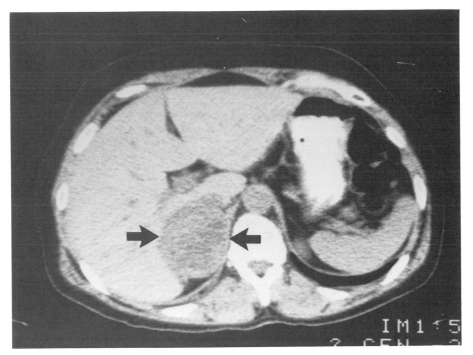

Figure 14-54. CT scan of patient with a large right adrenal pheochromocytoma (*arrows*).

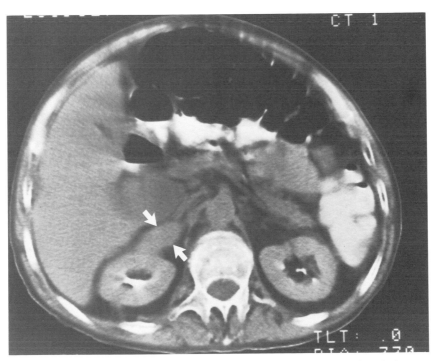

Figure 14-55. Enlarged right adrenal gland (*arrows*) due to a metastatic deposit from a bronchogenic carcinoma of the lung.

263

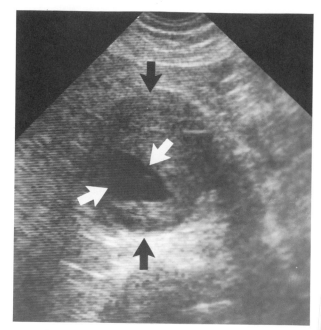

A

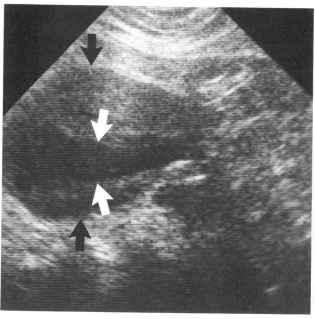

B

Figure 14-56. A patient with an abdominal aortic aneurysm. A: Transverse ultrasound identifies a large aneurysm. The *black arrows* delineate the overall size of the aneurysm; the *white arrows* indicate the lumen containing flowing blood. The space between the two represents thrombus. B: Midline sagittal ultrasound of the same patient. The patient's head is to your left, his feet to your right. Again, the *black arrows* indicate the overall size of the aneurysm and the *white arrows* the lumen. C (*opposite page*): Lateral aortogram shows that the aneurysm begins below the superior mesenteric artery (*sma*), coursing anteriorly, and the renal artery branches (*arrows*), coursing posteriorly.

Aortic Aneurysm

Atherosclerotic disease is the primary cause for imaging the abdominal aorta, either for evaluation of lower-extremity ischemic symptoms or for evaluation of suspected aortic aneurysm. In the former condition, sites of arterial stenosis and occlusion causing ischemia may be located anywhere from the aorta down to the pedal arteries. Those patients whose symptoms warrant treatment are usually investigated by an arteriographic examination commonly referred to as an *aortogram and runoff*.

To perform this procedure, an angiographic catheter is inserted percutaneously into a femoral artery and advanced proximally within the aorta to the level of the twelfth thoracic vertebra. Bolus injections of angiographic contrast material are administered while films are obtained of the arterial tree of the abdomen, pelvis, and legs. The vascular surgeon can then determine which occlusions or stenoses need to be circumvented with bypass grafts. Patients with short arterial stenoses or occlusions may be candidates for an angiographic dilatation of the lesion with a balloon catheter.

An abdominal aortic aneurysm is suspected when a midline, palpable, and pulsatile abdominal mass is discovered on physical examination. It may be asymptomatic, or it may be associated with pain or be tender on examination. This is an important differentiation, because it will alter the initial imaging workup. Asymptomatic aneurysms are usually not emergencies, and the clinically suspected aneurysm can be confirmed with a quick, accurate, and inexpensive ultrasound examination.

Figure 14-56 gives an example, a 69-year-old man with a large pulsatile abdominal mass. Note that ultrasound (A and B) can differentiate thrombus within the aneurysm from the patent lumen containing free-flowing blood. In addition, ultrasound can determine the overall size of the aneurysm. The aortic branches, however, are not well seen by ultrasound and any free blood in the retroperitoneum that may result from a leak cannot be as accurately identified by ultrasound as it can by CT. In most individuals an abdominal aortic diameter at ultrasound larger than 4 centimeters is consistent with an aneurysm.

A patient with a symptomatic or tender aneurysm should be examined with an emergency CT scan, as illustrated in Figure 14-57. This man presented with sudden back and right flank pain. On physical examination a tender, pulsatile abdominal mass was discovered. CT not only confirmed the presence of aneurysm but showed free blood in the retroperitoneum consistent with an acute leak. The patient was taken immediately to the operating room, where the leaking aneurysm was successfully resected.

Remember that a patient with a clinically obvious aneurysmal leak or rupture should be taken to the operating room, not to the CT scanner. The latter examination is reserved for stable patients whose diagnosis is uncertain. In this group a large number of patients may be saved from an unnecessary laparotomy when no leaking aneurysm is seen at CT. Also, CT may be helpful in the asymptomatic patient with a suspected aneurysm when copious bowel gas interferes with ultrasound imaging.

You may wonder why patients with abdominal aortic aneurysm are still examined by angiography if so much information is provided by CT. What angiography offers is a road map showing how the aneurysm relates to the aortic branches. This information will expedite aneurysm surgery. The lateral aortogram depicted in Figure 14-56C shows that the ultrasound-diagnosed aneurysm begins below the superior mesenteric artery, coursing anteriorly, and also below the renal arteries, coursing posteriorly. Patients having asymptomatic aneurysms are routinely referred for a preoperative aortogram. Symptomatic aneurysms may or may not have arteriography, depending on the individual clinical circumstances. You should remember that angiography only shows the lumen of the aneurysm and cannot determine overall size. Also, angiography will not show free blood in the retroperitoneum. CT is the procedure to perform if a leak is suspected and an imaging test is required. One final point: do not forget that many abdominal aortic aneurysms are calcified and can be identified on plain films.

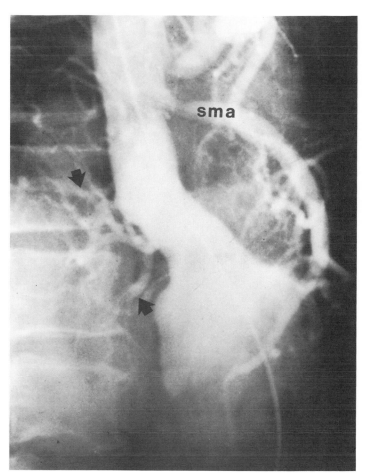

C

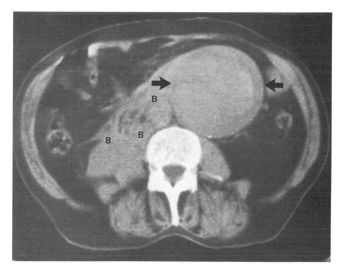

Figure 14-57. CT scan of a patient with a leaking abdominal aortic aneurysm. *Arrows* delineate the overall size of the aneurysm. *B* indicates free blood within the retroperitoneum. This patient, taken directly to the operating room for aneurysm resection and graft placement, made a good recovery.

265

The Inferior Vena Cava

The inferior vena cava may be imaged with a variety of techniques including ultrasound, computed tomography, magnetic-resonance scanning, and inferior vena cavography. By now you are quite familiar with its teardrop shape on CT, located in the prevertebral retroperitoneum, just to the right of the aorta. To perform an inferior vena cavagram, an angiographic catheter is inserted percutaneously via a femoral vein puncture and advanced proximally into a common iliac vein. A bolus of angiographic contrast material is then injected while x-ray films are taken overlying the abdomen. The contrast material ascends passively within the inferior vena cava, carried by the flowing blood. Consequently, the veins draining *into* the inferior vena cava are not opacified as are the branches of the aorta on an aortogram.

The two most common indications for imaging the inferior vena cava are suspected tumor invasion from an adjacent neoplasm, and suspected caval thrombosis from extension of lower extremity or pelvic vein thrombosis. Although both of these caval conditions may be diagnosed by ultrasound, CT, and MR scanning, inferior vena cavography is often performed because it shows the cava in greatest detail.

A tumor which frequently invades the inferior vena cava is renal cell carcinoma. Figure 14-58 illustrates such a case, a 62-year-old man with right flank pain and hematuria. He also noted recent onset of ankle swelling. His intravenous

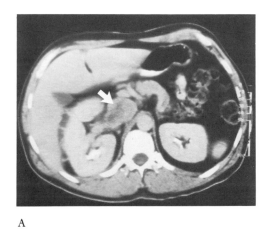

A

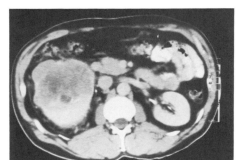

B

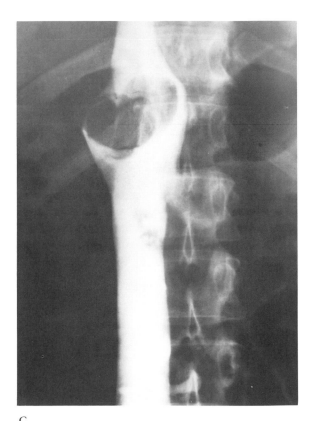

C

Figure 14-58. Renal cell carcinoma invading the inferior vena cava. A: CT scan showing a low-density tumor within the right renal vein and cava (*arrow*). B: Lower CT scan showing maximal diameter of tumor and necrotic center. C: Inferior vena cavagram showing invasion of the upper cava with a tumor mass extending from the right renal vein.

266

urogram showed a right renal mass, and a CT scan was requested. The CT scan, shown in Figures 14-58A and B confirmed a tumor in the lower pole of the right kidney, which appeared to be growing into the inferior vena cava (*arrow*). Note the low-density center typical of central tumor necrosis. His cavagram, Figure 14-58C, clearly delineates tumor extension which not only expands the inferior vena cava, but almost entirely occludes it. This explains his ankle swelling.

In addition to imaging the inferior vena cava, the radiologist may be involved in a therapeutic caval procedure: placement of an inferior vena cava filter. This technique is performed in patients with deep venous thrombosis of the lower extremities or pulmonary embolism, who have an absolute contraindication to anticoagulation. The filter will prevent life-threatening emboli from reaching the heart and lungs. There are several types of filters; one of the most popular, the Kimray-Greenfield filter, is shown in Figure 14-59. They are all collapsible, and are inserted into the inferior vena cava via a venous catheter under fluoroscopic control.

Deep venous thrombosis is most accurately diagnosed by leg venography, which requires only a needle stick of a dorsal foot vein with a small-gauge needle and hand injection of contrast medium. Figure 14-60 is from a venogram showing a normal femoral vein. In Figure 14-61, another patient, the popliteal and femoral veins are filled with thrombus.

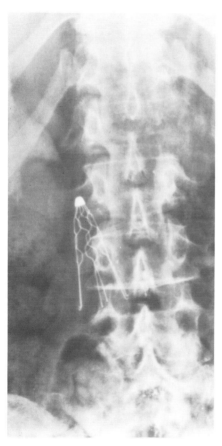

Figure 14-59. Abdominal plain film of a patient with an inferior vena cava filter in place.

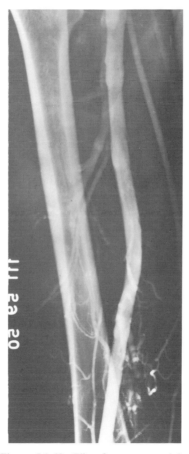

Figure 14-60. Film from a normal leg venogram, showing opacification of the femoral and popliteal veins.

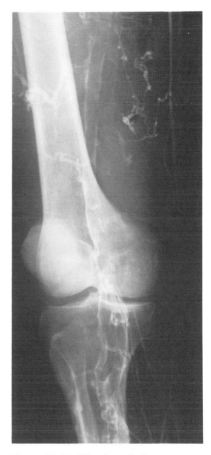

Figure 14-61. Film from the leg venogram of a patient with deep venous thrombosis; it shows extensive blood clots (long filling defects) within the femoral and popliteal veins.

Retroperitoneal Adenopathy

The retroperitoneal lymph nodes may be imaged by lymphangiography or computed tomography. Because CT is faster, easier to perform, less expensive, and better tolerated by patients, it has replaced lymphangiography as the initial procedure for staging malignancies that involve the retroperitoneal nodes. Although CT can readily demonstrate enlarged nodes (Figure 14-64), it cannot detect lymphomatous or metastatic disease involving normal-sized nodes. Consequently, lymphangiography is still indicated in staging lymphomas and genitopelvic malignancies, such as cervical and testicular carcinomas, when the CT examination is normal. Generally speaking, retroperitoneal lymph nodes measuring less than 1.5 centimeters in diameter at CT are considered to be normal sized.

Lymphangiography is a delicate procedure requiring the efforts of both the patient and the radiologist. In order to radiographically opacify the iliac and para-aortic nodes, the radiologist must cannulate a lymphatic channel on the dorsum of each foot with a tiny 30-gauge needle via a small cutdown. An iodinated, oily contrast medium is then slowly injected. This agent is transported passively, with normal lymphatic flow, through the lymphatic channels of the legs, pelvis, and retroperitoneum. Within the first hour or two, only the lymph channels are opacified (channel phase); later the nodes are opacified (nodal phase).

But how does the radiologist find a transparent lymph channel to cannulate within each cutdown? After sterilely prepping and draping each foot, he injects a tiny volume of blue dye intradermally into the first and fourth toe web spaces. Within 10 to 20 minutes the blue dye is picked up by the lymphatic system, visually revealing the lymph channels for cannulation and injection of x-ray contrast medium. The entire procedure takes about 2 hours. Channel phase films are taken during the infusion of contrast medium or immediately afterward; nodal phase films are taken the next day.

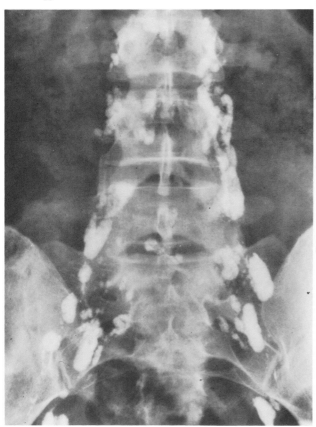

A

B

Figure 14-62. Normal lymphangiogram. A: Initial lymphatic, channel phase. B: Nodal phase, obtained 24 hours later.

Figure 14-62 illustrates the two stages in the lymphangiogram filming of a patient with normal nodes. A is the channel phase film, when the lymphatic channels are best opacified, but the lymph nodes are barely seen. Note the multiple small-diameter iliac and para-aortic lymph channels that follow the course of their associated blood vessels. At the level of the first lumbar vertebra the para-aortic channels drain into the cisterna chyli. B is a nodal phase film taken 24 hours later. The lymphatic channels are clear of contrast medium and the lymph nodes are better seen. Normal nodes are oval in shape with a homogeneous distribution of contrast medium. You will remember that the cisterna chyli empties into the left subclavian vein, so that any oily contrast medium not retained by the nodes will flow into the venous system to the pulmonary capillary bed. Ultimately the residual oily material will be coughed up by the patient. This is no problem for normal, healthy individuals, but you should be aware that lymphangiography *is* hazardous for patients with severely compromised pulmonary function and those with a right-to-left cardiac shunt. The radiologist performing the procedure always limits the amount of contrast medium for each individual patient.

Lymph nodes with lymphomatous involvement are uniformly enlarged, with a "foamy" appearance as in Figure 14-63. With metastatic involvement, single or multiple "punched-out" focal defects are seen in normal-sized or enlarged nodes. In addition, metastases may occlude lymph channels so that blocked channels with collateral circulation may be seen on the channel phase films, and the nodes supplied from the blocked channels may not be opacified at all. In the staging of malignant disease, if an abnormal nodal defect is identified it can be biopsied percutaneously by the radiologist for cytologic examination. Of course, nonneoplastic conditions such as infections may also cause lymph node enlargement.

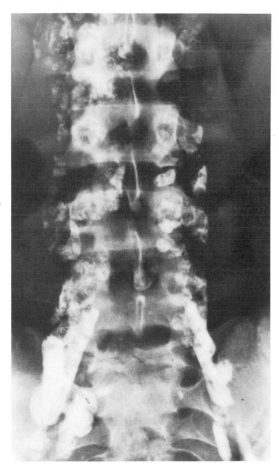

Figure 14-63. Abnormal nodal-phase lymphangiogram showing enlarged periaortic lymph nodes containing filling defects. This patient had widespread lymphoma.

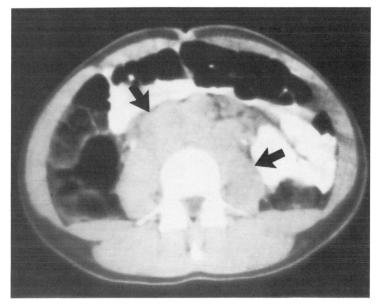

Figure 14-64. CT scan of a patient with extensive lymphadenopathy. The aorta, inferior vena cava, and psoas muscles are surrounded by a thick layer of enlarged lymphomatous nodes (*arrows*).

Angiographic Diagnosis and Control of Acute Gastrointestinal Hemorrhage

In patients with acute, unremitting, and life-threatening gastrointestinal hemorrhage, angiography offers a technique for both localization and treatment of bleeding. After selective arterial catheterization of the artery supplying the responsible lesion, sites of GI hemorrhage can be determined by injection of contrast medium and angiographic hemostasis accomplished with vasoconstrictor infusion or, for some bleeding sites, embolic occlusion of the arterial supply. Figure 14-65 depicts a patient with an acutely bleeding gastric ulcer, and Figure 14-67, a patient with an acutely bleeding colonic diverticulum.

Angiography is indicated in patients who are *actively* bleeding, as the angiographic demonstration of hemorrhage requires radiographic depiction of contrast medium extravasation from the arterial lumen into the bowel. Documentation of *active upper GI bleeding* is generally provided by observation of the nasogastric tube aspirate; if vigorous iced saline lavage fails to clear a patient's bright red bloody aspirate, then active bleeding is usually occurring proximal to the ligament of Treitz. Documentation of *active lower GI bleeding* is somewhat more difficult. A patient with a slowly bleeding small or large bowel source may have intermittent movements of bloody stool; in the interim, whether or not bleeding has stopped may be unclear. The usual measures include monitoring the patient's vital signs, blood requirements, and frequency of hematochesia.

In uncertain cases a radioisotope bleeding scan is performed (Figure 14-66). For this procedure a sample of the patient's own red blood cells is labeled with a radioisotope and reinjected into the patient. Scans of the abdomen are then obtained at frequent intervals. Normally, activity is shown only overlying the major blood vessels; positive scans are usually positive within 10 to 15 minutes and show pooling of radioactivity outside the vascular system and overlying the bowel. A positive bleeding scan calls for emergency angiography, whereas a negative scan informs us that angiography is not indicated at this time.

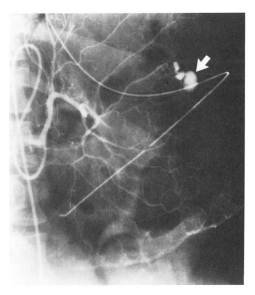
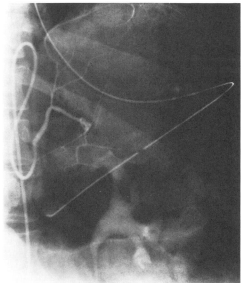

A   B

Figure 14-65. Left gastric arteriogram of a patient with a bleeding gastric ulcer. A: *Arrow* indicates extravasation of contrast medium at the bleeding site. B: Repeat arteriogram after treatment with a left gastric artery infusion of vasoconstrictor shows decreased caliber of the left gastric artery and its branches, and no further bleeding.

Acutely bleeding *upper* GI lesions which can be localized with selective arteriography include esophagitis, Mallory-Weiss tear, esophageal tumors, gastritis, gastric tumors, ulcers, and duodenal diverticula. *Lower* GI lesions include colonic diverticula, neoplasms of the small and large bowel, and vascular malformations. As angiography primarily localizes bleeding sites rather than characterizing the causes of bleeding, patients may be candidates for endoscopic and barium examinations for definitive diagnosis once hemostasis is achieved. Although gastroesophageal varices can be identified at angiography, *extravasation* from varices is not seen. Ideally, patients with acute upper GI bleeding are endoscoped prior to angiography to rule out varices, and patients with acute lower GI bleeding are sigmoidoscoped to rule out rectal causes, such as hemorrhoids. If angiography is available, *barium examinations should not be performed* initially in the acutely bleeding patient, as residual barium may interfere with angiographic visualization.

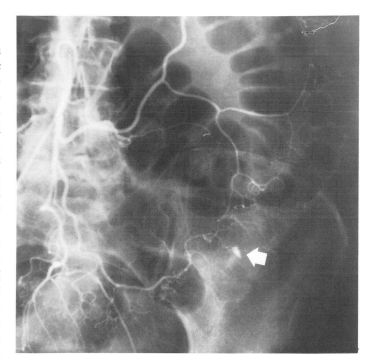

A

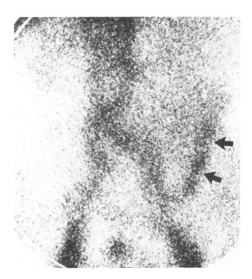

Figure 14-66 (*above*). Positive radioisotope bleeding scan, showing accumulation of isotope overlying the course of the distal descending colon (*arrows*).

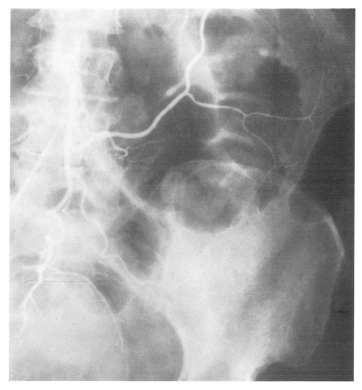

B

Figure 14-67 (*at right*). Inferior mesenteric arteriogram of a patient with a bleeding colonic diverticulum. A: *Arrow* points to the site of active bleeding (contrast medium extravasation) in the distal descending colon. B: Repeat arteriogram after treatment with vasoconstrictor shows no further bleeding.

271

CHAPTER 15   Bones

How to Study Radiographs of Bones

Bones are much more interesting than most students realize during their years in medical school. Probably no segment of medical information could seem fascinating during the tedium of memorizing the origins and insertions of muscles, and perhaps the remembrance of that tiresome and difficult task continues long afterward to cloud the subject of bone, even at a time when the metabolic disease processes in which bone shares as an organ are being studied.

The student cannot afford to neglect the bones—their function and change, their growth and mature microscopic structure in health and disease. He must be able to imagine what is going on in the bony skeleton of the immobilized patient with a healing fracture of the femur, not just at the site of the fracture but throughout the body as a result of enforced inactivity. The physician must be able to predict the degree to which invasion of his patient's bones by metastatic tumor will alter his blood chemistry. One

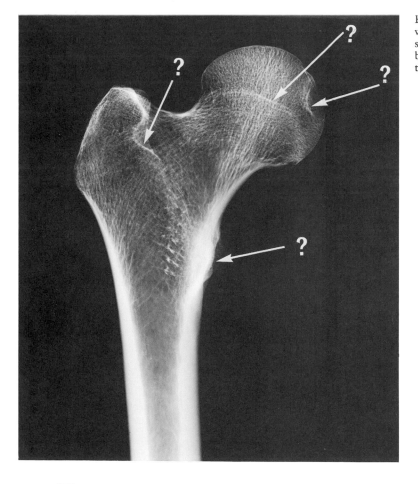

Figure 15-1. Can you explain precisely why the details of the radiographic shadows marked with arrows should have been produced by the anatomic structures they represent? (See text.)

272

must understand the metabolic reasons for the formation of kidney stones in hyperparathyroid patients in whom there is a marked increase in the rate of bone breakdown and a significant increase in serum calcium and calcium excretion.

The bony skeleton must not be thought of as a static and principally structural fabric. It is constantly changing throughout life, and since the functional lifetime of any microscopic plate of spongy bone or any osteone (Haversian) segment of compact bone is only about seven years, there is continuous bone breakdown and replacement. The rate of turnover may vary somewhat normally; bone production is more rapid than bone breakdown in children because their skeleton is increasing in size constantly. In the elderly the rate of bone replacement lags and the bones gradually become thinner and more fragile.

While these changes are all appreciable to the trained eye and intellect by means of a variety of imaging procedures, the degree to which they may be noted on radiographs is an important part of your training in radiology and medicine. Begin by examining the two radiographs on this page spread, which focus on the anatomic structure of bone.

You will have identified the fovea capitis in Figure 15-1, but did you account for the white streak that you see in the depth of that hollow in the femoral head as the cortical bone there caught tangentially by the ray? Similarly, the white line crossing the neck of the femur just where the epiphyseal line used to be is the tangentially viewed plate of somewhat more densely crowded trabecular plates that developed there as the growth plate fused when growth was complete. Another *arrow* indicates the tangentially viewed ridge of bone of the intertrochanteric line on the posterior surface of the femur, and it is being projected superimposed on all the spongy bone and cortex anterior to it. One must think of radiographs of bones as summation shadowgrams just as one does when looking at chest films. Finally, the fourth *arrow* points to the lesser trochanter, the surface of which is compact bone seen tangentially. Thus you can carry forward to your detailed examination of bone films what you learned in the first chapter about curving sheets of rose petal.

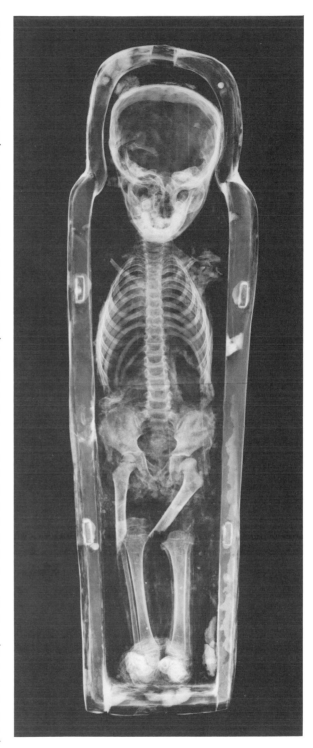

Figure 15-2. Radiograph of the mummy of a child. What can you determine about the remains? How do you know it is a child? How could experts determine his age at death? (See text.)

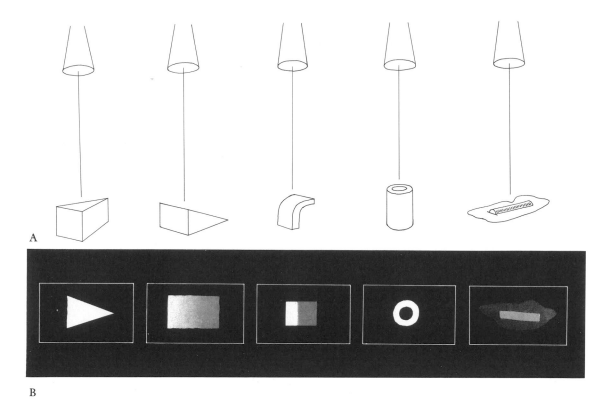

A

B

Figure 15-3. (See text.)

The legs of the mummy in Figure 15-2 were broken postmortem by an ancient Egyptian funeral director in order to make the body fit into a burial case the embalmer had on hand. The lower femurs have been removed, and the arms also are missing.

You can tell the mummy is that of a child because there are as-yet-unfused epiphyses present at the femoral heads and proximal ends of the tibias. The secondary centers of ossification at the ends of long bones appear on radiographs when mineralized bone forms at the center of the cartilaginous anlage of those epiphyses. The growth and development of the epiphyses and the ultimate fusion to their growth plates have been radiographically documented, both first appearance and fusion occurring at predictable ages, so that the age of unidentified skeletons can be easily determined.

Examine the several hypothetical examples of details of bony structure (A) and their approximate radiographic images (B) in Figure 15-3. By

a simple rule of summation the wedge casts a different shadow according to the direction in which the ray traverses it. The curved sheet of bone obeys the same principles as the curved rose petal and leaf in Chapter 1. The cylinder seen end-on becomes a dense circle in the radiograph, and if it were radiographed from the side would produce two parallel lines of tangentially projected "cortex," just as you see in the lower part of Figure 15-4C. Finally, the sheet of bone with a thicker ridge across it will x-ray as a gray area with a streak of white across it. Realize too that in Figure 15-4C at the level of the lesser trochanter you are seeing the x-ray shadows of the tangentially viewed lateral and medial compact bone on either side, and, between them, two layers of compact bone viewed en face—the anterior and posterior cortex, superimposed on the network of spongy bone inside.

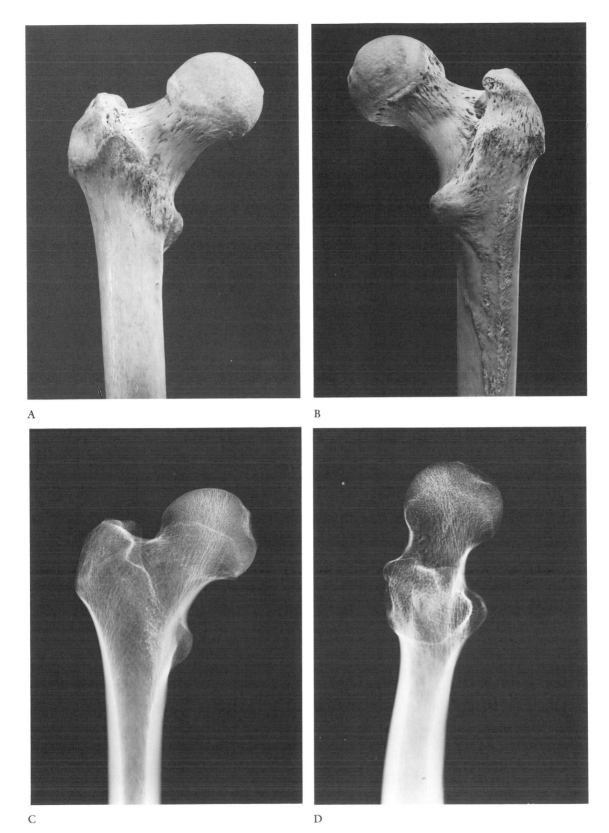

A

B

C

D

Figure 15-4. Anterior and posterior photographs of the upper femur (A and B) to help you account for details in the AP and lateral radiographs in C and D.

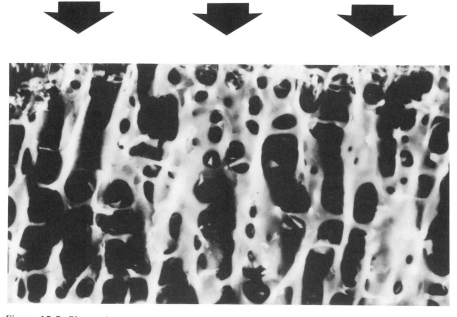

Figure 15-5. Photomicrograph showing trabecular arrangement developed with weight bearing (*arrows*).

You will have noticed on the films you have just seen of the upper femur that the cortical bone is very thick in the shaft or diaphysis, and that it thins out around the upper femur, where the bone is filled with trabeculae of spongy bone. These arch in parallel struts, which closely follow the lines of stress developed within this part of the bone in man, who stands erect and carries the weight of his trunk upon the two femoral heads. The arrangement of these struts to bear weight differs slightly from that of similar spongy bone in quadrupeds, and it is interesting to reflect how those trabeculae must have adapted themselves when our distant ancestors first stood to walk on their hind legs.

Figure 15-5 is a photomicrograph of the trabeculae in a coronal 3-millimeter slice of bone from the upper tibia showing adaptation to weight bearing being delivered from above. Note that the vertical struts are heavier and thicker, and that they are joined by much lighter and thinner ones called secondary trabeculae, which reinforce them structurally. In areas having spongy bone which is not so directly weight bearing, such as the central parts of the vertebral bodies or the scapula, for example, the size and thickness of the trabeculae are more uniform, the marrow spaces between being enclosed in a bony sponge which does not show any thicker struts. Try applying these observations to the lateral radiograph of the foot in Figure 15-6, identifying the stress vectors in the talus and calcaneus.

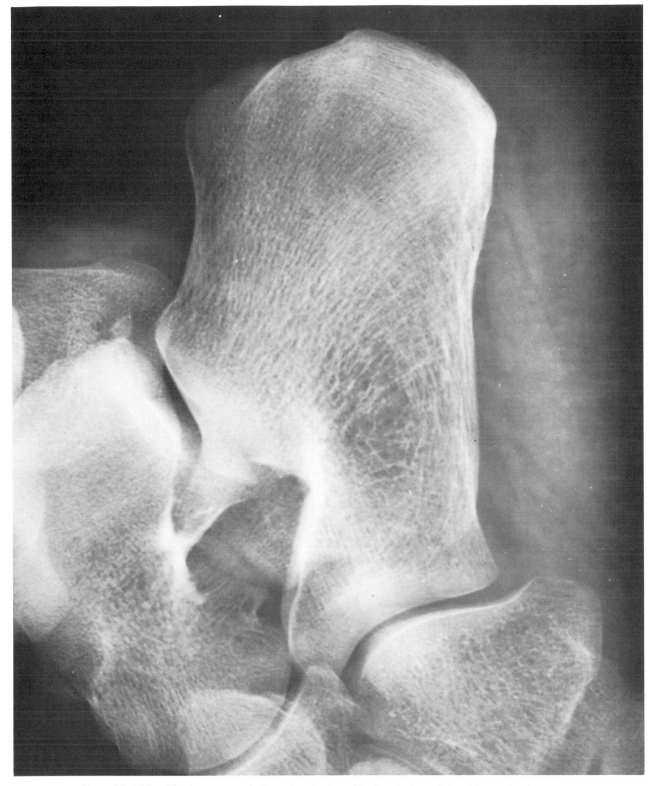

Figure 15-6. Magnification x-ray study. Lateral projection of the foot (sole parallel to side margin of page). Note the trabeculae, which arch backward and downward from the calcaneotalar joint toward the weight-bearing point under the heel.

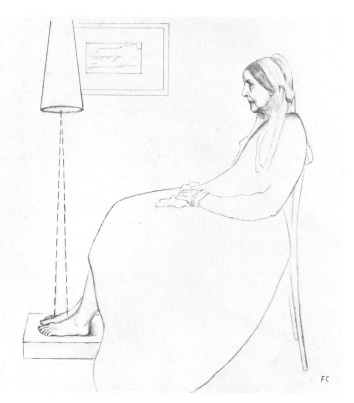

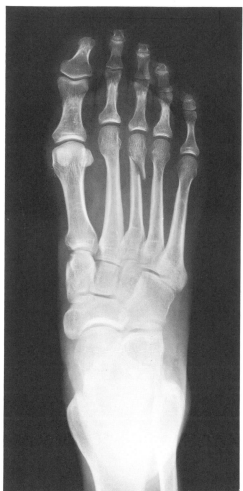

Figure 15-7. Mother Whistler has her foot x-rayed.

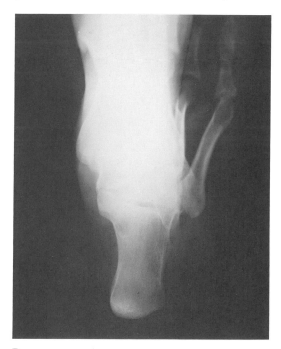

B

A

Figure 15-8. Two different views of the foot. How would you have to rearrange Mother Whistler's comfortable position to obtain B?

278

Requesting Films of Bones

The various projections in which films of the bones are made are largely a matter of convention based upon which ones produce the most information. You will easily become accustomed to the AP and lateral views, which are routine—two films made at 90 degrees being essential in almost all bone filming. Additional views often have to be designed by the radiologist to show to best advantage a particular lesion in a particular patient.

It will be a relief to you to know that you do not have to request particular views, therefore, since there are routine sets of views taken anyway by the radiologic technologist. You should *indicate on the requisition only the area to be filmed and the location of the pain or other symptoms*. Thus you would have requested "films of the foot" in Mother Whistler, since the pain was located in the midfoot, where you see the fractured metatarsal. If she had complained of pain farther up, you might have requested "films of the foot and ankle," and then additional routine films would have been obtained, including obliques of the ankle joint. Note that in Figure 15-8A the lower parts of the tibia and fibula are superimposed on the proximal part of the foot. Thus, a radiographic examination of the foot is inadequate for diagnosis of possible fracture of the ankle. Precise location of the pain and point tenderness often helps you to decide, therefore, whether you need films of foot or ankle or both.

X-rays of injured parts are usually obtained after fractures have been reduced and set in plaster casts, to determine the position and alignment of fracture fragments. With the superimposition of the cast material, of course, much less detail of the bones will be seen. For this reason, during the healing period of fractures films are generally made when the patient is out of plaster, between cast changes, in order to appraise the presence and integrity of callus and so on.

You will have to develop a familiarity with the details of the anatomy of bones on radiographs, anticipating that when bones are unavoidably superimposed (as are the femoral head and the acetabulum in Figure 15-9) you must account for every detail in the roentgen image by subtracting intellectually the parts that belong to one bone from the superimposed images of parts that belong to the other.

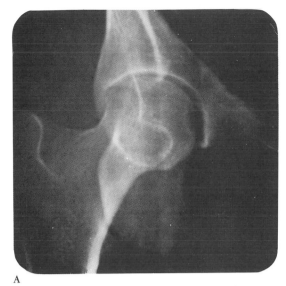

A

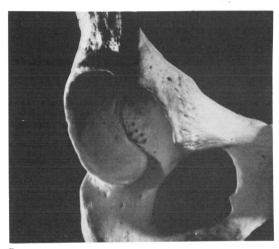

B

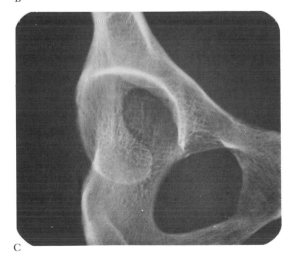

C

Figure 15-9. The shadow of the acetabulum superimposed on that of the upper femur. A: Radiograph of a patient. B: Photograph of specimen of another patient. C: Radiograph of acetabulum of specimen.

279

Trauma to Bones and Joints: Fractures

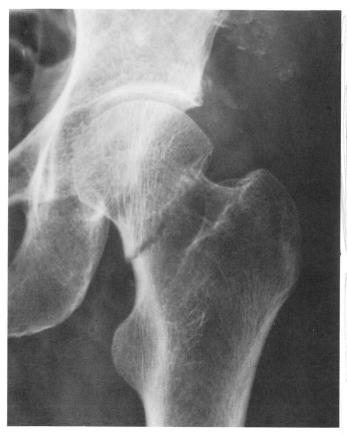

Figure 15-10

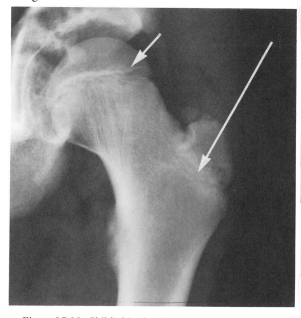

Figure 15-11. Child's hip showing growth plates (*arrows*) to be distinguished from fractures. The ossification of the epiphysis for the femoral head appears before 8 months and fuses at about 18 years. The one for the greater trochanter appears at around 2 years and fuses to its metaphysis at about 16 years.

Various types of fractures demand variations in filming. Fractures may be *transverse, spiral, oblique, simple, comminuted* (when there are several fragments and intersecting fracture lines), *impacted,* or *pathological* in the presence of underlying disease. Because of twisting types of trauma, it is wise to radiograph an entire bone you believe to be fractured. This is particularly true of the paired bones of the lower leg and the forearm. Obvious fracture of the lower tibia is quite often accompanied by a subtle fracture of the fibula near the knee, and films to include both knee and ankle should be requested. Of course, if you have examined the patient carefully, you will have observed point tenderness in both locations.

You will have no difficulty in recognizing the simple fracture of the neck of the femur in Figure 15-10. Fractures appear on radiographs as dark streaks across the bone where the continuity of both cortical bone and spongy bone is interrupted. Hemorrhage and soft tissue, torn and injured in the area, are often interposed to some extent between the fractured fragments. If the fracture is comminuted, several fragments and several separate but communicating fracture planes must be present (as in Figure 15-12). Sometimes one of these planes of fracture will not be obvious on the films obtained because it is oblique to the ray. In Figure 15-12 three planes of fracture may be seen and one more supposed—that for the greater trochanter.

In examining films for fracture you should look closely everywhere for interruption of the normal line of the periosteal surface of the cortex, as it may be the only indication of fracture if there is no separation of fragments. Remember that spongy bone is also fractured and close examination may show discontinuity of major trabeculae with only slight separation of the plane of the undisplaced fracture. Depending on the direction and character of the trauma, spongy bone may be impacted. The trabeculae will have become enmeshed so that innumerable fragments of bone across the plane of the fracture lie closer together than normally and produce an abnormally dense white area across the bone where the *impacted* plane of fracture is seen tangentially.

You will not mistake the similar white boundary of an epiphyseal growth plate like that in Figure 15-11 for a fracture, once you have studied a few of them. The linear dark area crossing the bone is the tangentially viewed cartilaginous growth plate, and its margin does not show an abrupt interruption of cortex, but a smoothly curved one at an expected location.

Computed tomography is the best way to assess injury to curving bony surfaces—for instance, about the acetabulum, where it is essential to evaluate both injury to the roof (weight bearing) and the stability of the rest of the acetabulum. CT, now employed in many emergency rooms, can reveal a three-dimensional array of fracture fragments, the orientation of fracture lines, and the degree of comminution better than any other imaging procedure. In addition, it can be done quickly, without uncomfortable positioning of the patient, and with less radiation than conventional tomograms. Today CT is widely used to evaluate fractures through complex bony areas such as the pelvis, spine, and base of the skull. MR imaging will not show fractures as well as CT because there is no signal from cortical bone.

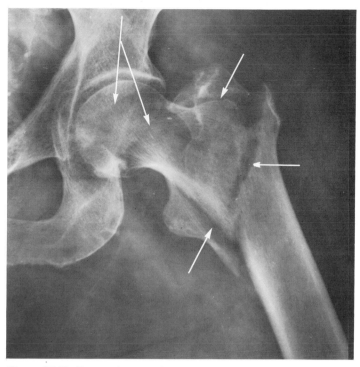

Figure 15-12. Intertrochanteric fracture of the left femur. *Longer arrows* indicate the overlapping margins of the anterior and posterior rims of the acetabulum. *Shorter arrows* indicate three communicating fracture planes.

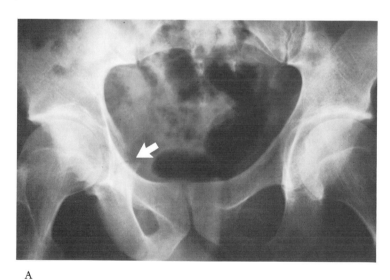

A

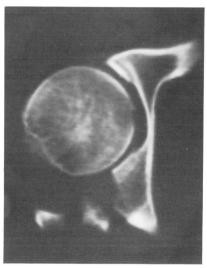

B

Figure 15-13. A: Pelvic fracture (*arrow*), which in B, the CT study, is shown to involve the posterior rim of the acetabulum.

Fracture Clinic

The illustrations on the next few pages constitute an exercise in fracture diagnosis, framed for you as unknowns because they are more interesting so. Not every film shows a fracture, as would be the case if you had seen these patients at random in the emergency room. All these patients *had* been injured. (Answers at back of book.)

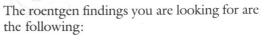

The roentgen findings you are looking for are the following:
(1) Breaks in the continuity of cortex
(2) Radiolucent fracture lines
(3) Overlap of both cortical bone and spongy bone creating an abnormally white area
(4) Unexplained fragments of bone, even in the absence of a visible fracture
(5) Denser areas where impaction of bone has occurred, seen in two views
(6) Flocculent density in soft tissues adjoining bone in healing fractures (callus), visible only after it calcifies

Remember that in describing these films to the attending physician over the telephone, for example, you would not only state the location and type of fracture, but also comment on alignment of the fracture fragments and any overriding that is present. Open or compound fractures may not be apparent at all radiographically unless there is obvious lucent air in the soft tissues.

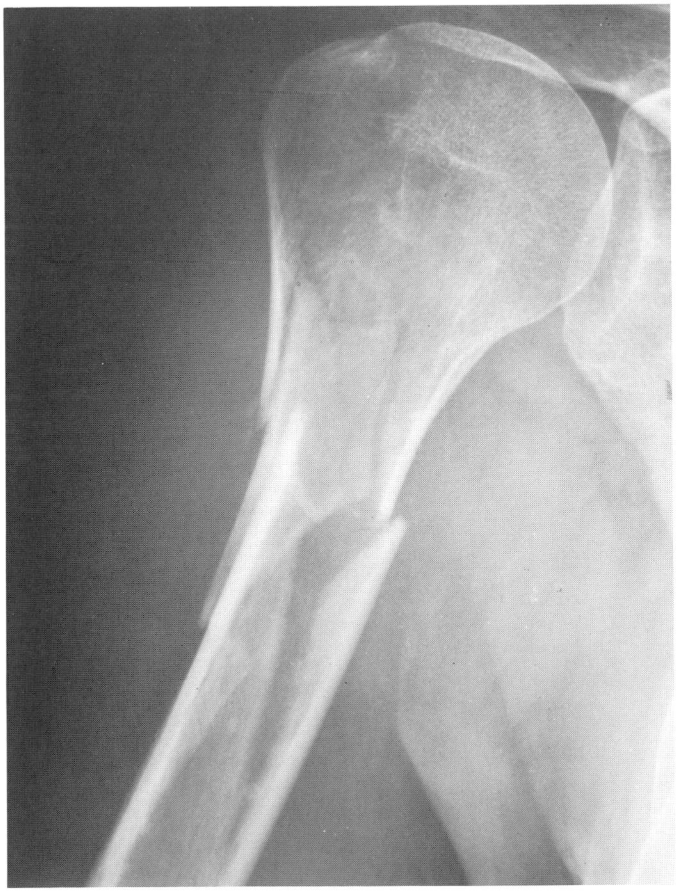

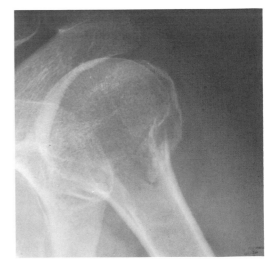

Figure 15-14 (*Unknown 15-1*)

Figure 15-15 (*Unknown 15-2*)

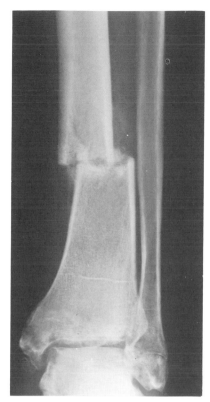

Figure 15-16 (*Unknown 15-3*)

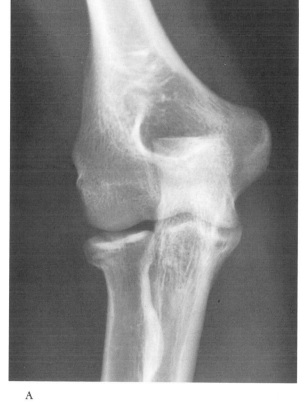

A

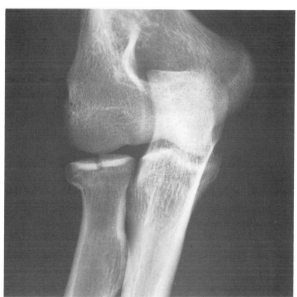

B

Figure 15-17 (*Unknown 15-4*)

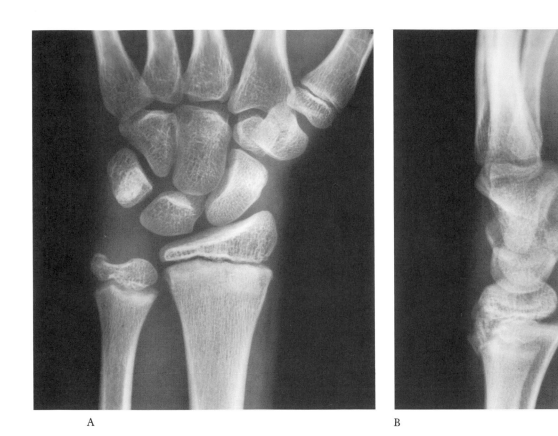

A   B

Figure 15-18 (*Unknown 15-5*)

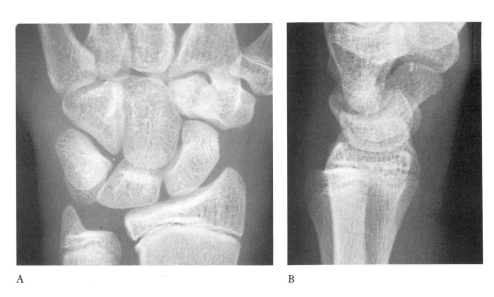

A   B

Figure 15-19 (*Unknown 15-6*)

284

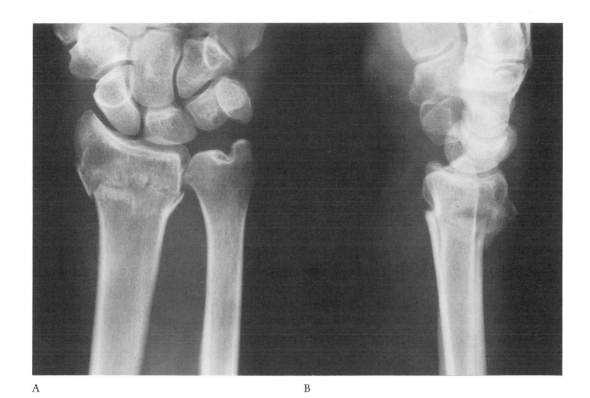

A   B

Figure 15-20 (*Unknown 15-7*)

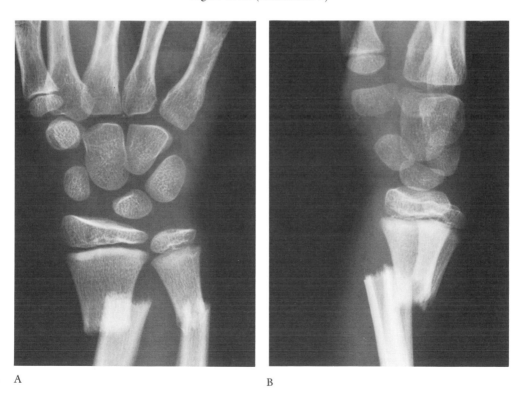

A   B

Figure 15-21 (*Unknown 15-8*). Patient fell out of an apple tree.

285

When a fracture appears to have occurred through bone which was already abnormal and may therefore have been unusually fragile, it is called a *pathological fracture*. Figures 15-22 and 15-23 are examples.

In Figure 15-22 a cylindrical cuff of bony cortex has been eroded by pressure from within. You observe the thinning best where you see cortex in tangent medially and laterally, although you know it has occurred anteriorly and posteriorly as well. The bone looks expanded, subperiosteal new bone having been added as the endosteal layers were removed by pressure. Across the thinned segment of bone a jagged fracture has occurred and is seen on the lateral margin as a distinct interruption of cortex. This is an example of a *unicameral bone cyst* in a child. It was fractured by a very trivial trauma, that of throwing a ball. The fact that the bone looks expanded is an indication of its benign nature, since there has been time for such change to occur. Malignant tumors are aggressively destructive and usually produce new bone in the soft tissues.

Figure 15-23 is the upper femur of a patient with Paget's disease. A transverse fracture has occurred across the shaft several centimeters below the lesser trochanter. Although it characteristically thickens bone, Paget's disease also weakens its structure, and the bone withstands stress less well than normal tubular long bone does. It is also more usual for normal upper femur to fracture irregularly in ragged points and with comminution; this bone has fractured transversely. Paget's disease typically produces enlargement of the bone, thickening of cortex, and grotesque disarrangement of trabecular pattern.

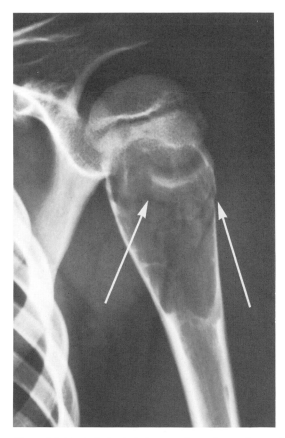

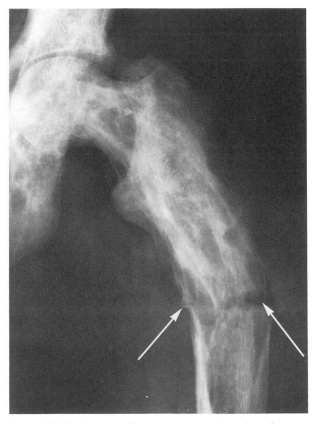

Figure 15-22. Pathological fracture through a unicameral bone cyst in its classic location in the metaphysis of a growing bone.

Figure 15-23. Transverse fracture, also pathological, in the upper femoral shaft of a patient with Paget's disease.

Dislocations

Fractures are often accompanied by dislocation of joints, or dislocations may occur without fracture. A partial dislocation is called a *subluxation*. Figure 15-24 shows you a dislocation of the shoulder and its appearance after reduction. Nearly all shoulder dislocations are anterior, with the humeral head displaced anteriorly and medially so that it is easy to diagnose clinically. The rare posterior dislocation may be missed on AP films since the displacement is much less, and often only special views can establish its presence. Acromioclavicular dislocations are easy to recognize when films are made of the two shoulders with weights in the patient's hands, a procedure that increases the separation on the side involved.

Infection

Osteomyelitis occurs most frequently in the long bones near the metaphysis and is usually blood borne. It is seen today in drug addicts, and the most common causative organism is the *Staphylococcus aureus*. The changes which are seen in osteomyelitis (bone destruction and periosteal reaction) unfortunately are not likely to be present for two weeks after the start of the process. Accordingly, in patients clinically suspected of having osteomyelitis an early bone scan is in order; it will indicate the presence of acutely reactive bone turnover within 48 hours so that therapy can be started. A more chronic, smoldering form of osteomyelitis is seen with the tubercle bacillus as the causative organism. It too produces bone breakdown, but much more gradually and with less acute clinical symptoms.

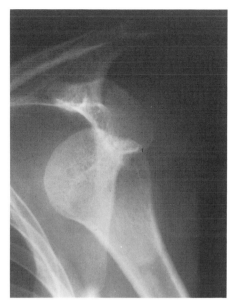

A

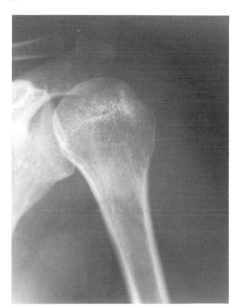

B

Figure 15-24. Anterior dislocation of the shoulder before and after reduction.

287

Arthritis

Most patients who present with a complaint of "arthritis" can be diagnosed clinically, and the radiographs of painful areas will help to confirm the clinical impression. Although you will refer many patients to a rheumatologist for differentiation of the rare forms of arthritis, it is important and easy for you to have good general information about the common forms yourself.

Degenerative arthritis is common in older patients but may occur following repeated trauma, for example, in younger people. In older patients it is often called *osteoarthritis*. It is frequently seen in weight-bearing joints such as the hip and knee and is characterized by narrowing of the joint space, productive bone of increased density on both sides of the joint, and small cysts in the bone near the joint. These result from fractures of the joint cartilage and penetration of the joint fluid into the juxta-articular bone.

Osteoarthritis also commonly involves the hands, which are not weight-bearing joints and which may have a different pathogenesis entirely. It too is quite characteristic radiologically and shows narrowing of the distal interphalangeal joints most commonly, with the middle interphalangeal joints next most frequently showing changes. The metacarpophalangeal joints are infrequently involved.

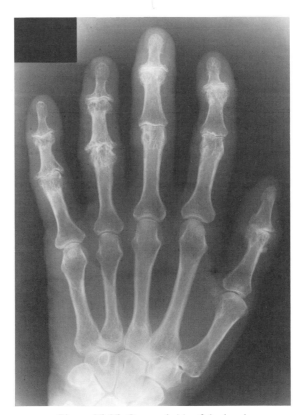

Figure 15-25. Osteoarthritis of the hand.

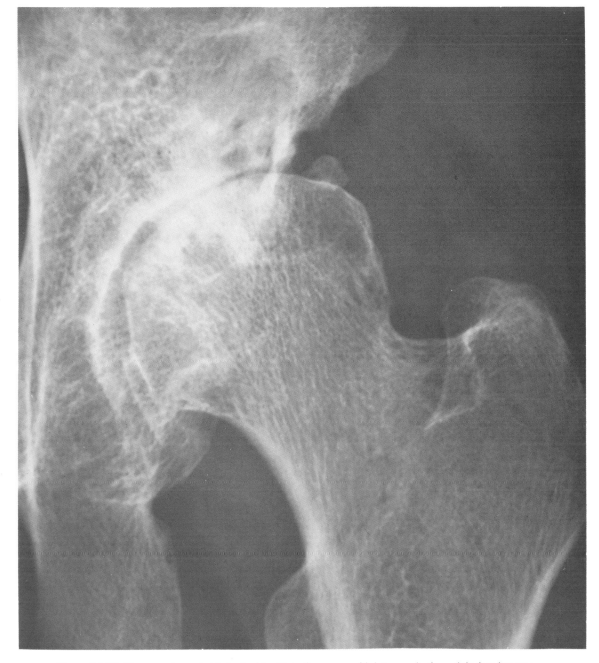

Figure 15-26. Degenerative arthritis in the hip. Note the narrowed joint space in the weight-bearing area, where the cartilage must be very thin and deteriorated. There is reactive eburnation of bone on both sides of the joint, with cysts forming in the juxta-articular bone.

Classically, *rheumatoid arthritis* occurs in women from 24 to 45 years of age. The patients complain of stiffness, swelling, and pain in the joints, especially the hands, although other joints as well are commonly involved. It is usually bilateral and symmetrical, and by x-ray soft-tissue swelling about the metacarpophalangeal and proximal interphalangeal joints is the rule. There are juxta-articular erosions of bone produced by hypertrophied synovium. Ultimately there will be destruction and even subluxation of the joints. The disease affects the carpal joints, and the wrist is classically seen to be fused in advanced states. Late in rheumatoid disease some of the findings of osteoarthritis may be superimposed. This confuses the picture unless one remembers that it may happen.

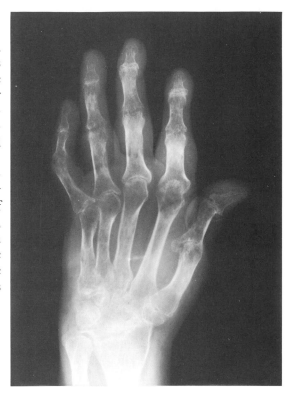

Figure 15-27. Rheumatoid arthritis of the hand.

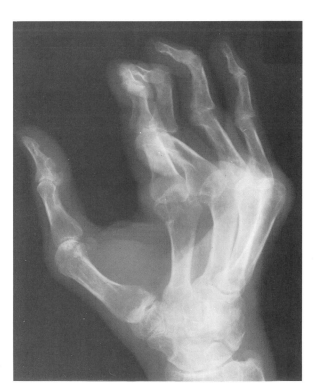

Figure 15-28. Rheumatoid arthritis, late, with subluxation of joints.

290

Gout is seen in errors of purine metabolism and involves many tissues including synovium, bone, soft tissues, and cartilage. It should not be thought of as a joint disease. It is at least ten times as common in men as it is in women and is seen most commonly in hands and feet, especially in the first metatarsophalangeal joint, in which extremely painful soft-tissue swelling accompanies the joint involvement, classic podagra. Radiologically the typical findings are large erosions of bone, often with hooklike margins where they adjoin a soft-tissue swelling (the tophus). No particular *group* of joints is affected, and many may be completely normal in appearance. The tophi may or may not calcify. The carpus is often involved with intraosseous cysts.

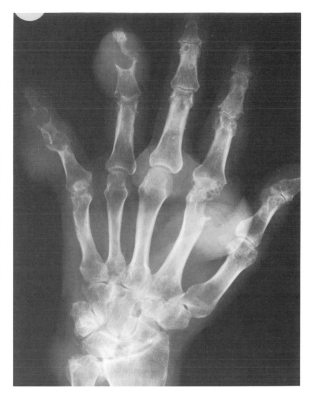

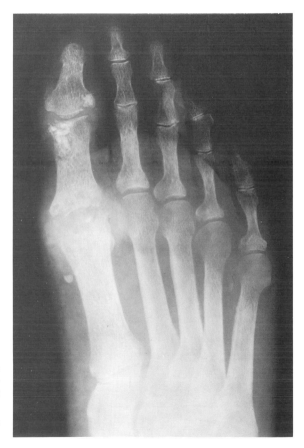

Figure 15-29 (*above*). Gout of the hand. Note classic tophi in the soft tissues, scattered rather than regular joint destruction, endosseous tophous inclusions, and hooklike bone spiccules remaining near the larger tophi.

Figure 15-30 (*below*). Gout involving the great toe (classic podagra).

291

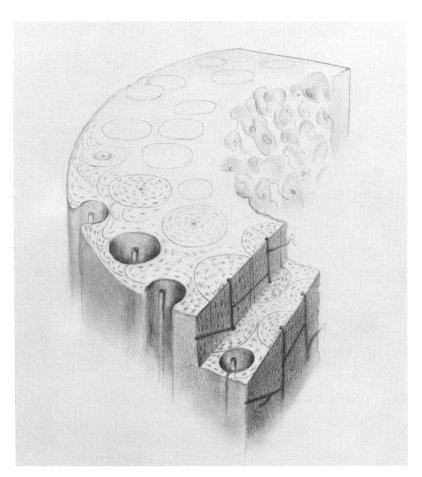

Microscopic
Bone Structure
and Maintenance

Figure 15-31. Knowledge of the structure of compact bone is important to an understanding of bone disease. This diagram, adapted from Ham, shows both horizontal and vertical cut faces of the femoral cortex. The diagram has been simplified for clarity; of course there are many more osteones in the full cortical thickness (see Figure 15-32).

Focus down intellectually on a cross section of the full thickness of the cortex of the femoral shaft you were looking at in Figure 15-1, and you will see the structure diagramed above in Figure 15-31. The cross-cut face reveals numerous sectioned *osteones* (or Haversian systems) with their central vessels. The vertical cut enables you to recall that the basic functioning adult bone unit is a cylinder of very minute dimensions. These cylinders, the osteones, are connected with one another via their branching central arteries and compose, in effect, a "breccia," units mortared together to form a mass. They are of a high order phylogenetically and do not exist in the bones of many lower animals. Structurally they produce a type of bone (and there are several types, remember) which is of excellent resilience and beautifully designed for adaptation to changing needs.

Such a composite of arterially connected units begins to be laid down in the bones of a human infant. This replaces a far less well designed type of immature bone, phylogenetically much earlier in type and resembling a woven fabric rather than a masonry wall. Even in the infant, osteones are found to be concentrated in regions of particular stress such as important tendon insertions. Eventually in the adult, most compact bone is composed of osteones mortared together by a lamellar bone matrix—as you can see in Figure 15-32, a microradiograph of a thin-ground cross section of the shaft of a long bone, which might have been sliced off the face of the diagramed bone wedge in Figure 15-31.

The osteones in such microradiographs are seen as rings of varying density about dark central holes which once contained arteries. Osteones vary in radiodensity because they are of different ages and therefore contain somewhat different amounts of mineral apatite. Mineral is precipitated very rapidly into the organic collagen bone matrix when it is first laid down, and after that more slowly, over several years.

The useful life expectancy of an individual osteone is around seven years, at the end of which it is removed by erosion from within until an empty cylinder exists where once it was traversed by the central artery and lined by sheets of

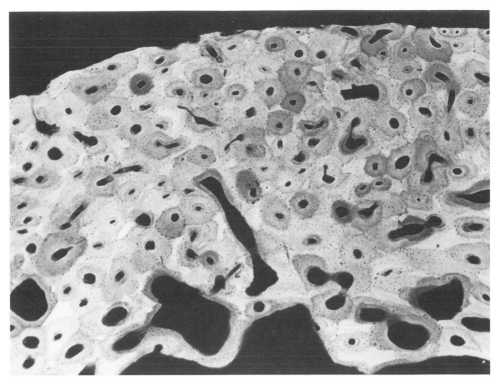

Figure 15-32. Microradiograph of a transverse section of the normal femoral cortex. The specimen was not prepared by sectioning decalcified bone but was sawed off and then ground down to a thickness of a few microns in a fresh state, retaining its normal calcium content. Radiograph made with specimen in close contact with photographic film.

mesenchymal cells. These differentiate into osteoblasts and lay down concentric new layers of bone matrix, one within another, until the central artery is again surrounded by a new osteone. The osteoblasts become engulfed in the bone matrix they elaborate (after which they are called osteocytes), continuing to function via minute canaliculi which radiate from their surfaces in all directions like the spines of a burr. These communicate with the canaliculi of other osteocytes nearby, so that the bone is able to be perfused with fluid and electrolytes, functioning throughout life as an organ no less important than the liver or kidney.

Because the osteoblasts become engulfed in concentric cylindrical layers of matrix, *in cross section* they will appear to be arranged in concentric circles about the artery, just as you see them in the diagram and in the microradiograph. You would *expect* the cells to be radiolucent compared with the mineralized matrix around them and could predict that in the microradiograph they would appear as minute black dots. Note

that some of the osteone circles in the microradiograph are very dark; these are the younger ones, less completely mineralized than their white, denser, older neighbors.

If the patient in Figure 15-32 had recently been given an injection of tagged (artificially rendered radioactive) calcium, the younger osteones which you have just identified would now contain much larger amounts of that calcium load, since they are mineralizing at a more rapid rate than their seniors. An *autoradiograph*, made by placing a fine-grained photographic film in close contact with a section of bone like the one x-rayed to produce Figure 15-32, would show darker spots in the precise locations of the younger osteones, because radioactivity of the calcium isotope produces silver precipitation in the film. When microradiographs, autoradiographs, photographs made with polarized light, and special stain studies of the same bone section are matched in register, an invaluable means of studying bone pathophysiology at the microscopic level emerges.

293

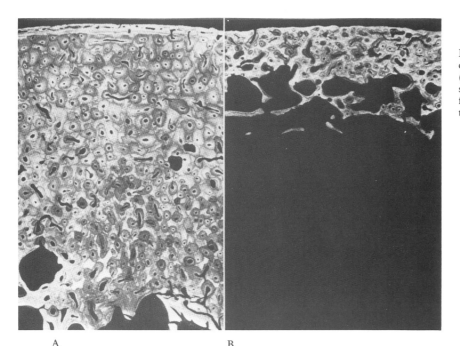

Figure 15-33. Microradiograph of normal cortex (A) and the cortex in an elderly woman (B) taken during autopsy from precisely the same location on the lateral surface of the femur. The periosteal surface is at the top and the medullary surface below. (See text.)

A   B

By means of *serial* studies of these types, the rate at which osteones form, are mineralized, removed, and restored can be recorded for healthy as well as abnormal bone. The gross appearance of a bone is so suggestive of permanence and durability that it is difficult to accept intellectually the degree to which bones are being constantly changed and remodeled throughout life, and the extent to which they do reflect and share in virtually every disease condition. In learning to comprehend these changes, you will find it essential to think clearly of the "flow" prevailing normally in the bones at various periods of life. The infant and young child grow in many ways and at different speeds from year to year, and their growth bonewise has been charted and documented extensively. Most of us fail to comprehend fully, however, that bone laid down in one site this year *may* begin next month to be removed, to accommodate developing changes.

Take any given tendon insertion site as an example. During childhood growth spurts, when the long bones are increasing in length very rapidly, an important muscle tendon inserted at one point soon functions at a disadvantage unless it is moved again close to the joint it subtends. The adductor muscles, arising from the pubis and inserting into the femur posteriorly along its entire length, powerfully adduct the thigh. The adductor longus inserts into the linea aspera on the posterior surface of the bone about midshaft, a location at which little or no change is occur-

ring, while the adductor magnus inserts farther down into a more limited area by means of a heavy aponeurosis and just above the margin of the epiphyseal growth plate. Here new bone is forming and extending the length of the femur at a very rapid rate indeed. If the tendon insertion of the adductor magnus remained attached at one point, it would soon be inserting farther up the femur and would adduct the thigh much less efficiently.

The concentration of osteones along the linea aspera in early childhood and at all tendon sites allows for a mechanism of adaptation. By destruction and reconstruction of osteones at slightly different locations, it is possible to maintain in an area optimal for function the heavy cortex into which the tendon fibers insert. Thus the bones, like every other tissue, adapt and change with growth until maturity. Through the prime years many individual osteones doubtless manage to live out their seven-odd years of usefulness in the same location, but others are removed before that time in order to accommodate to changes pertinent to the habits or activity or health of the individual patient. If a carpenter gives up his trade and learns another more sedentary one, the heavy concentrations of osteones under the tendon insertions in his dominant right arm will gradually be decreased. The young mental patient who recovers after several years of depression and inactivity and takes up the latest dance step must increase the rate of bone building throughout his body.

The Development of Metabolic Bone Disease

With the advent of postmaturity and the waning years, the process of bone replacement flags. The normal stimuli to the maintenance of healthy bone begin to diminish. Activity decreases. The appetite declines and less adequate supplies of proteins, vitamins, and minerals essential to proper bone building are available. Hormonal stimuli to bone maintenance gradually abate with advancing years in both men and women, although these changes, occurring earlier in women, have time to produce in them the atrophy of bone known as postmenopausal osteoporosis, which might best be thought of as the *net decrease in bone mass prevalent in old age*. Needless to say, such decrease is also partly vascular; all tissues as well as bone are less well repaired and maintained when endarterial disease occurs.

In Figure 15-33 you can judge for yourself the lengths to which this decrease in bone mass may be carried. The cortex of the elderly woman in B has gradually been decreased to one-fourth the normally maintained cortex in A, taken from exactly the same location on the femur. As osteones fail to be replaced, the juxtamedullary part of the cortex is gradually converted into a mesh of thin bone segments, which are then removed altogether.

Cancellous bone also shares in this attritional process. The high-magnification photographs in Figure 15-34 will give you an unforgettable concept of net decrease and increase in bone mass of *cancellous bone*, which is composed not of osteones but of sheets of lamellar bone, laid down or removed by the surface activity of osteoblasts and osteoclasts.

When you consider that bone mass may be decreased either by failure to replace it when it is removed in the course of normal bone maintenance (osteoporosis) or by some extraordinary process of bone destruction, you will understand that the *radiographs* of bones in both conditions will look similar: thin cortex and thinner, fewer plates of spongy bone are more radiolucent. The acceleration of bone destruction in hyperparathyroidism is an excellent working example to contrast with the much more gradual reduction in bone mass occurring in osteoporosis. In hyperparathyroidism, of course, a distinctive (in

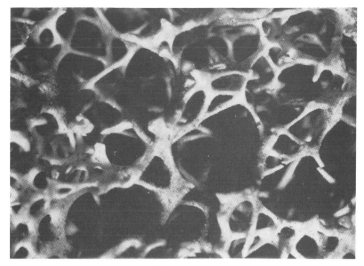

A

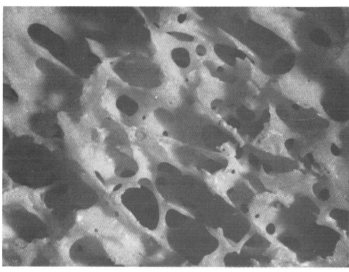

B

Figure 15-34. Cancellous bone, porotic (A) and sclerotic (B). The normal would be somewhere in between. Osteoporotic spongy bone should be thought of as composed of connecting threads of bone, whereas normal bone is composed of intersecting plates of bone.

fact, pathognomonic) x-ray finding is *subperiosteal erosion of bone*. This is often best appreciated in bones of the hands, where a very thin piece of bone, the phalanx, can be studied in tangent. Of course, the process of accelerated bone destruction is going on throughout the bony skeleton and may also be seen in large bones examined closely.

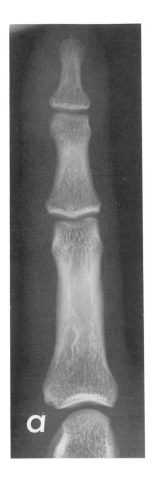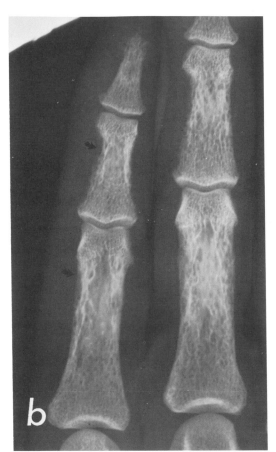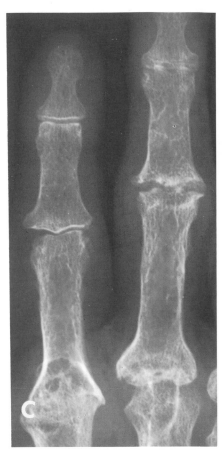

Figure 15-35. (See text.)

Variations in the appearance of cortical and cancellous bone which can be recognized from radiographs may be gauged from the six magnification studies of fingers on this page and the next. The engravings you see here were reduced by about half from the original magnification prints, and you are therefore seeing the details as though you were looking at a routine radiograph of the hand through a low-power magnifying glass.

The finger in A is from a normal young man. The relative thickness of compact bone in midshaft in the proximal phalanx, as well as the size of the individual trabeculae and the marrow space intervals between them, are to be compared with the abnormal bones in the other five radiographs.

In B, you can recognize the bone destruction (*black arrows*) occurring subperiosteally in hyperparathyroidism, which we were just discussing. Note the erosion of the terminal tuft of the distal phalanx as well as the appearance of destruction

in the subperiosteal compact bone, effectively thinning the cortex.

In C, the fingers of an elderly man whose activity had been limited for a prolonged period of time by generalized rheumatoid arthritis, the destructive joint changes are the finding which first strikes you. But look at the cortex and note how thinned it is even in midshaft well away from the joints. In any severe generalized illness in which activity is sharply reduced, the gradual development of osteoporosis is inevitable, since the normal stimulus of stress, weight bearing, and muscle pull is so much decreased. In the case of very sudden and almost total interruption of activity, as in the patient who is put into traction in bed after a fracture of the femur, disuse osteoporosis occurs and may become appreciable radiographically; about half the bone must be lost before this occurs. Thus in many painful bone conditions the typical radiographic picture is seen and, *superimposed on it,* a degree of disuse osteoporosis, with thinned cortex and trabeculae.

296

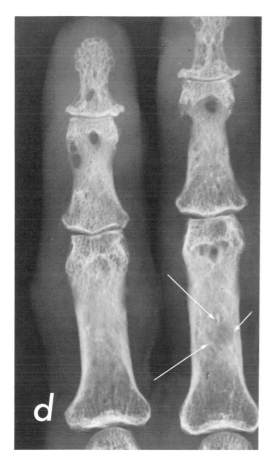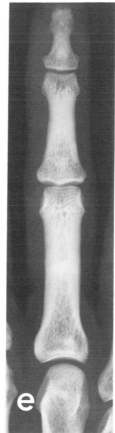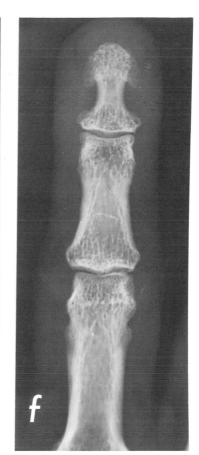

Figure 15-36. (See text.)

In D, sharply margined areas of bone destruction are seen scattered throughout the bones, pressure erosion from granulomatous foci in a patient with sarcoidosis. Note that where these involve principally the cortical bone, they are easier to recognize. When the destruction is mainly of trabecular bone (*white arrows*), a good deal more bone must be missing before that loss is apparent radiographically. The reason is of course that the areas of loss are masked by normal bone in front of and behind the destroyed area. In a lateral radiograph of the spine, areas of destruction in the body of the vertebra up to 1 centimeter in diameter may be invisible even in retrospect when their presence has been established at autopsy. It is for this reason that today isotope bone scans are used early to screen for metastases in bone; they are apparent much earlier in scans than on regular bone films.

The patient in E had osteopetrosis, or marble bones, an inherited fault in which reconstruction of bone is impaired and old bone accumulates. The cortex is abnormally thick and marrow cavities may be obliterated, so that patients die of failing hematopoiesis. The net bone mass is strikingly increased.

In F, form is faulty. This finger would be recognized by experts as having the typical alteration in form seen in acromegaly. Compare the widely flanged tuft of the terminal phalanx with the others on these two pages. The bones are broad and the bases of the phalanges splayed. Note the distinctive abundance of soft tissues. Roentgen findings of this sort may suggest a diagnosis not suspected clinically, or confirm one which is.

297

The Spine: Osteoporosis

The spine poses special problems in radiologic diagnosis because it is so complex in structure, with so many overlapping bony parts of diverse shapes. Computed tomography is, as we have said, of immense help in pinpointing obscure sites of fracture, or in confirming (or excluding) clinically suspected disease where regular bone films have shown no abnormality. CT is also used to measure the degree of osteoporosis, and serial CT scans can evaluate response to therapy.

In patients with back pain, routine films of the thoracic and lumbar spine would include AP and lateral views, but the lateral films often give most information about alignment, form, density, fracture, and the like.

In Figure 15-37 you see lateral films of the thoracic and lumbar spine of an older woman with pronounced osteoporosis. She has a marked kyphosis in the thoracic spine, produced over the years by gradual loss of bone mass with thinning of both cortical and spongy bone. This has produced anterior wedging—actually impaction fractures of the anterior parts of the bodies of the vertebrae, the posterior parts being better supported by their complex structure.

In her lumbar vertebrae, although there is little change in alignment there is marked thinning of cortex and radiolucency of the bodies of the vertebrae, largely the result of loss of spongy bone within them.

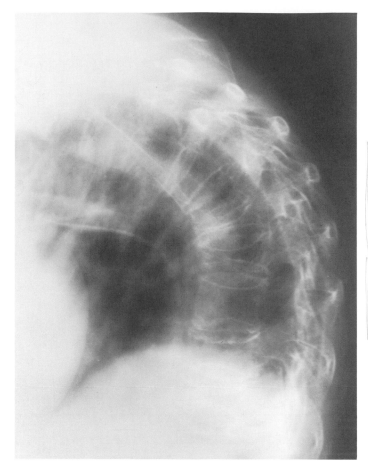

A

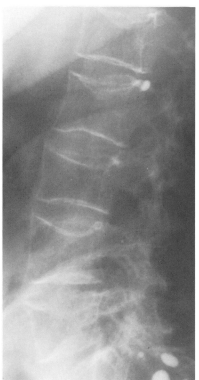

B

Figure 15-37. Osteoporosis of the thoracic and lumbar spine of an elderly woman. Note the extreme kyphosis in the thoracic region.

Compare them with the normal lumbar vertebrae of the young man in Figure 15-38; those appear much more dense, with a thicker surface investment of compact bone and denser central spongy bone. Observe also that the normal vertebrae have flat parallel endplates on either side of the lucent intervertebral discs. Now compare these spaces with the lozenge-shaped disc spaces in Figure 15-37B. Here, because of decreased bone mass, the discs have herniated into the endplates, producing a shape for the vertebral bodies that is roughly a biconcave disc. This has been termed a fish vertebra because many of the larger fishes normally have vertebrae that shape.

Of course the deformity of vertebrae produced in this way is not unique to osteoporosis, for it can occur whenever there is a decrease in bone mass—as, for example, in Cushing's disease, hyperparathyroidism, or prolonged therapy with steroids. Always remember as you examine this kind of change in vertebral body shape that the metabolic process by which it is produced varies from the slow failure of replacement of bone in osteoporosis to the rapid destruction of bone in hyperparathyroidism.

You can use Figure 15-38 as a normal for comparison with the cases of spine pathology to follow. Although the bones are normal, there *is* some narrowing of the L4-L5 disc space, which proved to have been caused by a ruptured intervertebral disc.

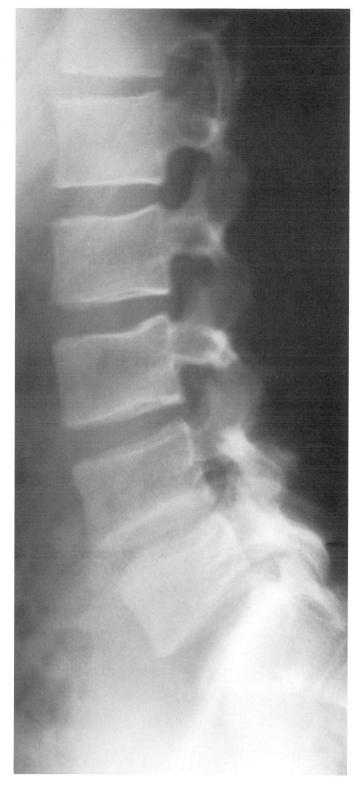

Figure 15-38. A young patient's lumbar spine, for comparison with preceding figures and those to follow.

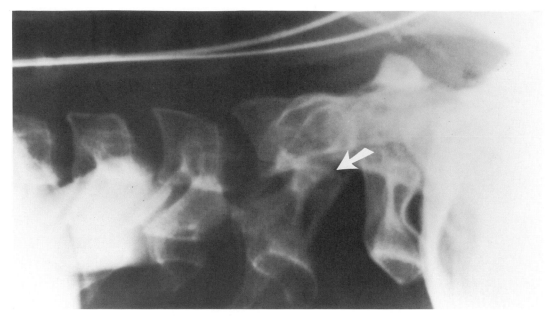

A

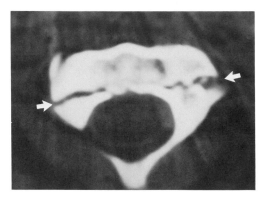

B

Figure 15-39. A: Hangman's fracture (see text). B: CT study clearly delineates location and extent of fracture.

The Spine: Fractures

The patient in Figure 15-39 was involved in a posterior-impact motor vehicle accident. Whenever such a patient is seen in the emergency ward or at the scene of the accident, a complaint of pain in the cervical spine should occasion enormous care in handling and management in order to prevent injury to the cord if possible. *Regular films of the cervical spine should not be made in such cases until a screening cross-table lateral film like that in Figure 15-39A has been made,* usually on the trauma board, the patient having been transported with an immobilization collar in place. Once this film has been made, films of the cervical spine and/or CT studies may be obtained, cautiously if the screening lateral showed a fracture or dislocation.

Here, of course, a classic "hangman's fracture" is present, as affirmed in the CT study in B. Note that there is a transverse fracture through the pars interarticularis behind the dens.

Computed tomographic studies are indicated or helpful—

(1) When the plain films are suspicious for fracture, but not decisive;

(2) When the plain films show a complex fracture that needs further imaging for understanding;

(3) When the plain films are normal but the clinical findings remain suspicious for fracture (local pain, neurologic findings, hematoma).

Fractures of the spine are frequently obvious on the x-ray films, but prove to be more complex than first appreciated. In persons who jump or fall from a considerable height, fractures of feet, legs, and hips may be perfectly clear on first examination of the patient, but unsuspected spine fractures not infrequently accompany this kind of trauma. In the patient in Figure 15-40, the obvious (and painful) fracture of the spine resulting in compression of L1 was suspected clinically and proven with plain radiographs. She also complained of numbness in the perineum, however. Any unusual neurologic finding in apparently simple spine fracture warrants CT for better evaluation. This woman was found (see B) to have a burst fracture with a bone fragment (*arrow*) pushed back into the neural canal. Compare C, a nonfractured vertebra at CT. The fragment was removed surgically.

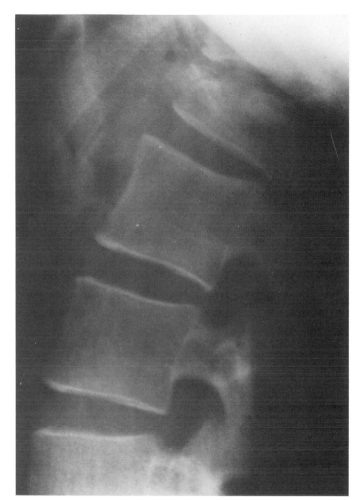

A

Figure 15-40. Burst fracture of L1 is seen in B, the CT study, to have a serious complication (see text). C shows a nonfractured vertebra for comparison.

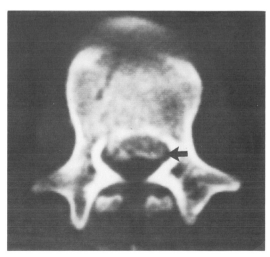

B

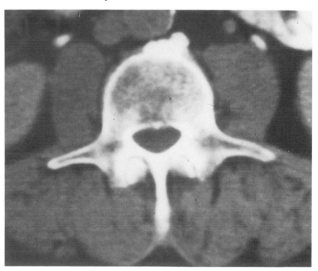

C

301

Osteomyelitis of the Spine

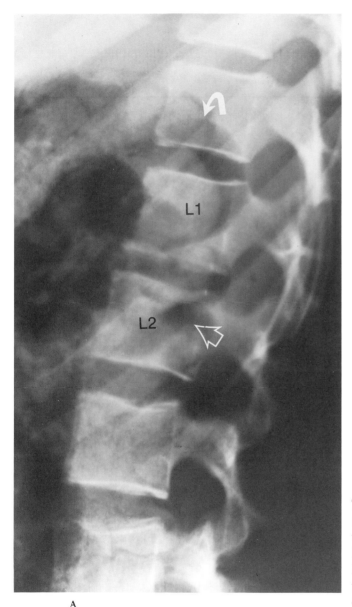

A

Figure 15-41. Osteomyelitis of the spine following pierced ears (see text). A, lateral plain film; B, conventional tomogram; C, MR image; and D, bone scan, same patient.

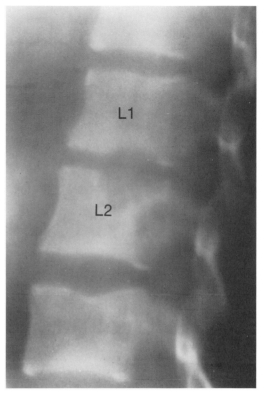

B

The young woman in the four illustrations above had had her ears pierced, and after two weeks developed pain in her back and a fever. Plain films of the spine centering across the L1-L2 area were suspicious for bone destruction in the posterior part of the body of L2. There is definite narrowing of the L1-L2 interspace. The *bent arrow* indicates air-in-gut overlying the body of the twelfth thoracic vertebra (T12), but the *open arrow* points to an area of questionable lucency, which is confirmed on the conventional tomogram in B, where areas of bone destruction are clearly seen on both sides of the disc space, typical of the bone destruction in osteomyelitis. In the magnetic-resonance image, C, one can

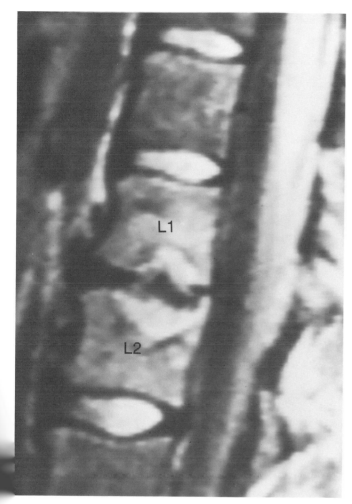

L1

L2

C

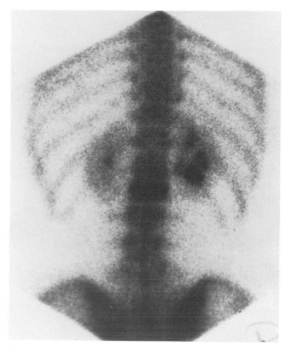

D

determine that there is no involvement of the spinal canal (no abscess). The cord is white and tapers off at the level of L2. Cerebrospinal fluid in the dural sac is black on this MR image. In D, the bone scan on this patient, much more signal is received from the area in question, and no similar intensity anywhere else, implying that the process is localized to the area seen by tomogram.

Bone Tumors: Metastatic

During your professional lifetime you will probably see 20 to 30 times as many patients with metastatic tumor to bone as with primary tumor of bone, for primary bone tumors are really very rare. You may not actually be responsible for making the diagnosis of either, which is in part radiological and in part a tissue diagnosis. However, you must be familiar with the role of imaging in making that diagnosis.

Almost any kind of malignant tumor may metastasize to bone, but the most common are five or six in number. They produce either *lytic* (lucent) or *blastic* (opaque) areas scattered through normal bone on routine bone films. Those that are characteristically lytic are from carcinoma of the lung, thyroid, and kidney, and metastases from carcinoma of the breast are usually lytic (Figure 15-42), although they may turn blastic with therapy. The common characteristically blastic spread to bone is seen with carcinoma of the prostate. It can be either spotty, as you see in Figure 15-43, or diffuse, as you see in Figure 15-44.

Long before such alterations in density in scattered areas in normal bone have grown large enough to be seen, they will be signaled in a bone scan at a time when the bone films look perfectly normal. For that reason it is common practice today to procure bone scans in patients known to have malignancy elsewhere who have bone pain, or in whom therapy might be altered if you knew there was already spread of the disease to bones. Generally, if there are "hot spots" in asymmetrical areas on the bone scans in such patients, it is assumed that they represent metastases—although the bone scan is not specific for tumor, and intense isotope signal only means augmented bone turnover, which can be present in infection and Paget's disease, for example, as well as in tumor. Both the patients in Figures 15-44 and 15-45 would have had widely positive bone scans, although only the former had tumor present.

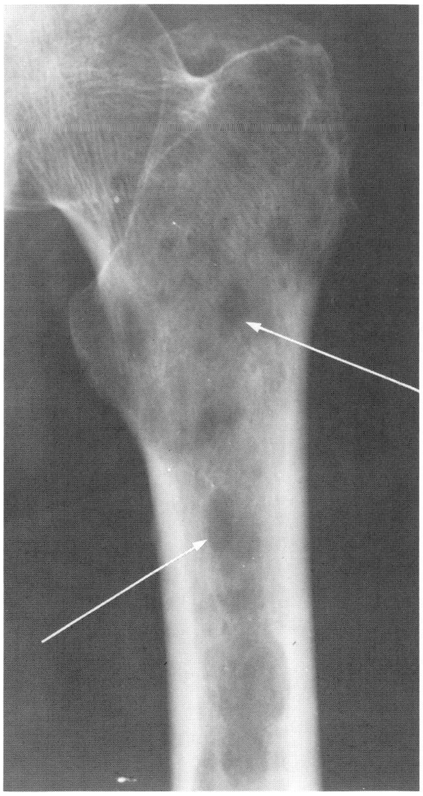

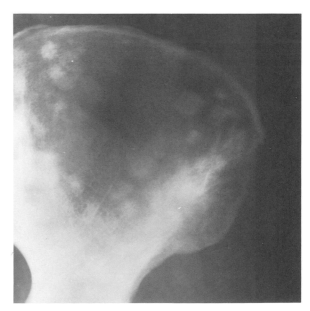

Figure 15-42. Osteolytic metastases. Lytic areas of destruction by growing tumor are the rule from *kidney, lung,* and *thyroid* carcinoma. Carcinoma of the breast may be lytic or blastic, or mixed.

Figure 15-43. Osteoblastic metastases from carcinoma of the *prostate.* New bone formation locally in areas of spread to bone may be spotty, as here, or diffuse, as in Figure 15-44.

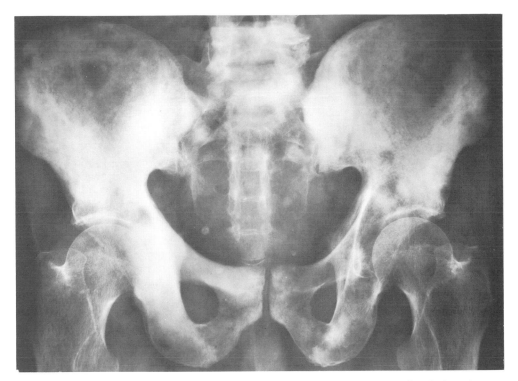

Figure 15-44. The pelvis in a patient known to have carcinoma of the prostate. Note that the bone is not enlarged as it is below in the patient with Paget's disease.

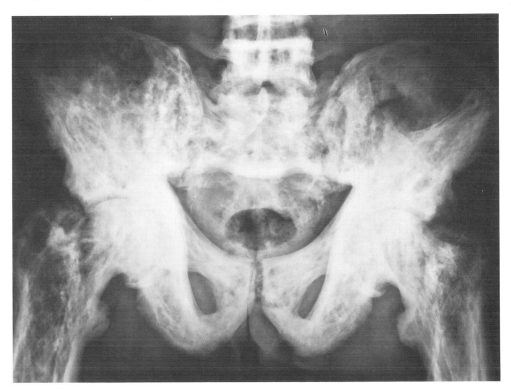

Figure 15-45. The pelvis in Paget's disease. Note the characteristic linear streaking of abnormal disarranged trabeculae and the enlargement of bone due to subperiosteal new bone added. This is an important distinction from the increased density in prostatic carcinoma metastases, because the two diseases are apt to be seen in the same group of patients (elderly men).

In Figure 15-46A you see the bone scan of a woman known to have had carcinoma of the breast with appropriate treatment sometime earlier. Her bone scan was negative at that time. Now she has new lower back pain, and this new bone scan shows multiple asymmetrical areas of uptake of isotope in the left hip, pelvis, thoracic and lumbar vertebrae, ribs, and left shoulder. Note that L2 and L4 are involved even though L1 and L3 appear to be clear.

The bone film (Figure 15-46B) showed pathologic compression fractures causing collapse of L2, but normal-appearing L1 and L3. It is difficult to be sure of abnormality in L4, which is partly overlapped on the density of the iliac wings. (*Arrow:* L2.)

Figure 15-46C gives you an MR image of the same segment of spine. The second lumbar vertebra gives off almost no signal, as its fatty marrow is replaced by tumor and bone itself gives no signal. In contrast, the bodies of L1 and L3 on either side of it give intense fatty bone marrow signal, but L4 and L5 are also seen to be involved. (*Arrow:* L2.)

Figure 15-47 is another patient with known breast carcinoma who had lower back pain in the sacral area but whose bone films did not show a definite lesion because of overlying gas in the bowel. This CT study across the sacrum shows the large area of destruction due to metastatic disease.

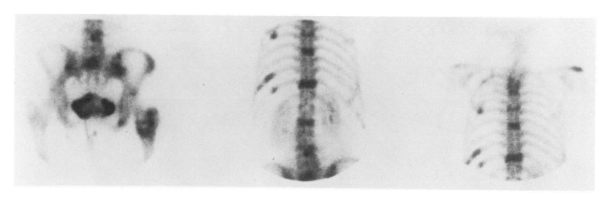

Figure 15-46A. Bone scan showing metastases in asymmetrical areas in many bones, in particular L2.

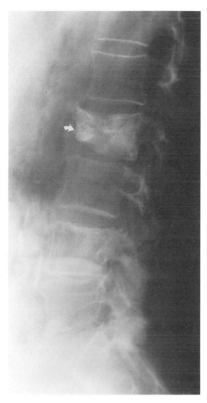

Figure 15-46B. Bone film, same patient (see text).

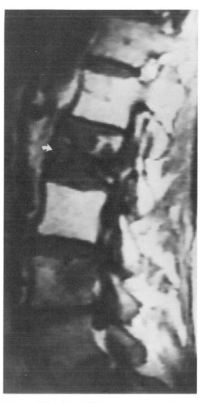

Figure 15-46C. MR image, same patient (see text).

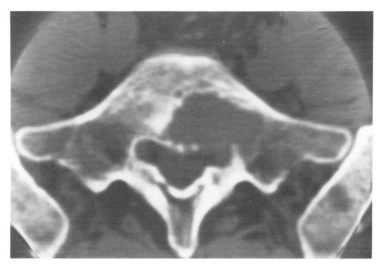

Figure 15-47. A different patient. Carcinoma of the breast, metastatic to the sacrum shown at CT, not visible on plain films.

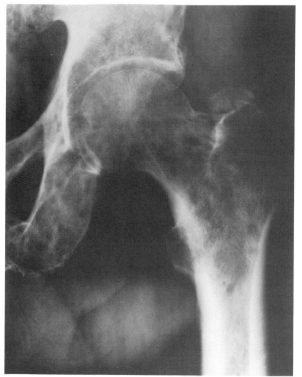

Figure 15-48. Multiple myeloma.

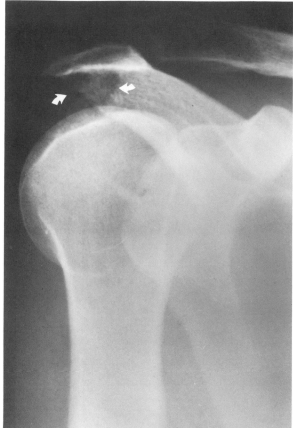

A

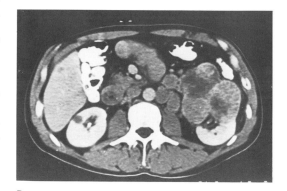

B

Figure 15-49. A: Solitary lytic lesion (*arrows*) in the acromion in a man with painful shoulder, fever, and anemia. B: CT, same patient.

However much the scattered lytic lesions in Figure 15-48 may resemble those you have been seeing, they are not from kidney, thyroid, lung, or breast cancer, but are the late "punched-out" areas of bone destruction in multiple myeloma. The patient was known to have myeloma chemically proven with Bence-Jones protein in the urine, and had this film made when he complained of hip pain. Such lesions occur rather late in the disease and often are preceded by years of bone pain in which regular bone films are entirely negative, showing only diffuse decrease of bone mass with loss of both cortical and spongy bone but no localized destruction. A diagnosis of osteoporosis is frequently offered on the basis of these films before the localized areas of destruction ultimately develop.

The man in Figure 15-49A was being studied because of an eight-week fever of unknown origin. He was 46 years old and also had anemia, but a normal urinalysis. He complained of vague shoulder pain. The plain film shows a lytic lesion in the right acromion. Bone scans showed this to

308

be the only such area of isotope activity (bone turnover). CT study through the area of the kidneys (Figure 15-49B) shows the primary tumor of the left kidney. Renal cell carcinomas are often locally asymptomatic but associated with anemia and fever.

Bone Tumors: Primary

Primary malignancies of bone fortunately are rare. Osteogenic sarcoma characteristically is seen in young males, 10 to 25 years old. Ewing's sarcoma is usually seen in younger children, and chondrosarcoma rarely before 40 and usually in older patients. There are several types of osteosarcoma, depending on the predominant malignant tissue (osteogenic sarcoma or fibrosarcoma). In Figure 15-50A you see the lower femur in a patient with osteosarcoma having the classic densely ossified soft tissue and intraosseous mass, thickening of the cortex from periosteal reaction, and raylike extension outward into the soft tissues. This patient was 22, complained of pain and swelling in the right knee, and a CT study (Figure 15-50B) made farther up the femoral shaft shows the intramedullary extension not suspected from the plain films.

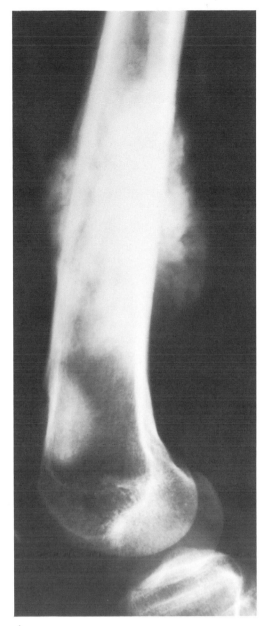

A

Figure 15-50. A: Osteogenic sarcoma. B: CT, upper shaft of the right femur shows intramedullary extension. Compare with the medullary canal of the normal left femur.

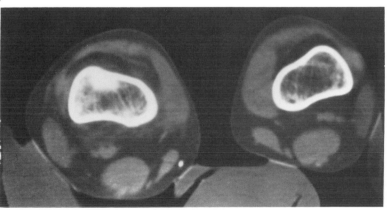

B

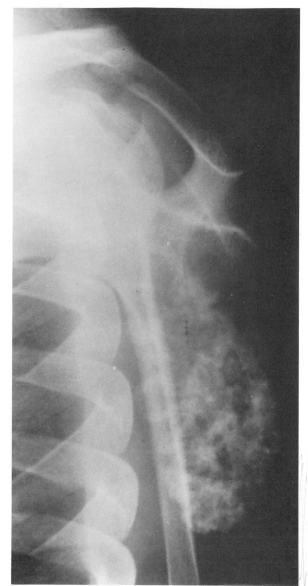

A

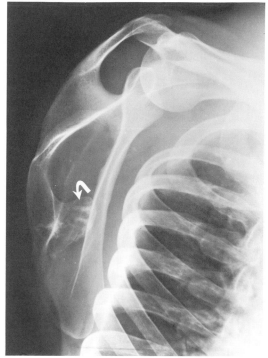

Figure 15-52. Another patient with osteochondroma (*arrow*) of the scapula.

Benign Bone Tumors

Many kinds of benign bone tumors also occur. Enchondromas are growing, expanding, cartilaginous tumors, common in the hands and ribs. Osteochondromas (often called exostoses) are discovered at any age, are more common about the knee, and may be multiple or solitary. Osteoid osteomas usually present in young males with intense bone pain, which responds dramatically to aspirin. They may not be tumors, in fact, but are inflammatory in origin and show a lucent area centrally with a surrounding shell of bony density. They must usually be differentiated from localized bone abscess.

The 24-year-old man in Figure 15-51A had a palpable but otherwise asymptomatic mass over his left scapula. The plain film shows an osseous mass associated with the scapula, which might be either benign (an osteochondroma) or malignant (an osteosarcoma). Fortunately, the CT study (Figure 15-51B) clearly shows it to be benign in character, an osteochondroma, with only normal muscles around it and no soft-tissue tumor mass. Figure 15-52 is another smaller osteochondroma of the scapula for you to compare.

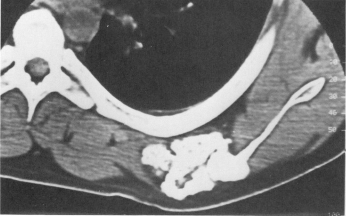

B

Figure 15-51. A: Osteochondroma of the scapula. B: CT, classic for benign tumor.

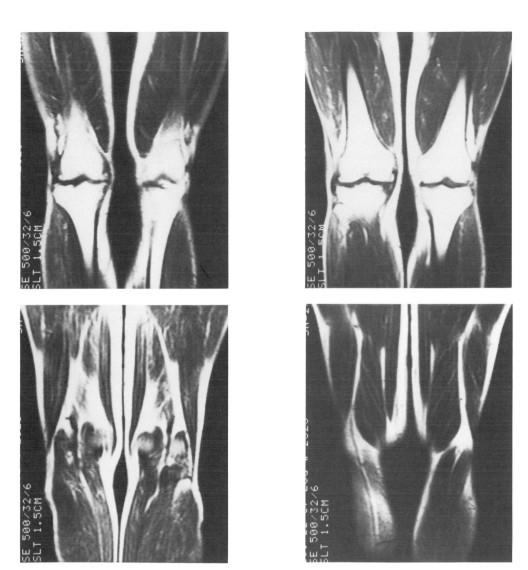

Figure 15-53. Four MR imaging studies of the region of the knee in the coronal plane (see text).

MR of Extremities

Finally, the four MR images in Figure 15-53 show you what can be done to demonstrate soft tissues in the extremities. The upper pair are anterior coronal sections and show symmetrical images of the extensor muscles of the knee, whereas the lower pair (slices behind the knee) show the flexors of the knee, and you can identify these muscles very easily. Magnetic resonance is a wonderful modality for identifying soft-tissue abnormalities such as a malignant muscle tumor. You may request MR when you are trying to differentiate a suspicious mass which may be either a hematoma or a malignant tumor, for example. MR scanning can show beautifully the soft-tissue structures associated with joints, including cartilages, ligaments, and tendons. In the knee, for example, MR is frequently requested to evaluate patients with suspected injuries of the menisci and cruciate ligaments.

Remember that subcutaneous fat and fatty bone marrow have a high signal and appear white, whereas compact bone gives no signal and is black on these images. Therefore the femur-shaped white shadows just above the knee are the fat-in-marrow, not bone.

CHAPTER 16 Neuroradiology

Techniques for Imaging the Central Nervous System

The term "neuroradiology" can be an intimidating one for medical students beginning their study of radiology. In truth, the central nervous system is very well organized, with little normal variation from patient to patient. The anatomy may be complex, but once the basics are learned, the student will become comfortable with the imaging techniques in common use.

In this chapter the major anatomic structures shown on skull films, facial films, CT scans, MR scans, cerebral arteriograms, and myelograms will be reviewed, and the diagnostic imaging of the more usual central nervous system conditions will be discussed. Before reading this chapter, you may wish to refresh your knowledge of the skull, brain, and spinal cord from a standard anatomy textbook or a review book of radiologic anatomy.

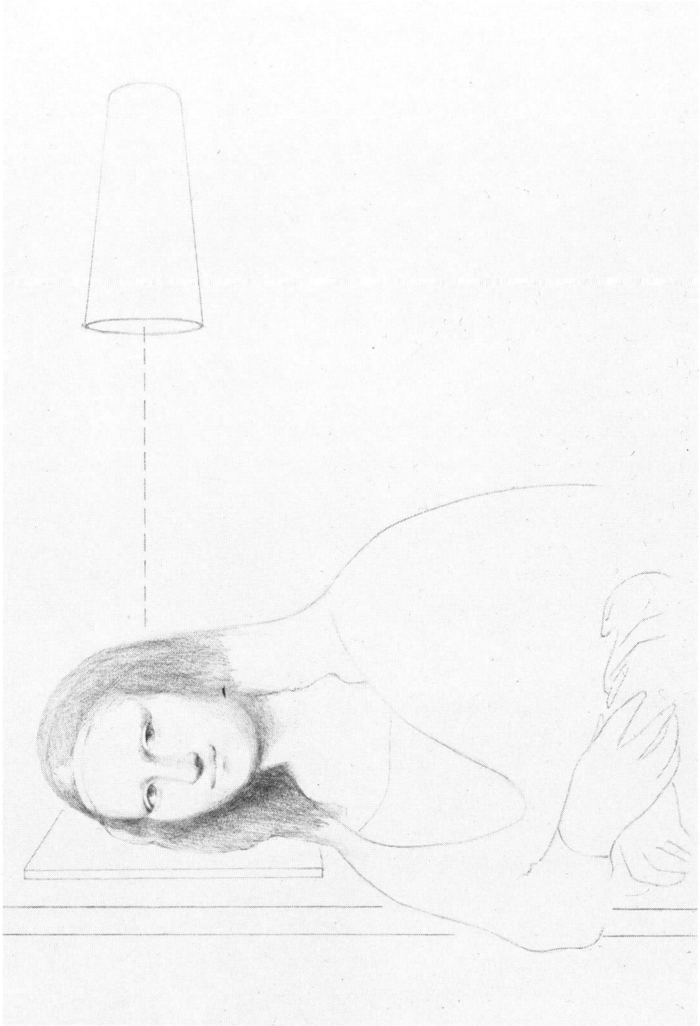

Skull films, like any other radiographic examination, must be viewed while thinking in three dimensions, and the superimposed bony parts must be subtracted one from the other. The usual skull film series comprises five views: AP, PA, both laterals (each side in turn close to the film cassette), and a Towne view (AP, with the x-ray tube angled caudad to show the occipital bone).

Study the lateral and PA skull films on the next two pages. The lateral view (Figure 16-2) shows the two halves of the coronal and lambdoid sutures superimposed. The sagittal suture is not seen, of course, and the face is "burned out"; facial fractures might be missed if you requested skull films instead of a facial series.

Skull films made PA and AP will look different to you, because in one the orbits are close to the film while in the other they are projected from far away and therefore magnified, showing larger round circles of bone. Each will depict best the details of the bony structures closest to the film. Figure 16-4 is a PA film of a patient with a skull fracture.

Sutures usually remain visible throughout life, distinguishable from fracture lines by their serpiginous character and white margins. A fracture will appear more linear, not at all marginated, and usually more radiolucent (blacker) than a suture line. Vascular grooves (middle meningeal artery branches and the like) are also not as black as fracture lines, and they are shown in their expected anatomic locations.

Plain skull films are not commonly requested today, as they show only the bony structures, intracranial calcifications, and pneumocephalus. We can see brain tissue directly with CT and MR scans, and these are currently the procedures of choice for patients who present with

Figure 16-1. Mona Lisa positioned for a lateral skull film.

acute or chronic central nervous system conditions that require imaging diagnosis. In fact, CT and MR show brain anatomy so well that these images are often used to teach neuroanatomy.

Radioisotope brain scans also are performed much less frequently these days because more detailed information is provided by CT and MR. In the neonate, the brain can be visualized with *ultrasound* through the still-open fontanels; this is not possible in the older child or the adult. *Cerebral arteriography* with contrast-medium injection into the carotid and vertebral arteries is most commonly utilized to evaluate cerebrovascular disease and better delineate cerebral aneurysms, arteriovenous malformations, and brain tumors.

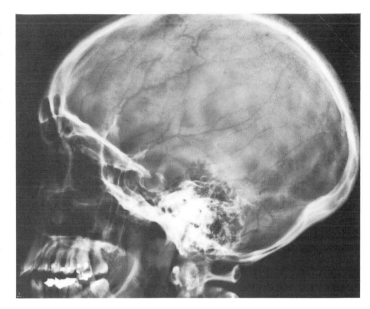

Figure 16-2. Normal lateral skull film.

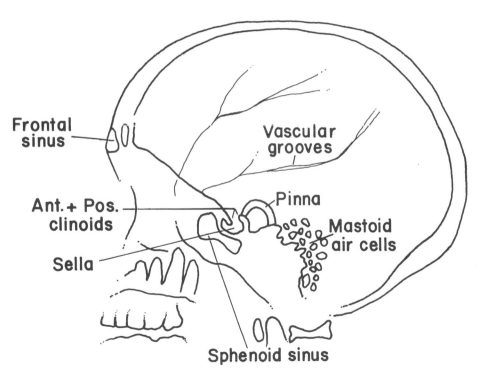

Figure 16-3. Labeled diagram to match Figure 16-2.

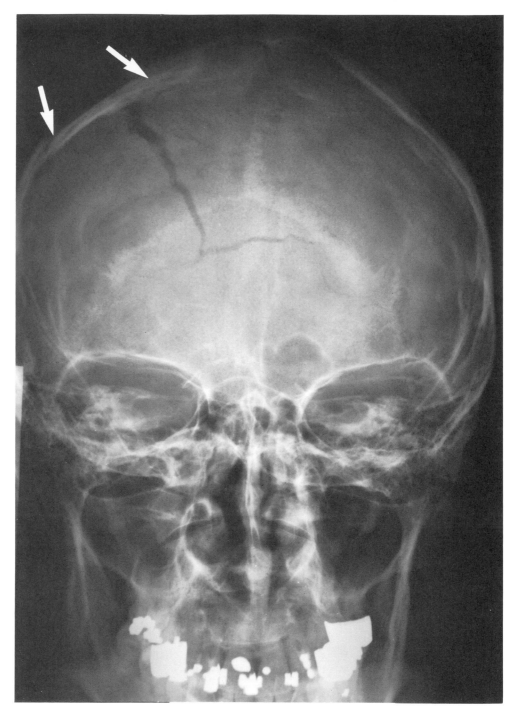

Figure 16-4. PA projection skull film with fractures both linear and depressed. A plate of bone seen in tangent (between the *arrows*) is slightly depressed. This is not a simple fracture, therefore, but a comminuted one. Note the metallic dental fillings and caps. Identify the orbits, frontal sinuses, mandible, and internal auditory canals.

314

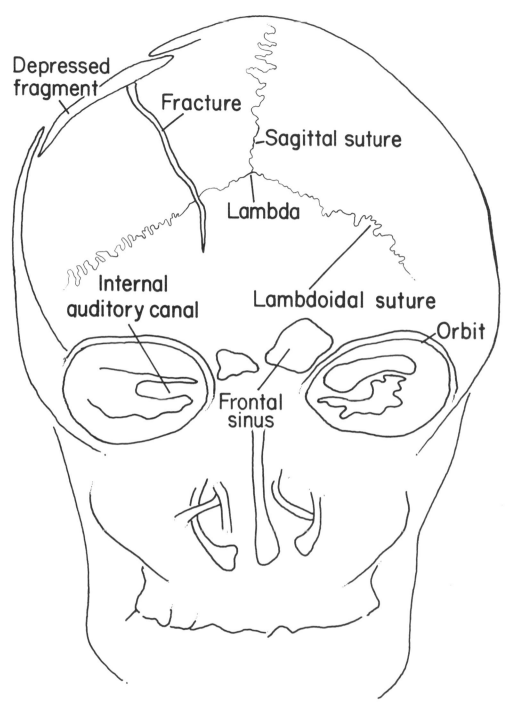

Figure 16-5. Labeled diagram to match Figure 16-4.

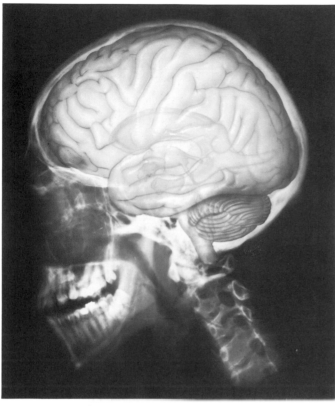

The Normal Brain: CT Anatomy

Study the CT scans of the normal head, performed after intravenous administration of contrast material, shown in Figure 16-8. They are a series of noncontiguous, 10-millimeter-thick axial scans, photographed with a "brain window," and obtained at intervals from the vertex of the skull down to its base. Compare the scans with the illustrations shown in Figures 16-6 and 16-7.

At CT cerebral white matter (shown centrally in the hemispheres) appears slightly less dense (blacker) than gray matter (shown peripherally) because the white-matter tracts contain more fatty tissue (myelin sheaths around neural processes). Cerebrospinal fluid (CSF) in the ventricles and subarachnoid spaces looks nearly black. The blood vessels and vascular structures (falx cerebri, choroid plexuses of the lateral ventricles, and so on) containing contrast substance are white. The bones of the calvaria and face also appear white but are poorly defined on these scans; the bony detail, of course, would be better shown with "bone-window" CT settings.

Figure 16-6. Superimposition of the apparently transparent brain and its ventricular system upon a lateral radiograph of the skull will help you to visualize the relationships and to think three dimensionally about skull films and brain anatomy. Identify the two lateral ventricles (superimposed in this projection), the third ventricle, the cerebral aqueduct (aqueduct of Sylvius) between the third and fourth ventricles, and the fourth ventricle. Note how the temporal horns of the lateral ventricles extend forward, appearing to cross the aqueduct, although intellectually you know the temporal lobes are lateral to the aqueduct, which is located in the midline.

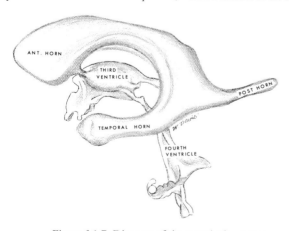

Figure 16-7. Diagram of the ventricular system.

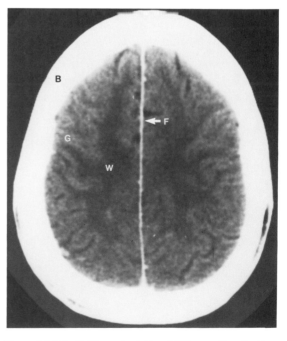

Figure 16-8 A–E. Normal axial head CT scans filmed with a brain window.

A: Upper scan obtained above the lateral ventricles. The falx cerebri (F) separates the two cerebral hemispheres. White matter (W) appears darker than gray matter (G). Note the sulci and gyri. The bony calvaria (B) looks very white.

316

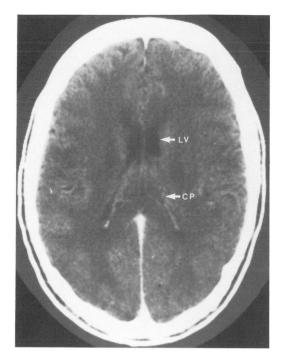

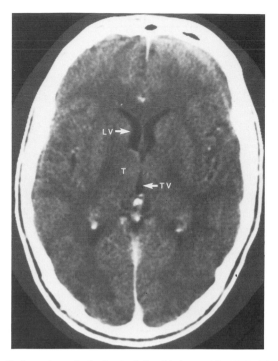

B: Scan through the bodies of the lateral ventricles. Cerebrospinal fluid within the lateral ventricles (*LV*) appears black, whereas the contrast-opacified choroid plexuses (*CP*) look white.

C: Scan through the level of the third ventricle (*TV*). The thalami (*T*) are seen immediately lateral to the third ventricle. The anterior horns of the lateral ventricles (*LV*) can also be seen on this scan, separated by the thin septum pellucidum.

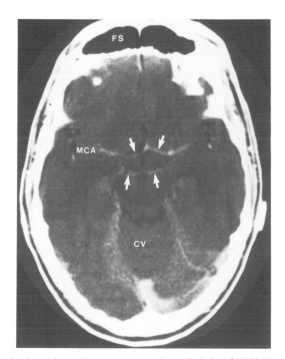

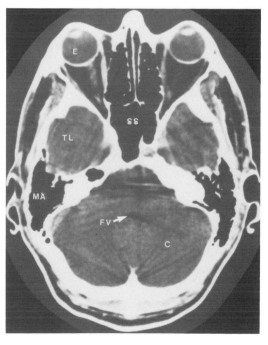

D: Scan through the contrast-enhanced circle of Willis (*arrows*). The middle cerebral arteries (*MCA*) can be seen coursing laterally within the sylvian fissures. This scan is low enough to show the cerebellar vermis (*CV*). Air within the frontal sinuses (*FS*) is very black.

E: Scan through the skull base. The eyeballs (*E*) and optic nerves are well shown, as are the sphenoid sinuses (*SS*), temporal lobes (*TL*), and mastoid air cells (*MA*). The fourth ventricle (*FV*) can be seen anterior to the cerebellum (*C*).

The Normal Brain: MR Anatomy

Magnetic-resonance scans of the brain allow even greater differentiation between gray and white matter than CT. In addition, MR scanning allows direct imaging in the coronal and sagittal planes. Study the axial and midsagittal scans shown in Figures 16-9 and 16-10. At the MR settings used, the CSF appears black, the gray matter gray, and the white matter white. Although cortical bone appears black (because of a lack of MR signal), fat (which has a strong MR signal) within the bone marrow and in the scalp appears very white.

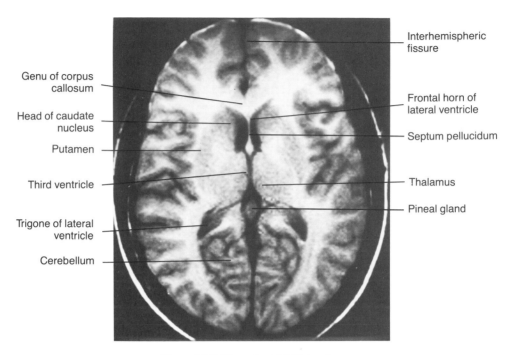

Interhemispheric fissure

Genu of corpus callosum

Head of caudate nucleus

Putamen

Third ventricle

Trigone of lateral ventricle

Cerebellum

Frontal horn of lateral ventricle

Septum pellucidum

Thalamus

Pineal gland

Figure 16-9. Normal axial MR head scan.

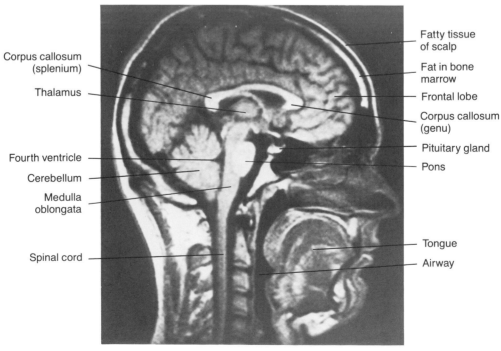

Corpus callosum (splenium)

Thalamus

Fourth ventricle

Cerebellum

Medulla oblongata

Spinal cord

Fatty tissue of scalp

Fat in bone marrow

Frontal lobe

Corpus callosum (genu)

Pituitary gland

Pons

Tongue

Airway

Figure 16-10. Normal midline sagittal MR head scan.

Hydrocephalus;
Brain Atrophy;
Intracranial Hemorrhage

Because CSF-containing spaces are so clearly shown at CT as low-attenuation areas, it is easy to identify conditions which alter their size and shape. With hydrocephalus the cerebral ventricles are shown to be enlarged, with brain tissue compressed against the inside of the calvaria, effacing the gyri and sulci. The child shown in Figure 16-11 had severe hydrocephalus caused by a tumor obstructing the fourth ventricle. In contrast, with brain atrophy the ventricles are also enlarged, but because of tissue loss the brain will be separated from the calvaria by CSF and the sulci will be prominent because of the decreased size of the gyri.

Intracranial fresh blood is readily apparent at CT. Because of the high concentration of protein constituents, it appears denser (whiter) than the adjacent brain tissue. Figure 16-12 shows a CT scan of a hypertensive patient with a spontaneous intracerebral hemorrhage. Note the large white collection of blood within the right cerebral hemisphere; blood can also be seen in both lateral ventricles. Old blood appears progressively less dense as a result of the metabolism of blood proteins, approaching the CT density of CSF within a few weeks. Figure 16-13 shows the CT scan of a chronic alcoholic with brain atrophy and a month-old right subdural hematoma. The crescent-shaped subdural hematoma has nearly the same density as the CSF.

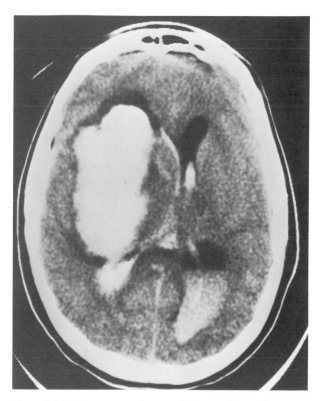

Figure 16-12. Spontaneous intracranial hemorrhage. There is a large collection of blood within the right cerebral hemisphere and smaller collections in the lateral ventricles, which are compressed and displaced to the left.

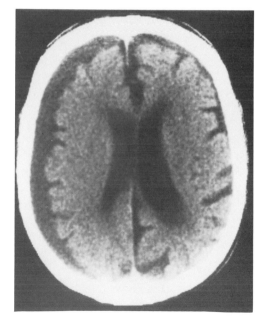

Figure 16-13. Old right subdural hematoma and brain atrophy. Compare this scan with Figures 16-11 and 16-12. (See text.)

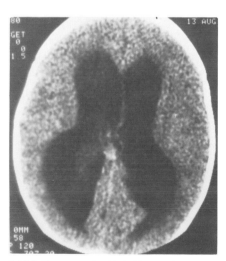

Figure 16-11. Four-month-old child with obstructive hydrocephalus. The lateral ventricles are markedly dilated.

319

Normal Cerebral Arteriography

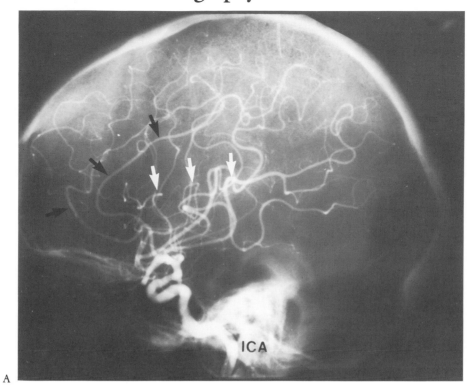

A

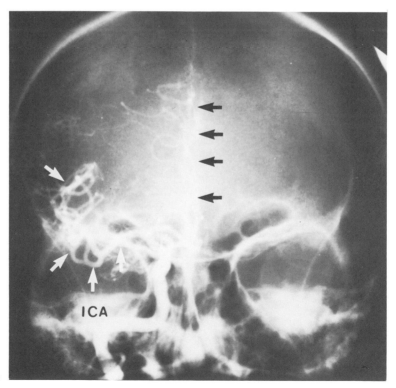

B

Figure 16-14. Normal selective right internal carotid arteriogram. A: Lateral view. *Black arrows* indicate anterior cerebral artery branches; *white arrows* indicate middle cerebral artery branches. *ICA* is the internal carotid artery B: Frontal view. *Black arrows* indicate the more medial anterior cerebral artery branches; *white arrows* indicate the laterally coursing middle cerebral artery branches.

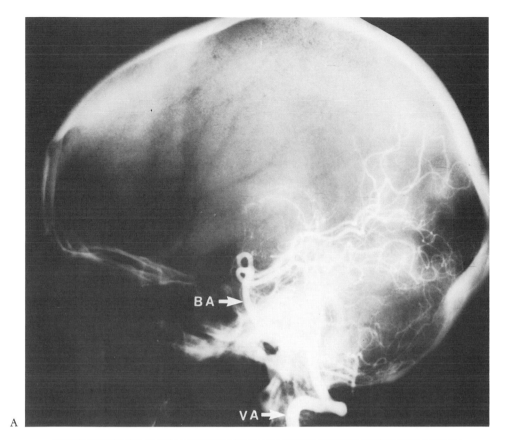

A

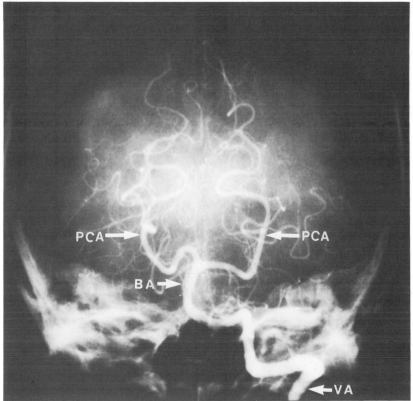

B

Figure 16-15. Selective left vertebral arteriogram. A: Lateral view shows the opacified left vertebral artery (*VA*) ascending superiorly into the skull. The left and right vertebral arteries join to form the basilar artery (*BA*), which divides into the two posterior cerebral arteries (overlying each other on the lateral view). B: Frontal view. The left vertebral artery and the basilar artery are again seen. The two posterior cerebral arteries (*PCA*) are shown separated from each other.

Head Trauma

CT has had a dramatic impact on the diagnostic workup of the head-trauma patient. When intracranial injury is suspected, CT can diagnose intracranial hemorrhage, brain contusion, pneumocephalus, foreign bodies, and skull fractures in an examination that is quickly and easily performed. Furthermore, CT can identify secondary effects of trauma such as edema, ischemia, infarction, brain shift, and hydrocephalus. In acute trauma, intracerebral hemorrhage and extracerebral blood collections (subdural hematoma and epidural hematoma) can be diagnosed by CT with nearly 100 percent accuracy. CT allows serial scanning without risk, in order that patients may be followed after trauma.

In any patient who has sustained head trauma and presents with signs of neurological dysfunction, CT is indicated. *It is not necessary to obtain plain films of the skull prior to CT examination, and precious time should not be wasted in obtaining them.* The radiation exposure to the patient with head CT is no greater than that of a plain skull film series. No intravenous contrast is required; in fact, it is contraindicated in the initial scan series, as the contrast enhancement of the cortical vessels can mask a diagnosis of subarachnoid hemorrhage. The images are photographed at both brain and bone windows. Extravasated blood has a high protein concentration and will appear white on the brain-window images, compared with the surrounding brain tissue. The bone-window images can show the presence and

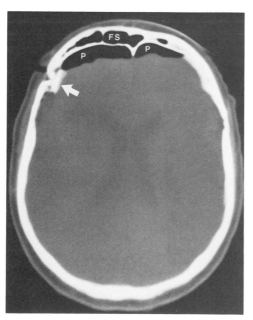

A

B

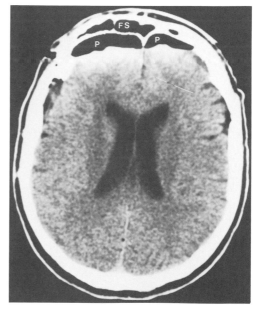

C

Figure 16-16. Depressed skull fracture with brain contusion. A: Lateral skull film shows a depressed fracture fragment (*arrows*). B: Bone window CT scan again shows the depressed fracture fragment (*arrow*) and pneumocephalus (*P*). Air is also seen within the frontal sinuses (*FS*). C: Brain-window CT scan at the same level shows brain contusion (increased whiteness) of the frontal lobe tips adjacent to the pneumocephalus.

configuration of skull fractures. Care should always be taken when transporting a head-trauma patient to the CT couch because of the high incidence of associated cervical spine and other injuries.

CT can depict depressed and basilar skull fractures better than plain films. A horizontal, nondisplaced linear fracture in the axial plane of section may be overlooked by CT, however; this is not as important as the brain injuries that are *not* overlooked by CT. If a head-trauma patient with no neurological dysfunction is initially studied with plain skull films, these are scrutinized for findings which might indicate the need for a CT examination. Such findings include displacement of a calcified pineal gland, pneumocephalus, an air-fluid level in the sphenoid or frontal sinuses, a depressed skull fracture, or a linear fracture crossing a meningeal artery groove or major venous sinus. Today most patients with an acute skull fracture on plain films are referred for a CT examination. Magnetic-resonance scanning can also show acute brain injuries. But during an MR scan the patient's entire body is positioned within the bore of an enormous magnet, so that observation and careful monitoring of an acutely injured patient is much more difficult than with CT.

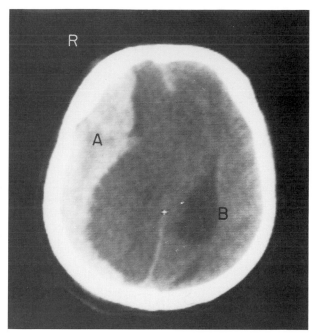

Figure 16-17. Acute subdural hematoma. Fresh blood in the subdural space appears white (*A*) and takes on a crescentic shape. Note that the anterior and posterior portions of the falx cerebri (normally midline) are displaced to the left. The dilated left lateral ventricle (*B*) reflects obstructive hydrocephalus.

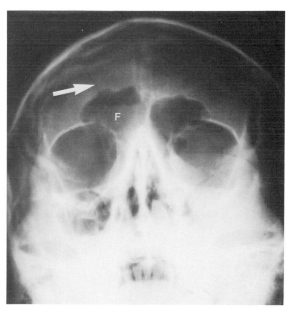

B

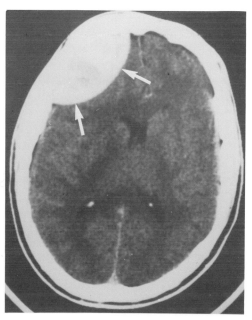

A

Figure 16-18. Acute epidural hematoma. A: *Arrows* indicate a lenticular-shaped, biconvex epidural hematoma. B: Upright skull film of the same patient shows a right frontal fracture (*arrow*) overlying the hematoma, as well as a collection of blood (*F*) in the right frontal sinus (note the fluid level).

Cerebrovascular Disease; Stroke

Cerebrovascular disease is a leading cause of death, and in the elderly, a major cause of disability. One of the most common manifestations is a *stroke,* which describes a syndrome characterized by the sudden onset of a neurologic deficit. Strokes are usually caused by acute cerebral ischemia (*cerebrovascular accident,* or *CVA*) resulting from thrombosis of a cerebral artery or a cerebral artery embolism. Emboli may arise from the heart or from atherosclerotic plaques, frequently located in and narrowing the carotid circulation at the level of the common carotid artery bifurcation (Figure 16-19). Less frequently, strokes are caused by acute subarachnoid or intracerebral hemorrhages.

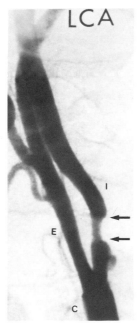

Figure 16-19. Selective left common carotid arteriogram (the arteries look black because of photographic subtraction) shows a stenosis (*arrows*) in the internal (*I*) carotid artery. The external (*E*) and common (*C*) carotid arteries are also visible.

Ischemic strokes usually cause brain *infarcts,* permanent areas of brain damage which can be detected by computed tomography and magnetic-resonance imaging. Strokes must be differentiated from *transient ischemic attacks (TIAs),* which are focal neurological deficits that develop suddenly, last for a brief period (minutes or hours), and then completely resolve; they are not associated with brain infarction and do not have detectable CT findings. TIAs are often a warning sign of an impending ischemic stroke, and they are regarded as cause for a diagnostic workup of correctable conditions leading to stroke, such as carotid artery stenosis or cardiac arrhythmia. The neurologic deficits with stroke last 24 hours or longer; they may be partially or fully reversible, or permanent.

CT can show the location and size of infarcts and can differentiate them from tumors, aneurysms, and other lesions which may mimic the clinical presentation of an ischemic stroke. The CT appearance of a brain infarct will vary with time. During the first few hours the CT scan may be entirely normal. At 12 to 24 hours the infarct will appear as a mottled or homogeneous area of diminished CT attenuation (Figure 16-20A), representing both interstitial and intracellular edema; generally there is no enhancement with intravenous contrast material. At one to four weeks the majority show patchy contrast enhancement (Figure 16-20B), representing breakdown in the blood-brain barrier (leak of contrast material from newly formed capillaries). One month later the density of the infarct will approach that of CSF, as the necrotic brain tissue is replaced by CSF. Recent investigations have shown that *MR* scanning may show an infarct earlier and better than CT (Figure 16-20C).

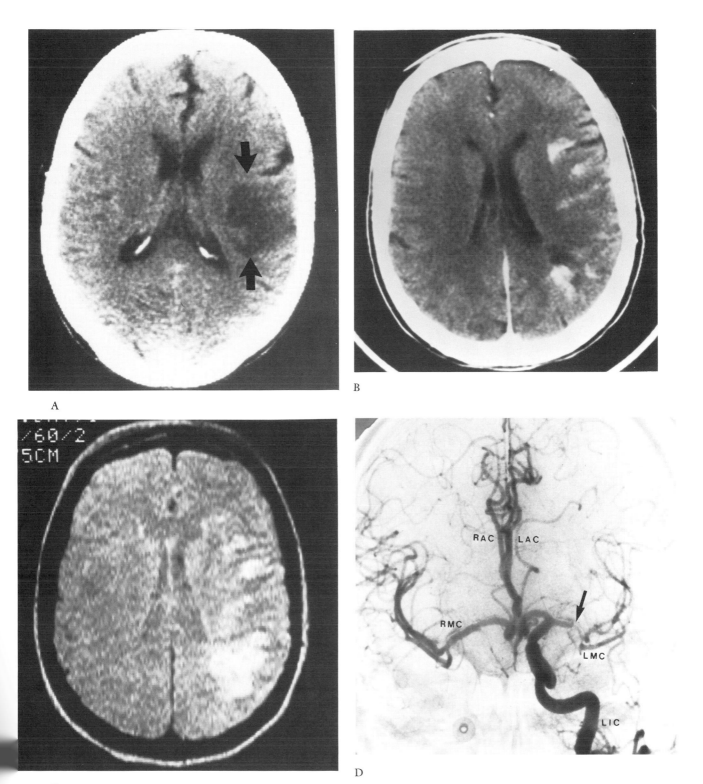

A

B

C

D

Figure 16-20. Stroke resulting from a left middle cerebral artery embolus. A: Early CT scan (12 hours after stroke) shows a low-density area of infarction (*arrows*) in the left hemisphere. B: Repeat CT scan with intravenous contrast one week later shows hyperdensity within the area of infarction. C: Axial MR scan one week after stroke shows increased MR signal (*white areas*) within the infarct. D: Frontal view of a selective left internal carotid arteriogram shows an embolus (*arrow*) almost totally occluding the left middle cerebral artery. The left internal carotid artery (*LIC*), right middle cerebral artery (*RMC*), left middle cerebral artery (*LMC*), right anterior cerebral artery (*RAC*), and left anterior cerebral artery (*LAC*) are clearly shown. The right middle and anterior cerebral arteries were opacified with contrast as the result of an angiographic maneuver in which the right carotid artery was externally compressed during injection of contrast medium into the left internal carotid artery.

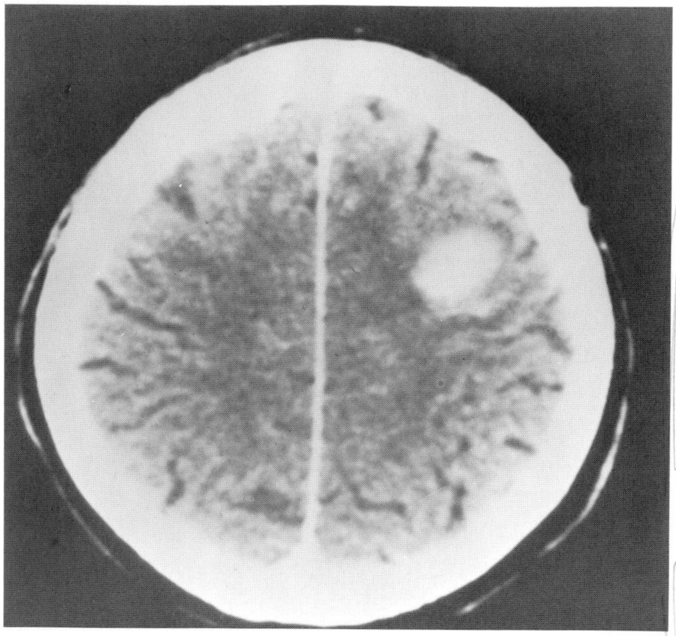

Brain Tumors

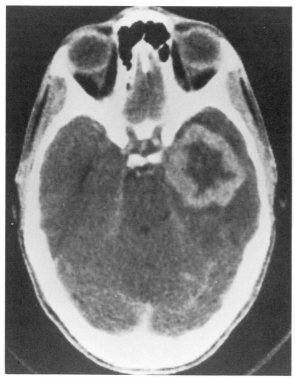

Figure 16-21. Contrast-enhanced CT scan showing a hyperdense small tumor located high in the left cerebral hemisphere. It proved to be an astrocytoma.

Figure 16-22. CT scan after intravenous contrast showing a metastasis from a primary lung cancer in the left temporal lobe. The irregular, contrast-enhanced edge is frequently seen in metastatic tumors.

Your search for a brain tumor may be precipitated by a variety of signs and symptoms of central nervous system dysfunction, including new seizures, headaches, personality changes, alterations in consciousness, visual changes, motor and sensory deficits, and papilledema. Brain tumors are most expeditiously diagnosed by CT, and with great accuracy. Skull films are usually normal with brain tumors, and skull abnormalities are seen only if the tumor contains calcifications, causes bony erosion or bony proliferation, or produces signs of increased intracranial pressure (enlarging the sella turcica, for example). Radioisotope brain scans lack the accuracy and specificity of brain CT. Angiography usually is performed only for surgical planning, to determine the vascularity of the tumor and to show its relation to adjacent vascular structures.

Not only can CT diagnose brain tumors with high accuracy, it can also localize them, determine their size, and show their effect on adjacent structures. In some cases CT can also suggest the histologic type. At CT most brain tumors, whether primary or metastatic, are radiolucent. Some have the same density as brain tissue itself. Nearly all show contrast enhancement in all or part of the tumor after intravenous contrast material (Figures 16-21, 16-22, 16-23). Frequently they are surrounded by a CT low-density area of edema, which may be massive in some patients. At magnetic-resonance imaging a tumor may appear whiter or blacker than the surrounding normal brain tissue, depending on the particular MR settings used (Figure 16-24).

Like other intracranial space-occupying lesions, brain tumors will compress, distort, and displace surrounding structures, and the clinical findings will be related to the location and size of the tumors. Intracranial calcifications are easier to see with CT than with plain films; consequently CT can better identify tumors containing calcifications, such as meningiomas, ependymomas, and oligodendrogliomas.

The CT appearance of a primary brain tumor varies with its degree of malignancy. Whereas grade 1 gliomas appear as low-attenuation masses with minimal contrast enhancement, grade 3 gliomas may appear cavitary, with thick walls and irregular, striking contrast enhancement.

Metastases are often multiple, and this is the most useful CT feature for distinguishing them from primary brain neoplasms, which are usually solitary. The features described above are common to both primary and metastatic brain tumors. Common sources for brain metastases are lung and breast cancers. Not infrequently, a patient is symptomatic from a brain metastasis before the primary tumor is detected. At CT, metastases are often characterized by extensive adjacent edema, irregular patterns of contrast enhancement, and indistinct margins reflecting their invasive nature. Edema appears less dense than normal brain tissue (Figure 16-23), because the increase in tissue fluid reduces the CT attenuation nearly to that of CSF.

A brain tumor may be clinically silent until there is a complication such as hemorrhage. In this situation CT is helpful in differentiating tumor from other conditions such as stroke that produce acute symptoms mimicking a tumor.

In medical centers where magnetic-resonance scanning is available, this procedure may be performed first in patients with suspected brain tumors. An advantage of MR over CT is its ability to yield multiplanar images such that the mass effect of the tumor on adjacent structures can be accurately delineated in the coronal and sagittal planes, in addition to the axial plane. Furthermore, no intravenous contrast material may be required.

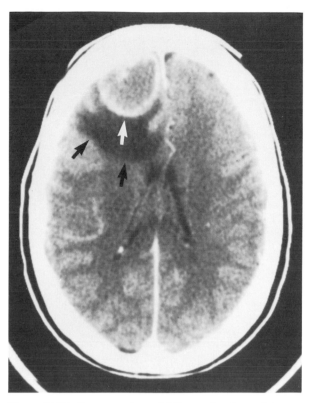

Figure 16-23. Contrast-enhanced CT scan showing a right frontal brain metastasis from a breast cancer. *White arrow* points to the metastasis itself; *black arrows* indicate a large area of low-density edema surrounding the tumor.

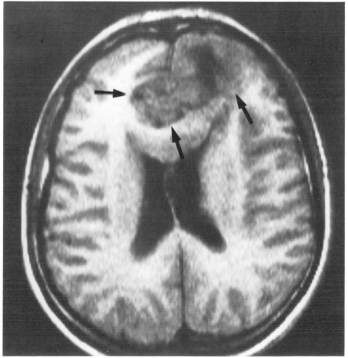

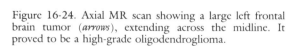

Figure 16-24. Axial MR scan showing a large left frontal brain tumor (*arrows*), extending across the midline. It proved to be a high-grade oligodendroglioma.

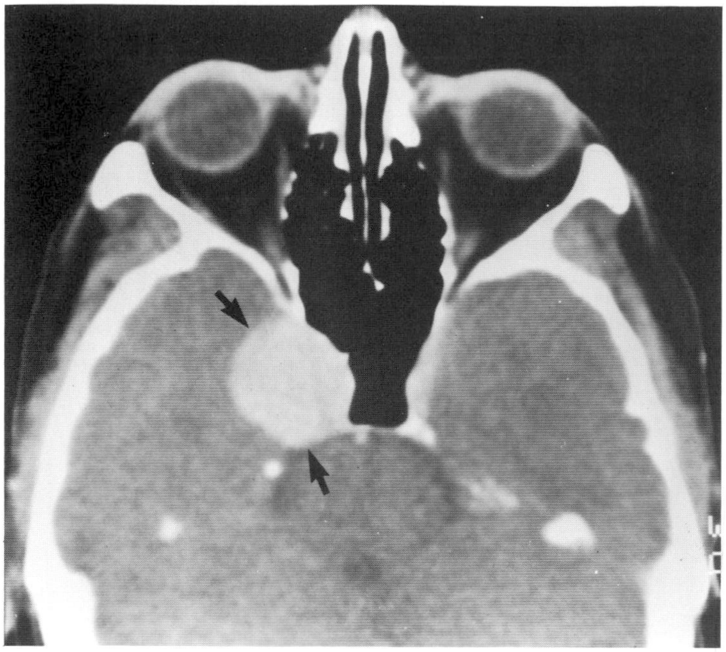

A

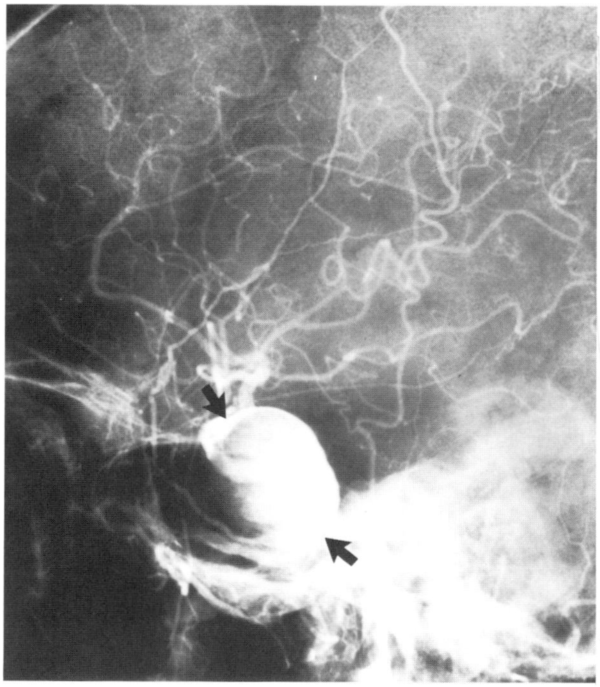

B

Cerebral Aneurysm and Arteriovenous Malformation

The physical signs and symptoms of brain tumors can be produced by two vascular lesions, cerebral aneurysm and cerebral arteriovenous malformation. Both can rupture and bleed intracranially, producing sudden deterioration in a patient's central nervous system function. In addition, symptoms can be produced simply by the mass effect of the vascular lesion itself.

Both can be diagnosed by CT and MR, although angiography is generally required for treatment planning. In recent years interventional angiography has been employed in the treatment of both lesions. A transcatheter approach makes it possible to occlude cerebral aneurysms and malformations with particulate material or detachable balloons. These techniques have been especially useful in cases where surgical access to the lesion would be difficult.

With intravenous contrast material an aneurysm will appear at CT as a smooth-margined, spherical mass of high CT attenuation (Figure 16-25). In fact, the attenuation will be the same as that measured in any major blood vessel, such as the patient's aorta. The aneurysm may contain thrombus, and hemorrhage may be seen around the aneurysm if rupture has occurred. Because of their location, aneurysms usually rupture into the subarachnoid space, producing a subarachnoid hemorrhage. Most large aneurysms can be seen at CT; however very small aneurysms may be overlooked by CT, requiring arteriography for their diagnosis.

Arteriovenous malformations are located within the brain parenchyma itself, and when they bleed, they produce intracerebral hemorrhage. At contrast-enhanced CT an arteriovenous malformation will appear as a tangle of blood vessels—some seen on end as high-attenuation dots, some cut through the side and

Figure 16-25. Cerebral aneurysm. A: CT scan with intravenous contrast identifies an aneurysm (*arrows*) just to the right of the sphenoid sinuses. B: Right internal carotid arteriogram shows the aneurysm (*arrows*) arising from this artery.

328

seen as high-attenuation serpiginous structures (Figure 16-26). Because of the arteriovenous shunting which takes place through these abnormal blood vessels, the blood flow itself is increased and the caliber of the supplying arteries is increased. Note the large-caliber left internal carotid artery branches in Figure 16-26B, compared to the normal internal carotid arteriogram of Figure 16-14A.

Arteriovenous malformations may produce local pressure effects on surrounding structures, may cause a "steal" of blood away from the adjacent brain, may become the foci of seizures, and of course may bleed.

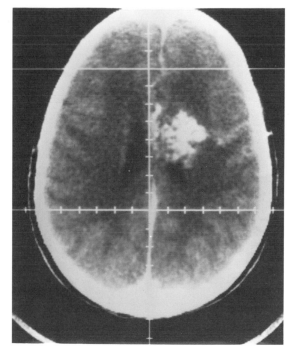

A

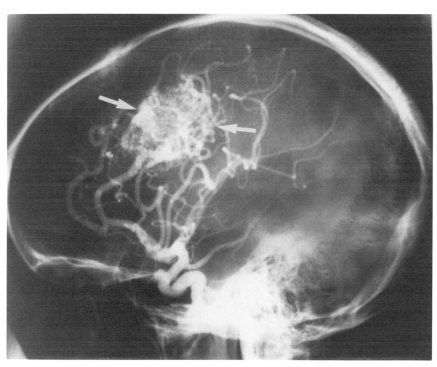

B

Figure 16-26. Cerebral arteriovenous malformation. A: CT scan, after intravenous contrast medium, of a patient with diplopia shows a tangle of abnormal blood vessels in the left cerebral hemisphere. B: Selective left internal carotid arteriogram shows the arteriovenous malformation (*arrows*) opacified with contrast material. The large caliber of the cerebral arteries reflects the increased blood flow passing through them to supply the arteriovenous malformation.

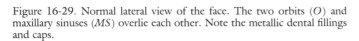

Figure 16-27. Normal Caldwell view of the face. The frontal sinuses (*FS*), ethmoid sinuses (*ES*), and orbits (*O*) are well shown.

Imaging the Face

The facial bones are not well seen on a routine skull film series. In fact, they are burned out because of the higher x-ray exposure necessary to see the skull. When your patient has a clinical condition requiring plain-film imaging of the face, you should request a *facial film series* which includes Caldwell, Waters, and lateral views of the face (Figures 16-27, 16-28, and 16-29). These are coned close to the margins of the face and taken with a PA technique (facial bones as close to the film as possible) and upright in order to show any sinus fluid levels.

Facial film series are most frequently requested to demonstrate or rule out facial fractures after trauma. They are also indicated for patients with suspected inflammatory conditions of the face, such as paranasal sinusitis and orbital cellulitis, or for patients with a suspected facial tumor.

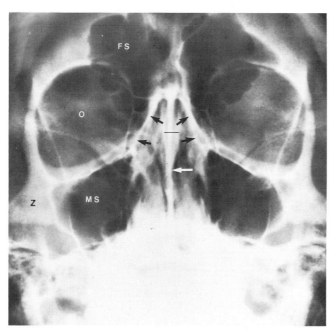

Figure 16-28. Normal Waters view of the face. The frontal sinuses (*FS*), orbits (*O*), maxillary sinuses (*MS*), and zygomas (*Z*) can be identified. *White arrow* indicates the nasal septum; *black arrows* show the margins of the nasal fossa.

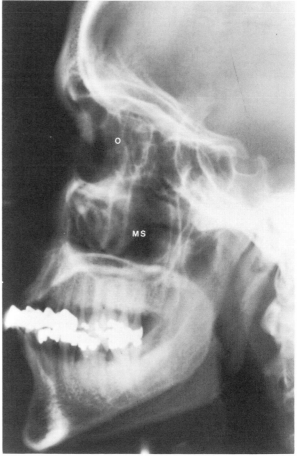

Figure 16-29. Normal lateral view of the face. The two orbits (*O*) and maxillary sinuses (*MS*) overlie each other. Note the metallic dental fillings and caps.

330

You are no doubt aware that the facial bones constitute one of the most complex arrangements of curving bony surfaces in the entire body, an arrangement that is often difficult to evaluate on plain-film x-rays. It is easy to understand why the advent of CT, with its ability to display and sort out complex anatomy in a variety of imaging planes, has provided such a major advance in facial imaging (Figures 16-30, 16-31, and 16-32).

CT can visualize soft-tissue structures directly and therefore can show disorders of these structures that would not be possible to image with plain films or conventional tomography. For example, with orbital trauma CT can show soft-tissue injuries such as extraocular muscle entrapment and impingement, orbital hematoma, globe rupture, lens dislocation, foreign bodies, and injuries to the optic nerve.

You should also know that nasal fractures may not be seen on facial films; a special *nasal film series* is usually required to detect them. Similarly, mandible fractures usually require examination with a *mandible film series*.

A *sinus film series* refers to a variation of the facial film series in which the x-rays are very tightly coned to the paranasal sinuses. With acute inflammatory or allergic sinusitis one may see thickening of the sinus mucosal membranes, air-fluid levels, and—rarely, in advanced cases—evidence of bony destruction.

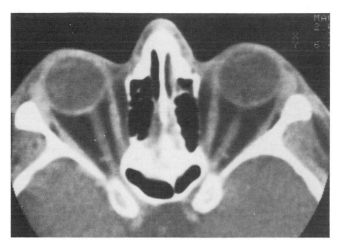

Figure 16-30. Normal CT scan through the midorbits. Note both eyeballs, the medial and lateral rectus muscles, and the optic nerves, all surrounded by orbital fat.

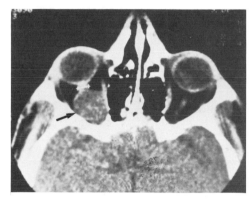

Figure 16-31. Right optic glioma. Notice that the right optic nerve tumor (*arrow*) has a spherical shape and its diameter is almost the same as that of the right eyeball.

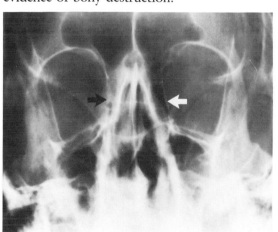

A

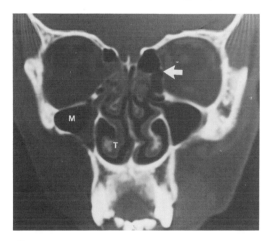

B

Figure 16-32. Right orbit medial blowout fracture. A: Plain film shows a fracture (*black arrow*) of the medial wall of the right orbit, with blood in the underlying right ethmoid sinus. Compare with the normal left medial orbital wall (*white arrow*) and normally aerated left ethmoid sinus. B: Coronal CT scan shows medial displacement of the right medial orbital wall. Note the position of the normal left medial orbital wall (*white arrow*). Blood can be seen in the right ethmoid sinus and also in the right maxillary sinus (*M*). The nasal turbinates are well seen (*T* indicates the right inferior turbinate). You may have noticed on the plain film that the right orbital floor appears to be lower than the left; CT shows that this is not a fracture, but instead an anatomic variant.

Lumbar Disc Syndrome

Low back pain is a very common problem, and you will no doubt see a large number of patients with this complaint during your professional training and career. In your emergency room, they may present with acute symptoms, after trauma or lifting a heavy object; in your office or clinic, they may present with subacute or chronic symptoms. You should remember that a plain-film series of the lumbar spine (AP, lateral, and coned-down lateral) are *only* helpful when the cause alters the radiographic appearance of the spine, as with fractures, primary and metastatic tumors, and arthritis. Evidence for degenerative disc disease may be shown by a narrowed intervertebral disc space. Young patients with low back pain caused by muscle strain will have normal lumbar spine x-rays, however. They should *not* be referred for radiologic examination unless you are seriously considering some other cause for their symptoms.

The spinal cord is *not* seen on plain spine films but can be visualized with computed tomography, magnetic-resonance scanning, and myelography. To perform a myelogram, the radiologist places a needle percutaneously into the lumbar spine, below the termination of the spinal cord (conus), with its tip in the thecal sac. Then, under fluoroscopic control, a myelographic contrast material is injected to allow visualization of the spinal cord, spinal nerve roots, and thecal sac. As the contrast material is radiopaque, the spinal cord and nerve roots will appear radiolucent.

One of the most common conditions requiring visualization of the spinal cord is lumbar disc syndrome. This diagnosis is considered in patients presenting with back pain that radiates to one or both legs. The pain may be associated with muscle weakness, a sensory deficit, or abnormal reflexes. In the majority of cases lumbar disc syndrome is caused by a herniated lumbar disc (nucleus pulposis), often at the L4–L5 level.

When patients present with their first episode of lumbar disc syndrome, they are customarily treated with a period of conservative therapy (bed rest, pain medication, and so on). They may be imaged with a lumbar spine film series, which usually shows disc space narrowing at the affected levels, but are not referred for special examinations to show the subarachnoid space, spinal cord, and spinal nerves unless surgery is planned. And patients do not become candidates for disc surgery until they have failed to improve with conservative therapy, or unless they present with unusually severe initial clinical manifestations such as loss of bowel or bladder control.

When surgery *is* planned, patients are most commonly imaged with computed tomography (Figure 16-33) or magnetic-resonance scanning. Myelography is usually reserved for cases in which the clinical findings are unusual or the scanning results uncertain.

Figure 16-33 (*opposite page*). Herniated L4–L5 lumbar disc. A: CT scan through the pedicles of the L4 vertebra shows herniated disc material (*black arrow*) extending posteriorly on the left side into the neural canal. B: CT scan through the pedicles of the L5 vertebra shows a normal portion of the neural canal, with black fatty tissue outlining the thecal sac centrally and nerve roots in both lateral recesses. C: Frontal view myelogram of the same patient shows bilateral compression of the opacified (*white*) thecal sac by herniated disc material (*black arrows*). There is more compression from the left side than from the right. Lumbar vertebrae 3 through 5 are shown; the sacrum (*S*) can also be seen. D: Oblique myelogram of the same patient. *White arrows* indicate the severe compression on the left side of the thecal sac. The *black arrows* indicate two radiolucent spinal nerves traversing the contrast-enhanced thecal space.

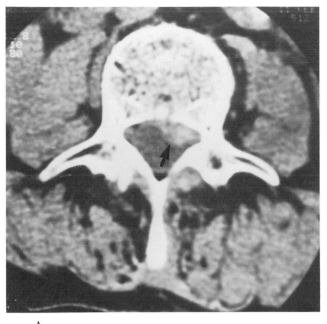

A

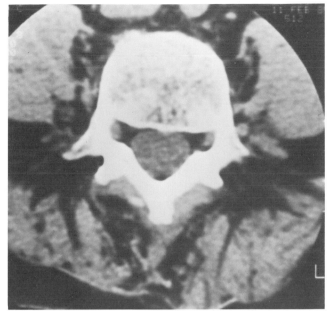

B

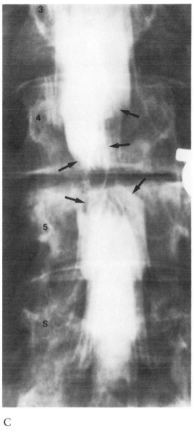

C

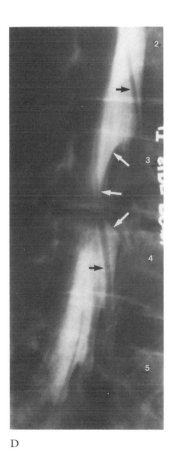

D

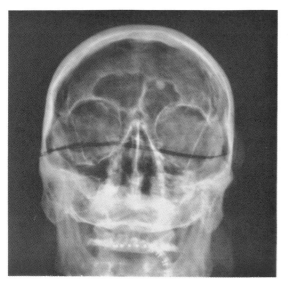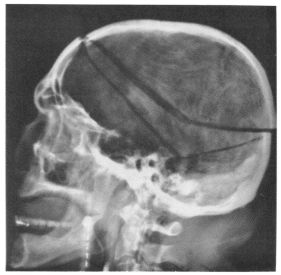

Figure 16-34 (*Unknown 16-1*). Try your hand at radiologic medicolegal detective work. These are radiographs made at the request of the coroner after autopsy had failed to establish the cause of death. The deceased had apparently been beaten to death in a drunken altercation. During the fight he had received multiple cuts from a soft-drink bottle, and at autopsy many contusions were seen about the face but there was no evidence of skull fracture or of intracranial hemorrhage. The lucency through the skull represents the saw cut made at autopsy. What cause of death, indicated by these films and noted by the radiologist, was confirmed upon reexamination of the corpse?

Answers to Unknowns

Unknown 1-1 (Figure 1-14)

The pair of dice on the right have been loaded by boring holes into the substance of each die, filling with lead, recapping, and repainting the dots. Bits of lead wire have been used. Of the loaded pair, the die on the left has been x-rayed with the loaded face down, as it would tend to fall. The die on the right has been turned on its side and then x-rayed. You are now looking through it from side to side. The loaded face is down and very dense. The upper part of the die has been evacuated and left empty, increasing its tendency to fall with the 2 facing up—or the 5, depending on which is chosen by the tamperer.

Unknown 1-2 (Figure 1-15)

No, not an egg with a nail in it. The oval object could not be an egg because its radiodensity falls away at the edge and is much greater and fairly uniform in the center. This must therefore be a solid oval body of considerable density and homogeneous composition—except for the nail, which actually was in the center of it. The dark streaks are air in the interfaces after it had been cracked open. The object was a mineral bolus found in the stomach of a horse. The nail, typical of those used in shoeing horses, had undoubtedly been swallowed many years ago and remained in the stomach. The "stone," a concretion like a gallstone, had built up around it gradually.

Unknown 3-1 (Figure 3-13)

The ribs are numbered correctly. The structures indicated by the white arrows are cervical ribs arising from the seventh cervical vertebra, a congenital aberration.

Unknown 3-2 (Figure 3-14)

The eighth rib on the left is fractured close to its vertebral end. There is also a fracture of the lateral margin of the scapula.

Unknown 3-3 (Figure 3-15)

Fractured clavicle. Air has infiltrated the soft tissues (subcutaneous emphysema).

Unknown 3-4 (Figure 3-19)

On mammography the suspicious mass palpated in the right breast (A) was clearly a fibroadenoma with characteristic calcifications. In the left breast (B), which seemed normal clinically, there is a spiculated tumor typical for carcinoma. Note the denser round nodule with minute central calcifications within it, and raylike extensions out into the breast in all directions. By obtaining the mammograms unnecessary surgery to the right breast was avoided and earlier treatment of the unsuspected carcinoma in the left breast was accomplished.

Unknown 3-5 (Figure 3-20)

The left shoulder girdle is missing, removed surgically because of a malignant bone tumor in the arm. Note that the medial part of the left clavicle is still present.

Unknown 4-1 (no figure in text)

Search the patient's clothing for a straight pin, specifying your reason for doing so. Having made sure no pin is present there, refilm the patient. It is not at all likely that this patient has aspirated a pin and can talk comfortably, but if she has, it will be present again on the second film. You might also study the lateral film.

Unknown 4-2 (Figure 4-26)

You see spotty densities out in the lung parenchyma which do not taper like vessels. They suggest both linear and punctate or nodular interstitial densities. Small clusters of air-space disease cannot be excluded. One small circular shadow with central lucency suggests a cavity.

Obviously at age 23 inflammation of some kind is more likely than tumor or lung insult through employment, neither of which is plausible from the history. Certainly tuberculosis, a strong possibility, must be ruled out, as it produces both air-space and interstitial changes. If the chest film made three months ago can be obtained for comparison, it may help to judge the age of the process. You can certainly discard consideration of an inflammation one day old or one week old, since the degree of involvement and the story of weight loss indicate a somewhat older process. The best choice would be subacute inflammation one month old.

Unknown 4-3 (Figure 4-27)

Multiple cavities with fluid-air interfaces in an intravenous drug abuser strongly suggest lung abscesses due to blood-borne septic material; they are not at all rare in large city hospitals.

Unknown 5-1 (Figure 5-13)

The superior segment of the right lower lobe is densely consolidated. This is clearly air-space disease of one bronchopulmonary segment of a lobe.

Unknown 5-2 (Figure 5-14)

The right middle lobe is consolidated. Clinically, the patient appeared to have pneumonia.

Unknown 6-1 (Figure 6-7)

The right diaphragm is that horizontal linear density overlapping the right ninth rib with air below it, pneumoperitoneum having been an older method of "putting the lung to rest" in patients with tuberculosis. You are seeing the crown of the diaphragm in tangent, but the part curving anteriorly and posteriorly is not well seen. Lung markings that seem to extend below the crown of the diaphragm are, of course, in the right lower lobe, posterior segment. The patient tried to take a deep breath but was unable to pull his diaphragm any farther down against the cushion of subdiaphragmatic air.

Unknown 6-2 (Figure 6-18)

The bones are normal, as are the soft tissues, in this male patient. The heart and mediastinum appear to be slightly deviated to the left. There is a right pneumothorax with pronounced collapse of the right lower and middle lobes and some degree of collapse of the upper lobe, which shows patchy densities. Similar lesions are seen in the left lung. There is a short horizontal fluid level blunting the right costophrenic angle, clear indication that there must be both fluid and air in the right pleural space. The most probable working diagnosis would be tuberculosis, and sputum examination revealed tubercle bacilli in this febrile patient.

Unknown 6-3 (Figure 6-19A)

Hydropneumothorax several days after pneumonectomy. The mediastinum is slightly shifted *toward* the side of the absent lung. Note missing sixth rib, and that the stomach bubble is located under a high (unseen) diaphragm. Thus that side of the thoracic cage is much smaller than the other (missing lung, crowded ribs, high diaphragm).

Unknown 6-4 (Figure 6-19B)

This fluid level extends beyond the bony thorax and was present inside a water-containing breast prosthesis used after mastectomy.

Unknown 8-1 (Figure 8-33)

Yes, the upper mediastinal mass to the right of the trachea certainly could be (and was) related to the small parenchymal lesion, and consisted of metastatic node masses compressing the superior vena cava. There is also a hilar mass of nodes, which is much more obvious in Figure 8-34 (a CT scan through the hilum) and can be seen flattening the superior vena cava.

Unknown 8-2 (Figure 8-35)

A large anterior mediastinal mass is flattening and displacing the trachea, and spreading the great vessels to each side. It is a goiter extending from the neck into the upper mediastinum. The mass was palpated in the neck.

Unknown 9-1 (no figure in text)

Bronchogenic carcinoma may first cause symptoms in a wide variety of ways. You probably have on your list all the following:

(1) Silent infiltration of the lung. Likely to be discovered only on routine physical examination or checkup chest film (for example, the solitary pulmonary nodule).

(2) Obstruction of a bronchus. May cause cough as the initial symptom, or occasionally hemoptysis. Radiograph may look entirely normal if the mass is small and close within the hilum. Will eventually appear on the radiograph as a mass of increased density within the lung or close to the hilum, and may appear at the time of the first examination as:

(3) Atelectasis of the segment of lung distal to the obstructed bronchus.

(4) Atelectasis with pneumonia distal to the obstruction.

(5) Pneumonia, apparently a simple inflammation clinically, but which does not clear and improve on schedule with appropriate treatment. (You must be very suspicious of repeated episodes of atelectasis in the same lung segment and of recalcitrant pneumonic infiltrations in the lung of patients in the cancer age group.)

(6) Bronchogenic carcinoma not infrequently metastasizes early to the pleura. The patient may therefore appear at your office for the first time complaining of symptoms and presenting signs of pleural effusion, without other complaints or findings.

(7) Bronchogenic carcinoma metastasizes to bone very commonly, and if such involvement occurs before other symptoms bring the patient to your office, he may be complaining of bone pain anywhere at all. You may see him because of a fracture which has occurred through bone invaded by tumor.

(8) Distant metastases to parenchymatous organs may occur early while bronchogenic carcinoma is still asymptomatic in the chest. Such a patient may therefore present himself for help with symptoms of a brain tumor or with almost total adrenal gland destruction, to mention only two possibilities. Radiographic study of his chest may reveal the shadow of the primary tumor, or if the tumor is small and has metastasized very early, the chest films may at first be entirely negative.

(9) Bronchogenic carcinoma may metastasize early to the lymph glands and bring the patient to you because of pressure from such glands on any of the mediastinal structures. Notable among these patterns of initial difficulty is one in which the trachea is surrounded and compressed by tumor nodes, resulting in dyspnea and wheezing. The vascular structures of the superior mediastinum may also be compressed, giving the symptoms of superior vena cava obstruction, for example.

(10) Bronchogenic carcinoma may invade the pericardium, presenting initial symptoms of pericardial effusion.

(P.S. There are still other possibilities!)

Unknown 15-1 (Figure 15-14)

Comminuted fracture of the humerus that extends into the base of the greater tuberosity.

Unknown 15-2 (Figure 15-15)

Impacted comminuted fracture of head and neck of humerus.

Unknown 15-3 (Figure 15-16)

Radiograph of a fractured tibia several weeks after the injury, made the day the initial plaster cast was removed. The shadowy flocculent white material (callus) is taking on mineral, which tells you that this is not a fresh fracture. The alignment and angulation of the tibial fracture fragments are not optimal.

Unknown 15-4 (Figure 15-17)

Fracture of the radial head is easier to see in B, an oblique view. Note the offset of white bone at the fracture point in A.

Unknown 15-5 (Figure 15-18)

Fracture of the distal end of the radial metaphysis at the wrist with displacement of its epiphysis (as seen in the lateral). Note the white overlap of bone in the AP view, often a clue to the presence of subtle fractures.

Unknown 15-6 (Figure 15-19)

No fracture is present. This is a normal immature wrist. In children it is the convention to radiograph the noninjured extremity also, as a mirror image for comparison with the injured part. A normal growth plate is always distinguishable from a fracture by its smooth, dense margination.

Unknown 15-7 (Figure 15-20)

Impacted fracture of the radius 1.5 centimeters from the radiocarpal joint. The typical Colles fracture adds a fracture of the styloid process of the ulna, not present here.

Unknown 15-8 (Figure 15-21)

Fracture of both bones of the forearm, with overriding due to muscle pull, which must be reduced, set end to end, and immobilized in good alignment in plaster. Trees are off limits for several months!

Unknown 16-1 (Figure 16-34)

Suffocation! The man was edentulous. A lower denture is in its normal place against the mandible, but the upper denture lies vertically behind the tongue. A large fragment of the soft-drink bottle was found lodged in the denture.

Credits

Chapter 1

Figure 1-1 The late Dr. Merrill Sosman brought this from Australia.

Figure 1-3 From *Medical Record* 149, February 15, 1896.

Figure 1-4 Courtesy Dr. W. Felts, Minneapolis, Minnesota.

Figures 1-5,11 From *Fundamentals of Radiography*, pp. 6, 25, published by Eastman Kodak Co., Rochester, New York.

Figure 1-8 Courtesy Dr. D. Eaglesham, Guelph, Ontario, Canada.

Figure 1-9 Courtesy Dr. E. Comstock, Wellsville, New York, and C. Bridgman, Rochester, New York.

Figure 1-10 Courtesy C. Bridgman, Rochester, New York, and S. Keck, New York, New York.

Figure 1-14 Courtesy C. Bridgman, Rochester, New York.

Chapter 2

Figure 2-1 Courtesy Dr. A. Richards and the publisher, *Medical Radiography and Photography* (hereafter *MR&P*) 32:28.

Figure 2-2B Courtesy Drs. W. Macklin, Jr., H. Bosland, and A. McCarthy and the publisher, *MR&P* 31:91.

Figure 2-4 Courtesy Dr. S. McPartland, Brooklyn, New York.

Figure 2-5 Courtesy C. Bridgman, E. Holly, and Dr. M. Zariquiey and the publisher, *MR&P* 32:49.

Figures 2-7,8 Courtesy Dr. H. Forsyth, Jr., and the publisher, *MR&P* 25:38.

Figures 2-10,12 Courtesy Dr. C. Behrens, Bethesda, Maryland.

Figure 2-13 Courtesy Dr. B. Epstein and the publisher, *MR&P* 34:60.

Figure 2-21 From *Fundamentals of Radiography*, p. 48, published by Eastman Kodak Co., Rochester, New York.

Figures 2-23,24,25 Courtesy Drs. A. Megibow and M. Bosniak, New York, New York.

Figure 2-26 Courtesy Drs. G. Leopold and B. Gosink, San Diego, California.

Chapter 3

Figures 3-3,16,17,18 From *Fundamentals of Radiography*, pp. 19,25,30,95, published by Eastman Kodak Co., Rochester, New York.

Figures 3-5,6 Courtesy Dr. O. Alexander and the publisher, *MR&P* 30:35,36.

Figure 3-7 Courtesy R. Phillips, Boston, Massachusetts.

Figure 3-9 Courtesy S. Forczyk, Fall River, Massachusetts.

Figures 3-11,12 Courtesy the late Dr. John Hope, Drs. E. O'Hare, T. Tristan, and J. Lyon, Jr., and the publisher, *MR&P* 33:30,31.

Figure 3-13 Courtesy Dr. J. Atlee, Lancaster, Pennsylvania.

Figure 3-15 Courtesy A. Dini, Rochester, New York.

Figure 3-19 Courtesy Dr. I. Andersson and the publisher, *MR&P* 62:cover.

Figure 3-20 Courtesy Dr. J. Jollman, Omaha, Nebraska.

Chapter 4

Figure 4-2 Courtesy R. Morrison and the publisher, *MR&P* 27:132.

Figures 4-4,5 Courtesy Dr. J. Harris and the publisher, *MR&P* 39:2,56.

Figures 4-9,11 Courtesy Drs. B. Felson, F. Fleishner, J. McDonald, and C. Rabin and the publisher, *Radiology* 73:744.

Figure 4-10 Courtesy Dr. C. Dotter and the publisher, *MR&P* 34:48, and Dr. J. Reed, Detroit, Michigan.

Figures 4-12,13 Courtesy Dr. B. Epstein and the publisher, *MR&P* 34:58,62.

Figure 4-14 Courtesy Dr. B. Epstein, New Hyde Park, New York.

Figures 4-15,22 Courtesy Dr. T. McLoud, Boston, Massachusetts.

Figures 4-16,17,18 Courtesy Drs. A. Bell, S. Shimomura, W. Guthrie, H. Hempel, H. Fitzpatrick, and C. Begg and the publisher, *Radiology* 73:566.

Figures 4-20B,21E   Courtesy Dr. R. Sherman, New York, New York.

Figure 4-21F   Courtesy Dr. R. Wagner, Detroit, Michigan.

Figure 4-26   Courtesy Dr. J. Tollman, Omaha, Nebraska.

Chapter 5

Figures 5-4,5   Courtesy Dr. M. Zariquiey and the publisher, *MR&P* 33:68–76.

Figures 5-11,13   Courtesy the late Dr. G. Simon, London, England.

Figure 5-16   Courtesy Dr. J. Woodring and the publisher, *MR&P* 62:1.

Chapter 6

Figure 6-2   Courtesy Dr. M. Strahl, Brooklyn, New York.

Figures 6-3,4   Courtesy Dr. J. Hope et al. and the publisher, *MR&P* 33:26,28.

Figure 6-5   Adapted from Sobotta-Uhlenhuth, *Atlas of Descriptive Human Anatomy,* 7th ed., 1957, Hafner Publishing Co., New York, New York.

Figure 6-6   Courtesy Dr. C. Dotter, Portland, Oregon.

Figure 6-7   Courtesy C. Brownell and the publisher, *MR&P* 27:114.

Figure 6-9   Courtesy Dr. W. Brosius, Detroit, Michigan.

Figures 6-12,17   Courtesy Dr. J. Petersen and the publisher, *Radiology* 74:36,40.

Figure 6-16   Courtesy Dr. E. Carpenter, Superior, Wisconsin.

Figure 6-18   Courtesy Dr. G. Schwalbach, Rochester, New York.

Figure 6-19   Courtesy Dr. H. Forsyth, Jr., and the publisher, *MR&P* 31:129.

Figures 6-20,21   Courtesy Dr. M. Fisher and the publisher, *MR&P* 46:2.

Figure 6-22   Courtesy Dr. N. Solomon, Brooklyn, New York.

Chapter 7

Figure 7-1   Courtesy Drs. I. Harris and M. Stuecheli and the publisher, *MR&P* 28:29.

Figures 7-2,3   Courtesy Dr. J. Hope et al. and the publisher, *MR&P* 33:26.

Figures 7-4,5,17,20   Courtesy Dr. G. Simon, London, England.

Figures 7-7,8,14,25   Dr. J. Woodring and the publisher, *MR&P* 62:1 (back), etc.

Figures 7-9,18,20,21,22,23,27,28,29,30,31   Courtesy Dr. D. Godwin, Seattle, Washington.

Figure 7-12   Courtesy Dr. W. Crandall, Sulphur, Oklahoma.

Figure 7-13   Courtesy Dr. H. Fulton and the publisher, *MR&P* 30:81,82.

Figure 7-16   Courtesy Drs. E. Uhlmann and J. Ovadia and the publisher, *Radiology* 74:269.

Chapter 8

Figure 8-1   Courtesy Dr. J. Woodring and the publisher, *MR&P* 62:1.

Figures 8-3,4   Courtesy Dr. C. Dotter and the publisher, *MR&P* 30:70.

Figures 8-5,8   Courtesy Drs. P. Markovits and J. Desprez-Curely and the publisher, *Radiology* 78:373, 377.

Figures 8-6,11,12,13,14,17,18,19,20,21,22,24,26,27, 28,29,30,31,32,33,34,35   Courtesy Dr. J. Woodring and the publisher, *MR&P* 62.

Figure 8-7   Courtesy Dr. G. McDonnell and the publisher, *MR&P* 30:84.

Figure 8-9   Courtesy Dr. T. Newton and the publisher, *American Journal of Roentgenology* 89:277.

Figure 8-10   Courtesy Drs. R. Ormond, A. Templeton, and J. Jaconette and the publisher, *Radiology* 80:738.

Figure 8-23   Courtesy Dr. J. Hope et al. and the publisher, *MR&P* 33:35.

Figure 8-25   Courtesy Drs. A. Megibow and M. Bosniak, New York, New York.

Chapter 9

Figure 9-3   Courtesy Dr. G. Schwalbach, Rochester, New York.

Figure 9-4   Courtesy Dr. G. Jacobson and the publisher, *MR&P* 44:21.

Figure 9-6   Courtesy R. Bottin, Indianapolis, Indiana.

Figure 9-9   Courtesy Dr. G. Baron, Rochester, New York.

Figure 9-10   Courtesy Dr. W. Brosius, Detroit, Michigan.

Figure 9-11   Courtesy Dr. B. Suster, Brooklyn, New York.

Chapter 10

Figures 10-1,3   Courtesy Dr. H. Forsyth, Jr., Rochester, New York.

Figure 10-8   Courtesy Dr. George Simon, London, England.

Figure 10-13   Courtesy Dr. B. Gosink, San Diego, California.

Figure 10-16   Courtesy Drs. M. Klein and E. Walsh and the publisher, *Radiology* 70:674.

Figures 10-18,19,20   Courtesy Dr. R. Kubicka and the publisher, *MR&P* 61:14–39.

Figure 10-21   Courtesy Dr. B. Epstein and the publisher, *MR&P* 34:68,69.

Figure 10-29   Courtesy Drs. A. Lieber and J. Jorgens and the publisher, *American Journal of Roentgenology* 86:1069–70.

Figure 10-37   Courtesy Dr. W. Tuddenham et al. and the publisher, *MR&P* 33:61.

Figures 10-40,43   Courtesy Dr. A. Strashun, Brooklyn, New York.

Figures 10-44,48   Courtesy Dr. R. Dinsmore, Boston, Massachusetts.

Figures 10-49,56   Courtesy Dr. M. Lipton and Imatron, Inc., San Francisco, California.

Chapter 11

Figures 11-2,3   Courtesy Dr. J. Hope et al. and the publisher, *MR&P* 33:37.

Figure 11-4   Courtesy Drs. B. Kalayjian and M. Sapula and the publisher, *MR&P* 30:57.

Figure 11-5   Courtesy Dr. J. McGillivray and the publisher, *MR&P* 30:27.

Figure 11-7B   Courtesy Dr. C. Stevenson, Spokane, Washington.

Figure 11-11   Courtesy Dr. G. Thompson and W. Cornwell and the publisher, *MR&P* 25:43.

Figure 11-15   Courtesy V. Yamamoto and the publisher, *MR&P* 26:121.

Figure 11-18   Courtesy Drs. R. Salb and G. Burton and the publisher, *MR&P* 33:106.

Figure 11-19   Courtesy Dr. F. Nelans, Wagner, Oklahoma.

Figure 11-21   Courtesy Dr. L. Cole, Blossburg, Pennsylvania.

Figure 11-23   Courtesy Dr. J. Wainerdi, New York, New York.

Figure 11-29   Courtesy E. Holly and G. Weingartner and the publisher, *MR&P* 29:91.

Figure 11-31   Courtesy Dr. W. Tuddenham and the publisher, *Radiology* 78:697.

Figure 11-32   Courtesy C. Bridgman and the publisher, *MR&P* 26:12.

Figure 11-39   Courtesy Dr. W. Irwin, Detroit, Michigan.

Figure 11-42   Courtesy Drs. G. Stein and A. Finkelstein and the publisher, *MR&P* 31:5.

Figure 11-43   Courtesy Dr. G. Schwartz and the publisher, *MR&P* 30:55.

Figure 11-45   Courtesy Dr. J. Becker, Brooklyn, New York.

Figure 11-50   Courtesy Dr. N. Alcock and the publisher, *MR&P* 23:27.

Figure 11-51   Courtesy J. Hill, Lancaster, England.

Figures 11-52,53   Courtesy Drs. A. Megibow and M. Bosniak, New York, New York.

Figures 11-54,55,62,64   Courtesy Drs. G. Leopold and B. Gosink, San Diego, California.

Figures 11-57,58   Courtesy of Dr. R. Filly and Acuson Corp., San Francisco, California.

Figure 11-59   Courtesy Dr. J. Birnholz and Acuson Corp., San Francisco, California, and the publisher, *American Scientist* 77:608.

Figure 11-60   Courtesy Dr. G. Grube and Acuson Corp., Loma Linda, California.

Figure 11-61   Courtesy Dr. E. Ferris and Acuson Corp., Little Rock, Arkansas.

Figure 11-62B   Courtesy Dr. C. Mueller and Acuson Corp., Columbus, Ohio.

Figure 11-63   Courtesy Dr. L. Berland and Acuson Corp., Birmingham, Alabama.

Chapter 12

Figure 12-2   Courtesy Dr. D. Haff, Northampton, Pennsylvania.

Figure 12-6   Courtesy Dr. C. Nice and the publisher, *Radiology* 80:44.

Figure 12-21   Courtesy Dr. J. McCort and the publisher, *Radiology* 78:51.

Figure 12-25   Courtesy Dr. E. Schultz and the publisher, *Radiology* 70:728.

Figure 12-26   Courtesy Dr. H. Welsh and the publisher, *MR&P* 34:78.

Chapter 13

Figure 13-3   Courtesy Dr. C. Nice and the publisher, *Radiology* 80:43.

Figure 13-4   Courtesy Dr. R. Sherman and Eastman Kodak Co., Rochester, New York.

Figures 13-8,34   Courtesy T. Funke, Lorain, Ohio.

Figure 13-9   Courtesy Dr. S. Wyman, Boston, Massachusetts.

Figure 13-10   Courtesy Drs. W. Horrigan, H. Atkins, and N. Tapley and the publisher, *Radiology,* 78:440.

Figure 13-11   Courtesy Dr. G. Joffrey, Olean, New York.

Figure 13-14   Courtesy Drs. J. Spencer and J. Schaeffer and the publisher, *MR&P* 29:22.

Figure 13-15   Courtesy Dr. M. Kulick, Brooklyn, New York.

Figure 13-16   Courtesy Dr. L. Cobbs and the publisher, *MR&P* 31:90.

Figure 13-19   From *Fundamentals of Radiography,* p. 6, published by Eastman Kodak Co., Rochester, New York.

Figure 13-20   Courtesy Dr. T. Orloff and the publisher, *MR&P* 35:53.

Figures 13-26,27   Courtesy Dr. S. Prather, Jr., Augusta, Georgia.

Figure 13-28   Courtesy Dr. G. Jaffrey, Santa Rosa, California.

Figure 13-29   Courtesy Dr. E. Ahern and the publisher, *MR&P* 30:9.

Figure 13-31   Courtesy Dr. J. Higgason and the publisher, *MR&P* 30:60.

Figure 13-32   Courtesy Dr. J. Dulin, Iowa City, Iowa.

Figure 13-33   Courtesy Dr. J. Reed, Detroit, Michigan.

Figure 13-38   Courtesy Dr. C. Cimmino and the publisher, *MR&P* 30:45.

Chapter 14

Figure 14-6   Courtesy Dr. J. Ferrucci, Boston, Massachusetts.

Figure 14-7   Courtesy Dr. J. Ferrucci et al. and the publisher, *Interventional Radiology of the Abdomen,* Williams & Wilkins Company, Baltimore, Maryland.

Figure 14-14   Courtesy Dr. J. Pepe, Brooklyn, New York.

Figures 14-16,17   Courtesy Dr. K. McKusick, Boston, Massachusetts.

Figure 14-18   Courtesy Drs. G. Stein and A. Finkelstein and the publisher, *MR&P* 31:12.

Figure 14-19   Courtesy Dr. E. Pirkey, Louisville, Kentucky.

Figure 14-21   Courtesy Dr. T. Van Zandt, Rochester, New York, and Eastman Kodak Company.

Figure 14-22   Courtesy Dr. C. Athanasoulis et al. and the publisher, *Interventional Radiology,* W. B. Saunders Company, Philadelphia, Pennsylvania.

Figure 14-24   Courtesy Dr. S. Dallemand, Brooklyn, New York.

Figures 14-36,37   Courtesy Drs. G. Leopold and B. Gosink, San Diego, California.

Figure 14-38   Courtesy Dr. J. Hope et al. and the publisher, *MR&P* 33:49.

Figure 14-39   Courtesy Dr. K. Fengler and the publisher, *Journal of Mount Sinai Hospital,* New York, New York.

Figure 14-43   Courtesy Drs. M. Bosniak and J. Becker, New York, New York.

Figure 14-45   Courtesy Dr. W. Foley and the General Electric Company.

Figure 14-47   Courtesy Drs. A. Waltman and C. Athanasoulis, Boston, Massachusetts.

Figure 14-50   Courtesy Drs. J. Edeiken, G. Strong, and J. Khajavi and the publisher, *Radiology* 79:88.

Figure 14-51   Courtesy Drs. J. Hope and C. Koop and the publisher, *MR&P* 38:47.

Chapter 15

Figure 15-2   Courtesy Chicago Museum of Natural History, Chicago, Illinois.

Figures 15-4,9   Courtesy C. Bridgman and the publisher, *MR&P* 26:4, 27:72.

Figure 15-5   Courtesy Dr. G. Mitchell and the publisher, *MR&P* 34:6.

Figures 15-6,26   Courtesy Drs. H. Isard, B. Ostrum, and J. Cullinan and the publisher, *MR&P* 38:97,101.

Figure 15-8   Courtesy J. Cahoon and the publisher, *Radiography and Clinical Photography* 22:4,6.

Figure 15-12   Courtesy Dr. L. Hilt, Eugene, Oregon.

Figures 15-14,16,17,18   Courtesy T. Funke and the publisher, *MR&P* 36:9,29.

Figure 15-22   Courtesy Dr. W. Irwin, Detroit, Michigan.

Figure 15-23   Courtesy Dr. D. Wilner, Atlantic City, New Jersey.

Figure 15-31   Adapted from A. W. Ham, *Histology,* 3rd ed., p. 295, published by J. B. Lippincott, Philadelphia, Pennsylvania.

Figure 15-32   Courtesy Dr. P. Lacroix, University of Louvain, Belgium.

Figure 15-33   Courtesy Dr. M. Urist, *Bone as a Tissue,* p. 37, and the publisher, McGraw-Hill Book Co., New York, New York.

Figure 15-34   Courtesy Dr. L. Luck, *Bone and Joint Diseases,* 1st ed., and the publisher, Charles C Thomas, Springfield, Illinois.

Figures 15-35,36   Courtesy Dr. J. Feist, Pittsburgh, Pennsylvania.

Chapter 16

Figure 16-6   Courtesy R. Matthias and the publisher, *MR&P* 28:cover.

Figures 16-8,14,15,18   From *Living Anatomy* by R. A. Novelline and L. F. Squire, Hanley and Belfus, Philadelphia, Pennsylvania.

Figure 16-17   Courtesy Dr. G. Hotson, Brooklyn, New York.

Figures 16-27,28   Courtesy Drs. G. Potter and R. Gold and the publisher, *MR&P* 51:2.

Figure 16-30   Courtesy Drs. A. Megibow and M. Bosniak, New York, New York.

Figure 16-34   Courtesy Dr. C. Dotter and the publisher, *MR&P* 37:19.

Index